T0362411

Pain Management in Plastic Surgery

Editors

MICHAEL W. NEUMEISTER
REUBEN A. BUENO Jr

CLINICS IN PLASTIC SURGERY

www.plasticsurgery.theclinics.com

April 2020 • Volume 47 • Number 2

ELSEVIER

1600 John F. Kennedy Boulevard • Suite 1800 • Philadelphia, Pennsylvania, 19103-2899

http://www.theclinics.com

CLINICS IN PLASTIC SURGERY Volume 47, Number 2
April 2020 ISSN 0094-1298, ISBN-13: 978-0-323-73284-0

Editor: Stacy Eastman
Developmental Editor: Nicole Congleton

Clinics in Plastic Surgery (ISSN 0094-1298) is published quarterly by Elsevier Inc., 360 Park Avenue South, New York, NY 10010-1710. Months of issue are January, April, July, and October. Business and Editorial Offices: 1600 John F. Kennedy Blvd., Suite 1800, Philadelphia, PA 19103-2899. Periodicals postage paid at New York, NY and additional mailing offices. Subscription prices are $543.00 per year for US individuals, $987.00 per year for US institutions, $100.00 per year for US students and residents, $607.00 per year for Canadian individuals, $1175.00 per year for Canadian institutions, $655.00 per year for international individuals, $1175.00 per year for international institutions, $100.00 per year for Canadian and $305.00 per year for international students/residents. To receive student/resident rate, orders must be accompanied by name of affiliated institution, date of term, and the *signature* of program/residency coordinator on institution letterhead. Orders will be billed at individual rate until proof of status is received. Foreign air speed delivery is included in all *Clinics* subscription prices. All prices are subject to change without notice. **POSTMASTER:** Send address changes to *Clinics in Plastic Surgery*, Elsevier Health Sciences Division, Subscription Customer Service, 3251 Riverport Lane, Maryland Heights, MO 63043. **Customer Service: 1-800-654-2452 (US and Canada). From outside of the United States and Canada, call 314-447-8871. Fax: 314-447-8029. E-mail: JournalsCustomerService-usa@elsevier.com (for print support); JournalsOnline-Support-usa@elsevier.com (for online support).**

Reprints. For copies of 100 or more of articles in this publication, please contact the Commercial Reprints Department, Elsevier Inc., 360 Park Avenue South, New York, New York 10010-1710. Tel.: +1-212-633-3874; Fax: +1-212-633-3820; E-mail: reprints@elsevier.com.

Clinics in Plastic Surgery is covered in *Current Contents, EMBASE/Excerpta Medica, Science Citation Index, MEDLINE/PubMed (Index Medicus), ASCA, and ISI/BIOMED.*

Contributors

EDITORS

MICHAEL W. NEUMEISTER, MD, FRCSC, FACS
Professor and Chairman, Department of Surgery, Institute for Plastic Surgery, SIU School of Medicine, Springfield, Illinois, USA

REUBEN A. BUENO Jr, MD
Professor and Chief, Institute for Plastic Surgery, Elvin G. Zook Endowed Chair of Plastic Surgery, SIU School of Medicine, Springfield, Illinois, USA

AUTHORS

AUSTIN M. BEASON, MD
Resident in Orthopaedic Surgery, Department of Surgery, Division of Orthopaedic Surgery, SIU School of Medicine, Springfield, Illinois, USA

SANDIP BISWAL, MD
Department of Radiology, Stanford University, Stanford, California, USA

KORY D. BLANK, MD
PGY-IV Orthopaedic Surgery Resident, SIU School of Medicine, Springfield, Illinois, USA

PAUL S. CEDERNA, MD
Chief and Robert O'Neal Collegiate Professor, Section of Plastic Surgery, Department of Surgery, University of Michigan, Ann Arbor, Michigan, USA

AVA G. CHAPPELL, MD
Resident, Division of Plastic Surgery, Department of Surgery, Northwestern University Feinberg School of Medicine, Chicago, Illinois, USA

JANA DENGLER, MD
Assistant Professor, Division of Plastic and Reconstructive Surgery, Department of Surgery, Sunnybrook Health Sciences Centre, Toronto, Ontario, Canada

GREGORY A. DUMANIAN, MD
Orion and Lucille Stuteville Professor of Surgery, Chief, Division of Plastic Surgery, Department of Surgery, Northwestern University Feinberg School of Medicine, Chicago, Illinois, USA

YOUSSEF EL BITAR, MD
Clinical Assistant Professor of Orthopaedic Surgery, Department of Surgery, Division of Orthopaedic Surgery, SIU School of Medicine, Springfield, Illinois, USA

NICHOLAS F. HUG, BA
Department of Neurosurgery, Stanford University, Stanford, California, USA

LAUREN JACOBSON, MD
Resident Physician, Division of Plastic and Reconstructive Surgery, Department of Surgery, Barnes-Jewish Hospital, Washington University School of Medicine, St Louis, Missouri, USA

JEFFREY E. JANIS, MD, FACS
Professor of Plastic Surgery, Neurosurgery, Neurology, and Surgery, Chief of Plastic Surgery, University Hospital, The Ohio State University Wexner Medical Center, Columbus, Ohio, USA

SUMANAS W. JORDAN, MD, PhD
Assistant Professor, Division of Plastic Surgery, Department of Surgery, Northwestern University Feinberg School of Medicine, Chicago, Illinois, USA

THEODORE A. KUNG, MD
Assistant Professor, Section of Plastic Surgery, Department of Surgery, University of Michigan, Ann Arbor, Michigan, USA

GREG I. LEE, MD, PhD
SIU School of Medicine, SIU Plastic Surgery, Springfield, Illinois, USA

MICHELE MANAHAN, MD
Department of Plastic and Reconstructive Surgery, Johns Hopkins Hospital, Baltimore, Maryland, USA

AMY M. MOORE, MD
Professor and Chair, Department of Plastic and Reconstructive Surgery, The Ohio State University Wexner Medical Center, Columbus, Ohio, USA

JOHN B. MOORE IV, MD, FACS
Director, Midwest Migraine Surgery Center & KS Hand Center, Assistant Clinical Professor Plastic Surgery, The University of Kansas Medical Center, Kansas City, Kansas, USA

EVYN L. NEUMEISTER, MD, MPH
Resident in Plastic Surgery, Department of Surgery, Institute for Plastic Surgery, SIU School of Medicine, Springfield, Illinois, USA

MICHAEL W. NEUMEISTER, MD, FRCSC, FACS
Professor and Chairman, Department of Surgery, Institute for Plastic Surgery, SIU School of Medicine, Springfield, Illinois, USA

JEREMIE D. OLIVER, BS, BA
Medical Student, Mayo Clinic School of Medicine, Rochester, Minnesota, USA

DANIELLE OLLA, MD
Resident Physician, Institute for Plastic Surgery, Southern Illinois University, Springfield, Illinois, USA

NORMAN Y. OTSUKA, MSc, MD, FRCSC, FAAP, FACS, FAOA
Professor and Chairman, Division of Orthopaedic Surgery, SIU School of Medicine, Springfield, Illinois, USA

SARAH PERSING, MD, MPH
Department of Plastic and Reconstructive Surgery, Johns Hopkins Hospital, Baltimore, Maryland, USA

DAVID A. PURGER, MD, PhD
Department of Neurosurgery, Stanford University, Stanford, California, USA

MICHAEL R. ROMANELLI, MD
Resident Physician, Department of Surgery, Institute for Plastic Surgery, SIU School of Medicine, Springfield, Illinois, USA

GEDGE ROSSON, MD
Department of Plastic and Reconstructive Surgery, Johns Hopkins Hospital, Baltimore, Maryland, USA

SARADA SAKAMURI, MD
Department of Neurology and Neurological Sciences, Stanford University, Stanford, California, USA

KATHERINE B. SANTOSA, MD, MS
House Officer, Section of Plastic Surgery, Department of Surgery, University of Michigan, Ann Arbor, Michigan, USA

JUSTIN SAWYER, MD
Resident Physician, Institute for Plastic Surgery, Southern Illinois University, Springfield, Illinois, USA

ANNA R. SCHOENBRUNNER, MD, MAS
Resident, Department of Plastic and Reconstructive Surgery, The Ohio State University, Columbus, Ohio, USA

NICOLE SOMMER, MD, FACS
Associate Professor, Program Director, Director of Cosmetic Center, Institute for Plastic Surgery, Southern Illinois University, Springfield, Illinois, USA

JACOB A. THAYER, MD
Resident Physician, Department of Surgery, Institute for Plastic Surgery, SIU School of Medicine, Springfield, Illinois, USA

LILY A. UPP, BS
Research Assistant, Michigan Opioid
Prescribing Engagement Network, Institute
for Healthcare Policy and Innovation,
University of Michigan, Ann Arbor, Michigan,
USA

JENNIFER F. WALJEE, MD, MPH
Associate Professor, Section of Plastic
Surgery, Department of Surgery, University
of Michigan Medical School, Michigan
Opioid Prescribing Engagement Network,
Institute for Healthcare Policy and Innovation,
University of Michigan, Ann Arbor, Michigan,
USA

THOMAS J. WILSON, MD
Department of Neurosurgery, Stanford
University, Stanford, California, USA

JAMES N. WINTERS, MD
Institute for Plastic Surgery, SIU School of
Medicine, Springfield, Illinois,
USA

LILY A. LAI, BS
Research Area and Michigan Center
for Value-Based Insurance Design
for Healthcare Policy and Innovation,
University of Michigan, Ann Arbor, Michigan,
USA

JENNIFER F. WALJEE, MD, MPH
Associate Professor, Section of Plastic
Surgery, Department of Surgery, University
of Michigan Medical School, Michigan

Institute for Healthcare Policy and Innovation,
University of Michigan, Ann Arbor, Michigan,
USA

THOMAS J. WILLICH, MD
Department of Neurosurgery, Stanford
University, Stanford, California, USA

JAMES R. WINTERS, MD
Institute for Plastic Surgery, SIU School of
Medicine, Springfield, Illinois,
USA

Contents

in such patients should aid the surgeon in his attempt to rid the patient of painful conditions through surgery.

Adequate pediatric pain management is difficult to achieve for a variety of reasons. Pain assessment is more difficult in the pediatric population. There are a variety of different tools that may be used to accurately assess pain. There are many modalities to achieve pain control, including pharmacologic and nonpharmacologic means. These different modalities should be used in unison to achieve pain control. Compartment syndrome is a surgical emergency, and pediatric patients present differently from adult patients. The 3 As (anxiety, agitation, increase in analgesia requirement) should be monitored in all pediatric patients.

The Enhanced Recovery After Surgery (ERAS) protocol is a multidisciplinary, multimodal, and evidence-based approach to perioperative management. The ERAS pathway has been applied to numerous major surgical procedures throughout various specialties and has shown reduced postoperative morbidity, reduced opioid use, higher patient satisfaction, and shortened hospital length of stay. In the current health care climate, there has been a growing focus on optimizing the quality of care for patients and reducing the overall cost burden of health care. In this article, the authors review the ERAS pathways for breast reconstruction procedures and discuss the outcomes of implementation of these pathways.

Nerve imaging is an important component in the assessment of patients presenting with suspected peripheral nerve pathology. Although magnetic resonance neurography and ultrasound are the most commonly utilized techniques, several promising new modalities are on the horizon. Nerve imaging is useful in localizing the nerve injury, determining the severity, providing prognostic information, helping establish the diagnosis, and helping guide surgical decision making. The focus of this article is imaging of damaged nerves, focusing on nerve injuries and entrapment neuropathies.

This article discusses the pathophysiology, presentation, cause, and treatment of ischemic pain in the surgical patient. Causes of ischemic pain vary but all fundamentally cause local acidosis in the peripheral tissues, which causes signals to be passed through ascending pain pathways to the thalamus and eventual cerebral cortex where it is interpreted as ischemic pain. Ischemic pain is classically associated with an insidious onset but can present in the acute or chronic setting. Treatments are aimed at improving perfusion to the affected tissue. Surgical options include repairing damaged vessels, bypassing diseased vessels, performing thrombectomy, or embolectomy. Numerous conservative therapies exist.

impairment, and eventual atrophy. This hyperalgesic disease affects musculoskeletal, neural, and vascular structures more commonly in the upper extremity than the lower extremity. Although the etiology behind the pathophysiology of CRPS is unknown, the pain pathway extending from peripheral nociception to central nervous system modulation of stimuli is highly sensitized and overactive, disrupting the surrounding autonomic response. The diagnosis and treatment of CRPS are reviewed.

Symptomatic neuromas are a common cause of postamputation pain that can lead to significant disability. Regenerative peripheral nerve interface surgery is performed to treat symptomatic neuromas and prevent the development of neuromas. This review delineates the clinical problem of postamputation pain, describes the limitations of the available treatment methods, and highlights the need for an effective treatment strategy that leverages the biologic processes of nerve regeneration and muscle reinnervation. The evidence supporting use of regenerative peripheral nerve interface surgery to mitigate neuroma formation is discussed and the rationale behind the efficacy of regenerative peripheral nerve interfaces is explored.

Perioperative pain management in surgery of the hand and upper extremity relies on a multimodal approach involving systemic, local, and presurgical considerations. A pain management plan should be tailored to each patient. Management of pain of patients undergoing upper extremity surgery begins before surgical intervention and continues postoperatively. Patient education, setting expectations, psychological interventions, and addressing risk factors associated with postoperative pain are critical to successful pain management. Intraoperative anesthesia is accomplished via a variety of means. Cryotherapy, transcutaneous electrical nerve stimulation, acupuncture, massage, and localized heat are used in concert with pharmacologic therapies postoperatively to continue pain management.

CLINICS IN PLASTIC SURGERY

ISSUE OF RELATED INTEREST

Facial Plastic Surgery Clinics
https://www.facialplastic.theclinics.com/
Otolaryngologic Clinics
https://www.oto.theclinics.com/

THE CLINICS ARE AVAILABLE ONLINE!
Access your subscription at:
www.theclinics.com

CLINICS IN PLASTIC SURGERY

Preface
The Maladies of Pain

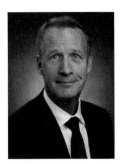
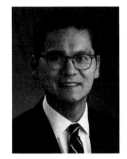

Michael W. Neumeister, MD, FRCSC, FACS   Reuben A. Bueno Jr, MD

Editors

In 1993, Paul Brand and Phillip Yancey wrote about the importance of pain in a book entitled, *Pain, The Gift Nobody Wants*. This was followed in 1997 by their book entitled, *The Gift of Pain*. Each book embraces the essential role that pain has in protecting the body from further harm. As an intensely unpleasant sensation, pain makes our bodies withdraw from the offensive malefactor to the security of an innocuous environment. So pain is good! Pain is a gift.

Unfortunately, cells, tissues, and organs within our bodies may incur insults that take advantage of "the gift of pain" to protect themselves, and the body as a whole, but lose sense of the inciting noxious stimuli and continue to propagate the pain signals to the central nervous system. The pain becomes chronic, giving no choice to the body but to react with defensive mechanisms that affect our activities of daily living and our psyche. We can then either live with the pain until it subsides, if ever, disrupt the pain pathway, or treat the pain with various modalities, including pharmacologic agents. The maladies of pain can be very difficult to manage, making patients suffer until a root cause is identified and treated. The treatment, however, may not be that easy.

This issue of *Clinic in Plastic Surgery* focuses on the anatomy, physiology, and management of various pain syndromes as they relate to patients seen in the plastic surgery practice. We thank all of the authors who contributed their time, effort, and expertise into creating this issue.

Michael W. Neumeister, MD, FRCSC, FACS
Department of Surgery
Institute for Plastic Surgery
SIU School of Medicine
747 North Rutledge, 3rd Floor
PO Box 19653
Springfield, IL 62794, USA

Reuben A. Bueno Jr, MD
Institute for Plastic Surgery at
SIU School of Medicine
747 North Rutledge, 3rd Floor
PO Box 19653
Springfield, IL 62794, USA

E-mail addresses:
mneumeister@siumed.edu (M.W. Neumeister)
rbueno@siumed.edu (R.A. Bueno)

Clin Plastic Surg 47 (2020) xiii
https://doi.org/10.1016/j.cps.2020.01.005
0094-1298/20/© 2020 Published by Elsevier Inc.

Pain: Pathways and Physiology

Greg I. Lee, MD, PhD, Michael W. Neumeister, MD, FRCSC*

KEYWORDS

- Pain • Neuropathic pain • Chronic pain • Acute pain

KEY POINTS

- Pain is a multifactorial process that may not always be linked to a stimulus and does not always directly correlate with the severity of injury.
- The pain pathways are constantly modulated through physical, biochemical, and psychological interactions.
- To optimize the treatment of pain, it is necessary to understand the anatomy and physiology of pain so that targeted therapies may be developed and used.

INTRODUCTION

The International Association for the Study of Pain defines pain as "an unpleasant sensory and emotional experience associated with actual or potential tissue damage".[1] Pain is often difficult to measure and assess accurately because of its subjectivity where sensation experienced by any one individual has both physical and emotional overtones. Pain, however, is a vital protective sensory phenomenon essential to survival. Patients with leprosy or congenital insensitivity to pain are prone to repeated tissue and organ injuries. Generally, pain is elicited from any stimulus that damages tissue or potentially damages tissue. Pain alerts the individual pathologic affronts on the body and possibly permits avoidance of the offending pathogen or stimulus. However, when the signaling becomes aberrant and chronic, the sensation of pain becomes detrimental to the individual, both physically and psychological. Although in this review the authors describe the physiologic pathways involved in pain, it is important to understand that pain is not always tied to a stimulus. In addition, there may be no direct correlation between the perceived intensity of pain and the severity of tissue damage.[2]

PAIN VERSUS NOCICEPTION

Pain refers to the conscious, subjective experience or perception of a feeling or sensation, which a person calls pain.[3] Nociception is the physiologic activation of neural pathways by stimuli (noxious, thermal, mechanical, or chemical) that are potentially or currently damaging.[4] A stimulus is deemed nociceptive if it results in a behavioral, withdrawal, or escape response. Proprioception is the awareness of oneself or one's body part relative to their environment. There are many types or descriptions of pain that are descriptive and to some degree may identify sources of ongoing stimulus (Table 1).

ANATOMY OF PAIN

In order to understand pain pathways, a brief description of normal anatomy and physiology of the sensory system is required. Afferent sensory nerves send various types of information to the brain. The sensory end organs are made of stimulus accommodating receptors within the skin and tissues (Fig. 1). The various receptors are activated by their stimulus to create an electrical impulse or action potential within the sensory nerve. The action potential is transduced to the nerve cell body within the dorsal root ganglion of the spinal cord. The nerves synapse with a spinal cord nerve that carries the action potential signal to the brain through the spinothalamic and spinoparabrachial tracts. The brain network of signal transduction includes synapses within the

Southern Illinois University School of Medicine, SIU Plastic Surgery, 747 North Rutledge 3rd Floor, PO Box 19653, Springfield, IL 62794, USA
* Corresponding author.
E-mail address: mneumeister@siumed.edu

Clin Plastic Surg 47 (2020) 173–180
https://doi.org/10.1016/j.cps.2019.11.001

Table 1
Pain terminology and definitions

Pain Terminology	Definition
Allodynia	Pain due to a stimulus that normally does not provoke pain
Causalgia	Syndrome of sustained burning pain, allodynia, and hyperpathia after a traumatic nerve lesions.
Dysesthesia	Unpleasant abnormal sensation, spontaneous or evoked
Hyperalgesia	Increased pain from a stimulus that normally provokes pain
Neuropathic pain	Pain caused by a lesion or disease of somatosensory system
Phantom pain	Perception relating to a limb or organ that is not physically part of the body
Nociceptive pain	Pain that arises from actual or threatened damage to nonneural tissue; due to activation of nociceptors
Acute pain	Pain that lasts less than 3–6 mo and is directly related to tissue damage and resolves as tissues heals
Chronic pain	Pain that lasts >3 mo and is primarily mediated by C fibers may have some element of central sensitization
Sensitization	Increased responsiveness of nociceptive neurons to their normal input resulting in recruitment of response to normally subthreshold inputs

parabrachial medulla oblongata, thalamus, amygdala and limbic system, and somatosensory cortex.

The pathway of pain begins at the periphery with the free nerve endings of primary afferent neurons whose peripheral terminal axons respond to different types of stimuli (mechanical, heat, cold, chemical)[5,6] and transduction occurs. The primary afferent fibers are classified based on their conduction velocity and the stimuli that results in their activation (**Table 2**). A-beta (Aβ) fibers are large-diameter myelinated fibers that are fast

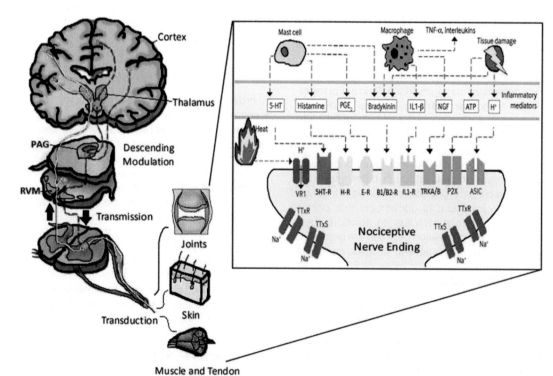

Fig. 1. Complex pain pathways: stimulation of nociceptive nerve endings from joints, muscles/tendons, and skin are transmitted from the periphery to the spinal cord to the cortex in a complex pathway involving transduction, transmission, and modulation of the pain signal.

Table 2
Characteristics of major fibers involved in pain transmission

	Fiber Type		
	Aδ	C	Aβ
Myelinated	Yes	No	Yes
Diameter	1–5 μm	0.02–1.5 μm	6–12 μm
Conduction speed	2–20 m/s	< 2 m/s	>20 m/s
Thermal sensitivity	Yes/No	Yes/No	No
Function	Nociception/Touch	Nociception/Touch	Proprio/mechanoreceptor
Modality	Mechanothermal and touch from skin	Polymodal (mechanical, thermal, chemical)	Touch and pressure from skin

conducting (>20 m/s) and activated and produce the sensation of light touch, pressure, or hair movement. A-delta (Aδ) fibers are thinly myelinated fibers that conduct at 2 to 20 m/s. C fibers, the predominant afferent fibers in peripheral nerves, are unmyelinated fibers that conduct at less than 2 m/s. Both Aδ and C fibers may respond to intense heat, cold, mechanical, and chemical stimuli and are subsequently called "polymodal."[6] Aδ activation elicits an intense, sharp, tingling sensation, whereas C fiber activation results in a dull prolonged burning sensation. Because Aδ fibers conduct at a higher velocity than C fibers, Aδ fibers are believed to convey the "first pain" sensation, whereas C fibers elicit the "second pain" burning sensation. Both Aδ and C fibers are found in skin and other superficial organs, whereas C fibers are the main suppliers of deep structures including muscles and joints.[6] These sensory neurons then synapse in the dorsal horn of the spinal cord in various areas called laminae[7] with second-order neurons. There are 3 types of second-order neurons, including nociceptive specific (NS), wide dynamic range (WDR), and low threshold (LR). NS respond to high-threshold noxious stimuli, WDR respond to sensory stimuli, and LR respond to innocuous stimuli only.[7] These second-order neurons then continue to transmit their signal to the thalamus via the spinothalamic and spinoreticular tracts. The thalamus processes somatosensory information, and neurons within the thalamus project to various regions of the brain including the primary and secondary somatosensory cortices, insula, anterior cingulate cortex, and the prefrontal cortex. The cortex is where the perception of pain (intensity, duration, location) is integrated.[2] The transmission of pain can be modulated throughout this pathway in various locations. Within the spinal cord itself, both excitatory and inhibitory interneurons are present that

can modify the pain signal. Within the dorsal root ganglion, the various sensory nerves are modulated by TrkA, TrkB, TrkC receptors, or c-Ret receptors. In fact, there are a multitude of receptors and neurotransmitters throughout the pain pathway that modulate the pain signal and are beyond the scope of this paper (see **Fig. 1**). There are also descending inhibitory tracts involved in reducing pain. The periaqueductal gray (PAG) and nucleus raphe magnus (NRM) are regions in the brainstem that work in concert to block pain transmission.

PHYSIOLOGY OF PAIN

There are four processes that occur in the perception of a painful stimulus. The first is transduction. This occurs in the peripheral axons where primary afferent neurons are activated by a noxious stimulus. Receptors found on these axons include vanilloid receptor 1, which responds to heat, capsaicin, and protons, and Mas-related G protein–coupled receptors, which are thought to mediate nociceptive behavior to mechanical stimuli. The next process of the pain pathway is transmission. During this process, pain impulses are transmitted by a 2-fiber system that includes the fast and sharp sensation of the Aδ fibers, and the slower sensation attributed to the C fibers. Both fibers end in the dorsal horn of the spinal cord where Aδ fibers synapse with neurons in laminas I and V and C fibers synapse in laminas I and II.[6] Because of the significant plasticity of the cells located in the dorsal horn, pain impulses can be modified or "gated" in this location. Transmission continues via second-order neurons to the central nervous system via the lateral spinothalamic tract and medial spinothalamic tract. The lateral spinothalamic tract projects to the ventral posterolateral nucleus of the thalamus and informs the brain regarding duration, location, and intensity of pain,[6] whereas the medial spinothalamic tract projects to the medial thalamus and carries the autonomic and unpleasant emotional perception of pain. Third-order neurons in the thalamus subsequently project to specific cortical regions that mediate the perception, localization, and emotional components of pain. Signal modulation is the third process and occurs peripherally, within the spinal cord, and in the brain. Altering neural activity along the pain pathway can result in the suppression or inhibition of pain.

MODULATION OF PAIN

The modulation of pain is an endogenous process that is thought to provide a survival advantage. Evidence of this was portrayed in a study by Beecher,[8] an anesthesiologist in World War II, in which they identified soldiers that suffered from severe battle wounds and found that they often experienced little or no pain. This signified that the body possesses an endogenous mechanism that dissociates and modulates (enhances or diminishes) the transmission of pain. Mechanisms responsible for this phenomenon include segmental inhibition, the endogenous opioid system, and the descending inhibitory nerve system. In addition, cognitive and coping strategies also play a role in altering pain perception. Segmental inhibition more commonly known and originally described by Melzack and Wall[9] as the "gate theory" infers that the synapses between afferent neurons that transmit noxious stimuli (Aδ and C fibers) and neurons in the dorsal horn of the spinal cord can be blocked. This occurs when large myelinated nerve fibers (Aβ) that sense touch (nonnoxious stimuli), stimulate the inhibitory nerve in the spinal cord, which in turn inhibits the transmission of the pain signal by suppressing transmission in small unmyelinated C fiber afferents. This explains why rubbing an injury reduces the sensation of pain. The mechanism behind transcutaneous electrical nerve stimulation for pain control is based on this theory. The endogenous opioid system arose when receptors to opium derivatives were found in the central nervous system (PAG, ventral medulla) and spinal cord (lamina I and II). Three groups of endogenous compounds were subsequently identified, and they include enkephalins, endorphins, and dynorphins. These endogenous compounds bind to the opioid receptors in the pain pathway and modulate the pain signal. Finally, the descending inhibitory nerve system controls the transmission of noxious signaling by using the neurotransmitters serotonin and norepinephrine. The limbic system projects to the PAG and medulla before synapsing in the dorsal horn of the spinal cord. Serotonin, synthesized from the NRM, and norepinephrine, synthesized from locus coeruleus,[4] are released to dampen the pain signal in the dorsal horn. These neurotransmitters work to diminish the transmission of pain by (1) direct inhibition of the dorsal horn cells transmitting pain, (2) inhibition of excitatory dorsal horn neurons that work to enhance/exacerbate the transmission of pain, or (3) excitation of inhibitor neurons in the dorsal horn. Collectively, they work to inhibit the transmission of pain through the pain pathways.

NEUROPATHIC PAIN

Defined as "pain caused by a lesion or disease of the somatosensory system"[10,11] has an estimated prevalence of 7% to 9.8% with up to 20% of patients with chronic pain.[12,13] Neuropathic pain arises from spontaneous activity or an aberrant response to normal stimulation.[14] It occurs in the presence of an abnormally functioning somatosensory system and can be present in the absence of obvious tissue injury. Unfortunately, it can be refractory to pharmacologic and noninterventional treatment resulting in severe disability and negative impacts on the quality of life. Examples of neuropathic pain include postherpetic neuralgia, postsurgical neuropathy, diabetic neuropathy, peripheral neuropathies, and complex regional pain syndrome. There are many factors that are attributed to neuropathic pain, but an essential component includes injury to the afferent pathway.[15] Other mechanisms include changes in ion channels (quantity and density), central and peripheral sensitization, cortical reorganizations, and disinhibition with cellular and molecular changes. It is also believed that the sympathetic nervous system plays a role in maintaining neuropathic pain.[16] Neuropathic pain is often associated with allodynia, which is a central pain sensitization due to repetitive nonpainful stimulation.[6] Sensitization at the periphery includes the formation of ectopic foci, whereas multiple changes occur centrally, including decreased nonnociceptive input, downregulation of opioid and GABA receptors in the dorsal horn, and death of dorsal horn interneurons in lamina II resulting in "disinhibition" of the pain stimuli. There are also changes in central modulation that result in hyperexcitability of injured nerves, loss of C fibers, as well as increased activity in the sympathetic nervous system. Effective therapies aim to target the receptors and neurotransmitters in these regions and therefore first-line drugs for neuropathic pain include tricyclic antidepressant, serotonin-norepinephrine reuptake inhibitors, gabapentin (best for postherpetic neuralgia and diabetic neuropathy), and pregabalin (shorter time to therapeutic effect and lower effective doses)[17] (**Table 3**). Second-line therapy includes tramadol, capsaicin patches, and 5% lidocaine patches.[18] Lastly, third-line medications include strong opioids (ie, oxycodone and morphine) and botox (neuropathic pain drugs; see **Table 2**).

ACUTE VERSUS CHRONIC PAIN

Acute pain is a natural and useful sensation that warns the individual of possible injury and usually results in behaviors that avoid further injury and is mediated by Aδ fibers.[6] It is often seen in the emergency room and is the most common reason for an emergency room visit.[19] Early control of acute pain reduces the incidence of chronic pain syndromes. With concerns increasing about the opioid epidemic, clinicians and patients are often fearful of creating addiction when managing pain. However, studies reveal that there is low risk of opioid addiction when treating acute pain.[20] Chronic pain, on the other hand, serves no benefit to the patient. Chronic pain can be defined as lasting more than 3 months and may have some element of central sensitization[21] and is primarily mediated by C fibers.[6] In fact in chronic pain, cognitive and emotional factors have a critical influence on pain perception due to the connectivity of brain regions controlling pain perception, attention or expectation, and emotional states.[21] Imaging studies have demonstrated alterations of afferent and descending pain pathways by attentional state, positive or negative emotions, and other nonpain-related stimuli. This state is termed centralized pain. There are many alterations in the normal physiology of pain in the chronic pain states. For example, chronic peripheral nerve injury results in both chemical and physical changes in the neural pathway for pain. These changes are seen in the periphery, dorsal ganglion, and central nervous system. Expression and distribution of ectopic sodium channels are altered in the periphery resulting in significant lowering of the depolarization threshold of nociceptors. Furthermore, ectopic sodium channels are known to spontaneously depolarize in chronically irritated or injured nerves. These nerves thus become "sensitized" to any stimuli. These alterations continue in the central nervous system including upregulation of pain receptors (N-methyl-D acetylate receptor), increased sprouting of A fibers in the dorsal horn lamina where C fibers terminate, and changes in the levels of neurotransmitters. Similarly, injured C fibers become sensitized and undergo similar chemical and biological changes. There is an increased production of adrenergic receptors in the C fibers that react to sympathetic release of norepinephrine resulting in vasoconstriction and pain. This may explain why stress, emotion, and cold are significant stimuli for the pain seen in Raynaud disease. Another pathway for chronic pain is from the stimulation of c-polymodal nociceptors that release substance P. Substance P, a neurotransmitter, acts on the central nervous system and is able to self-propagate. Both substance P and glutamate are neurotransmitters that act as positive feedback signals. Chronic pain can be categorized into broad groups: (1) those due to underlying disease, (2) those with known neuropathic pain syndromes, (3) those without an identifiable cause, and (4) those who seek personal gain.[22] Management of the last group requires patience and professionalism. It is important to remember that malingering is a diagnosis of exclusion and if it is determined, the patient should be referred to outpatient pain and psychiatric services for further evaluation and treatment. Nonsteroidal antiinflammatory drugs may be offered but often they will be refused or stated that they are unable to take them for some reason or another. Another cause of pain (acute or chronic) is postsurgical pain. It is estimated that 40 million surgical procedures occur annually in the United States and 10% to 15% will develop chronic pain 1 year after surgery.[23] A study by Katz and colleagues[24] reported that early severe postoperative pain significantly predicted development of long-term pain. Other risk factors include preexisting pain, psychosocial factors,

Table 3	
First-line drugs for treatment of neuropathic pain	
First-Line Drugs For Neuropathic Pain	
Tricyclic antidepressants (TCAs)	Amitriptyline
Serotonin-norepinephrine reuptake inhibitors (SNRIs)	Duloxetine
Gabapentin	Most studies based on immediate release
Pregabalin	All studies based on immediate release

age, gender, and potentially a genetic susceptibility. Prevention includes good surgical technique (care to protect nerves during surgery) and aggressive multimodal analgesia (use of opioids and nonopioids) before surgery,[25] as well as aggressive treatment of acute pain after surgery.

TREATMENT AND PREVENTION

As mentioned earlier, the best means to prevent chronic pain is to effectively treat severe acute pain or to prevent acute pain before it occurs, especially with regard to surgical procedures. Examples of effective treatment and prevention include nerve blocks either before or during surgery. For example, pectoral blocks (aka Pec blocks) described by Blanco and colleagues[26] are effective for perioperative pain control and management of chronic pain after breast surgery. There are 2 types of Pec blocks,[26,27] with type I best suited for tissue expander and prosthesis insertion, whereas type II block is effective for mastectomy and axillary dissection due to involvement of long thoracic and thoracodorsal nerves. Reports indicate that compared with control, blocks resulted in decreased use of intraoperative fentanyl usage, lower pain scores, less postoperative morphine usage, and decreased postoperative nausea and vomiting, with shorter postanesthetic care unit and hospital stays.[28] Another example is the Tap block, described in 2007 by McDonnell,[29] which is delivered through the triangle of Petit[30] and targets T7 to T12 and L1 nerves. This is well used in abdominal surgeries, and studies show decreased need for opioids and increased patient satisfaction. Tap blocks may also be effective in targeting visceral pain and have been used for acute flares of chronic pancreatitis.

Other treatment modalities in the armamentarium for pain treatment includes peripheral nerve stimulation, with studies showing promise for both acute and chronic pain of peripheral nerve origin,[31–35] peripheral neurolysis (chemical and surgical),[36] peripheral neurectomy/ganglionectomy,[37,38] sympathectomies, and radiofrequency and cryoablation,[39] which works by interrupting nociceptive pathway to reduce pain. Other nontraditional treatment modalities include Tai Chi,[40] shown to be effective in reducing pain in osteoarthritis, fibromyalgia, and chronic low back pain; acupuncture,[41] shown to only provide temporary benefits in chronic pain; as well as psychological interventions including behavioral and cognitive approaches to change the emotional and behavioral response to chronic pain. In fact, psychological interventions have been shown to be extremely beneficial and should always be a part of the treatment of chronic pain.[42,43] Notably, 60% to 80% of patients with chronic pain have concomitant psychiatric pathology; therefore concurrent treatment of psychiatric disorders will significantly improve pain symptoms. Currently studies indicate that cannabis is not effective for acute pain[44,45] but may show promise in chronic neuropathic pain[46] and mixed reviews for cancer pain.[47,48] Botox is believed to induce pain relief due to its paralytic effect but also in the reduction in peripheral and central sensitization through multiple mechanisms.[49] In light of the current opioid epidemic, it is important to understand that patients with chronic pain are at increased risk for substance use disorders and that active substance use disorder is a strong relative contraindication to chronic opioid therapy.[50] This necessitates the need for awareness of other treatment therapies available. Furthermore, it emphasizes the importance of preventing the development of chronic pain to avoid this complication altogether.

SUMMARY

Pain is a normal sensory function that is necessary for survival. It is intended to protect the individual from continued or current injury; however, when the sensation becomes aberrant and develops into a more chronic nature, it transitions into a dysfunctional sensation that handicaps the sufferer, severely affecting quality of life. To optimize the treatment of pain, it is necessary to understand the anatomy and physiology of pain so that targeted therapies may be developed and used. Furthermore, knowledge of the mechanism and pathways of pain will lead to the therapies that prevent the development chronic pain and its sequelae.

DISCLOSURE

No disclosures related to this topic.

REFERENCES

1. IASP. IASP terminology. 2017. Available at: https://www.iasp-pain.org/Education/Content.aspx?ItemNumber=1698. Accessed June 26, 2019.
2. Ringkamp M, Dougherty PM, Raja SN. Anatomy and physiology of the pain signaling process. In: Benzon HT, Raja SN, Liu SS, et al, editors. Essentials of pain medicine. 4th edition. Amsterdam: Elsevier; 2017.
3. Patel NB. Physiology of pain. In: Kopf A, Patel NB, editors. Guide to pain management in low-resource settings. Seattle: IASP; 2010. p. 13–7.

4. Leung E. Physiology of pain. In: Sackheim KA, editor. Pain management and palliative care: a comprehensive guide. New York: Springer New York; 2015. p. 3–6.

5. Sneddon LU. Comparative physiology of nociception and pain. Physiology (Bethesda) 2018;33(1):63–73.

6. Yam MF, Loh YC, Tan CS, et al. General pathways of pain sensation and the major neurotransmitters involved in pain regulation. Int J Mol Sci 2018;19(8) [pii:E2164].

7. Steeds CE. The anatomy and physiology of pain. Surgery - Oxford International Edition 2016;34(2):55–9.

8. Beecher HK. Relationship of significance of wound to pain experienced. J Am Med Assoc 1956;161(17):1609–13.

9. Melzack R, Wall PD. Pain mechanisms: a new theory. Science 1965;150(3699):971–9.

10. Treede RD, Jensen TS, Campbell JN, et al. Neuropathic pain: redefinition and a grading system for clinical and research purposes. Neurology 2008;70(18):1630–5.

11. Finnerup NB, Haroutounian S, Kamerman P, et al. Neuropathic pain: an updated grading system for research and clinical practice. Pain 2016;157(8):1599–606.

12. Bouhassira D, Lantéri-Minet M, Attal N, et al. Prevalence of chronic pain with neuropathic characteristics in the general population. PAIN 2008;136(3):380–7.

13. Yawn BP, Wollan PC, Weingarten TN, et al. The prevalence of neuropathic pain: clinical evaluation compared with screening tools in a community population. Pain Med 2009;10(3):586–93.

14. Endrizzi SA, Rathmell JP, RW. Hurley. Painful peripheral neuropathies. In: Benzon HT, Raja SN, Liu SS, Fishman SM, Steven P. Cohen, eds. Essentials of pain medicine. Vol. 4. Amsterdam: Elsevier; 2018. 273-282.e2.

15. Finnerup NB, Jensen TS. Mechanisms of disease: mechanism-based classification of neuropathic pain-a critical analysis. Nat Clin Pract Neurol 2006;2(2):107–15.

16. Lanz S, Maihofner C. Symptoms and pathophysiological mechanisms of neuropathic pain syndromes. Nervenarzt 2009;80(4):430–44 [in German].

17. Peterson S, Benzon HT, Hurley RW. Membrane stabilizer. In: Benzon HT, Raja SN, Liu SS, et al, editors. Essentials of pain medicine. 4th edition. Amsterdam: Elsevier; 2018. p. 437–44.e2.

18. Haroutounian S, Finnerup NB. Recommendations for pharmacologic therapy of neuropathic pain. In: Benzon HT, Raja SN, Liu SS, et al, editors. Essentials of pain medicine. 4th edition. Amsterdam: Elsevier; 2018. p. 445–56.e2.

19. Cordell WH, Keene KK, Giles BK, et al. The high prevalence of pain in emergency medical care. Am J Emerg Med 2002;20(3):165–9.

20. Porter J, Jick H. Addiction rare in patients treated with narcotics. N Engl J Med 1980;302(2):123.

21. Crofford LJ. Chronic pain: where the body meets the brain. Trans Am Clin Climatol Assoc 2015;126:167–83.

22. Mathews J, Moore A. Pain management in the emergency department. In: Benzon HT, Raja SN, Liu SS, et al, editors. Essentials of pain medicine. 4th edition. Amsterdam: Elsevier; 2018. p. 315–22.e1.

23. Crombie IK, Davies HT, Macrae WA. Cut and thrust: antecedent surgery and trauma among patients attending a chronic pain clinic. Pain 1998;76(1–2):167–71.

24. Katz J, Jackson M, Kavanagh BP, et al. Acute pain after thoracic surgery predicts long-term post-thoracotomy pain. Clin J Pain 1996;12(1):50–5.

25. McCartney CJL, Tremblay S. Chronic pain after surgery. In: Benzon HT, Raja SN, Liu SS, et al, editors. Essentials of pain medicine. Amsterdam: Elsevier; 2018. p. 147–54.e2.

26. Blanco R. The 'pecs block': a novel technique for providing analgesia after breast surgery. Anaesthesia 2011;66(9):847–8.

27. Blanco R, Fajardo M, Parras Maldonado T. Ultrasound description of Pecs II (modified Pecs I): a novel approach to breast surgery. Rev Esp Anestesiol Reanim 2012;59(9):470–5.

28. Bashandy GM, Abbas DN. Pectoral nerves I and II blocks in multimodal analgesia for breast cancer surgery: a randomized clinical trial. Reg Anesth Pain Med 2015;40(1):68–74.

29. McDonnell JG, O'Donnell BD, Farrell T, et al. Transversus abdominis plane block: a cadaveric and radiological evaluation. Reg Anesth Pain Med 2007;32(5):399–404.

30. Suresh S, Chan VW. Ultrasound guided transversus abdominis plane block in infants, children and adolescents: a simple procedural guidance for their performance. Paediatr Anaesth 2009;19(4):296–9.

31. Soin A, Shah NS, Fang ZP. High-frequency electrical nerve block for postamputation pain: a pilot study. Neuromodulation 2015;18(3):197–205 [discussion: 205–6].

32. Rauck RL, Cohen SP, Gilmore CA, et al. Treatment of post-amputation pain with peripheral nerve stimulation. Neuromodulation 2014;17(2):188–97.

33. Huntoon MA, Burgher AH. Ultrasound-guided permanent implantation of peripheral nerve stimulation (PNS) system for neuropathic pain of the extremities: original cases and outcomes. Pain Med 2009;10(8):1369–77.

34. Matharu MS, Bartsch T, Ward N, et al. Central neuromodulation in chronic migraine patients with suboccipital stimulators: a PET study. Brain 2004;127(Pt 1):220–30.

35. Deer T, Pope J, Benyamin R, et al. Prospective, multicenter, randomized, double-blinded, partial

crossover study to assess the safety and efficacy of the novel neuromodulation system in the treatment of patients with chronic pain of peripheral nerve origin. Neuromodulation 2016;19(1):91–100.

36. Saeed K, Adams MCB, Hurley RW. Central and peripheral neurolysis. In: Benzon HT, Raja SN, Liu SS, et al, editors. Essentials of pain medicine. 4th edition. Amsterdam: Elsevier; 2018. p. 655–62.e1.

37. Koch H, Haas F, Hubmer M, et al. Treatment of painful neuroma by resection and nerve stump transplantation into a vein. Ann Plast Surg 2003;51(1):45–50.

38. Williams HB. The painful stump neuroma and its treatment. Clin Plast Surg 1984;11(1):79–84.

39. Malik K. Pulsed radiofrequency, water-cooled radiofrequency, and cryoneurolysis. In: Benzon HT, Raja SN, Liu SS, et al, editors. Essentials of pain medicine. 4th edition. Amsterdam: Elsevier; 2018. p. 619–26.e2.

40. Flamer D, Peng P. Tai chi and chronic pain. In: Benzon HT, Raja SN, Liu SS, et al, editors. Essentials of pain medicine. 4th edition. Amsterdam: Elsevier; 2018. p. 551–8.e2.

41. Hsu ES, Wu I, Lai B. Acupuncture. In: Benzon HT, Raja SN, Liu SS, et al, editors. Essentials of pain medicine. 4th edition. Amsterdam: Elsevier; 2018. p. 545–50.e1.

42. Hosey M, McWhorter JW, Wegener ST. Psychologic interventions for chronic pain. In: Benzon HT, Raja SN, Liu SS, et al, editors. Essentials of pain medicine. 4th edition. Amsterdam: Elsevier; 2018. p. 539–44.e1.

43. Issa MA, Marshall Z, Wasan AD. Psychopharmacology for pain medicine. In: Benzon HT, Raja SN, Liu SS, et al, editors. Essentials of pain medicine. 4th edition. Amsterdam: Elsevier; 2018. p. 427–36.e2.

44. Beaulieu P. Effects of nabilone, a synthetic cannabinoid, on postoperative pain. Can J Anaesth 2006;53(8):769–75.

45. Buggy DJ, Toogood L, Maric S, et al. Lack of analgesic efficacy of oral delta-9-tetrahydrocannabinol in postoperative pain. Pain 2003;106(1–2):169–72.

46. Narang S, Gibson D, Wasan AD, et al. Efficacy of dronabinol as an adjuvant treatment for chronic pain patients on opioid therapy. J Pain 2008;9(3):254–64.

47. Staquet M, Gantt C, Machin D. Effect of a nitrogen analog of tetrahydrocannabinol on cancer pain. Clin Pharmacol Ther 1978;23(4):397–401.

48. Noyes R Jr, Brunk SF, Baram DA, et al. Analgesic effect of delta-9-tetrahydrocannabinol. J Clin Pharmacol 1975;15(2–3):139–43.

49. Nicol AL, Anitescu M, Benzon HT. Pharmacology for the interventional pain physician. In: Benzon HT, Raja SN, Liu SS, et al, editors. 4th edition. Amsterdam: Elsevier; 2018. p. 501–8.e2.

50. Hobelmann JG, Clark MR. Substance use disorders and detoxification. In: Benzon HT, Raja SN, Liu SS, et al, editors. Essentials of pain medicine. 4th edition. Amsterdam: Elsevier; 2018. p. 419–26.e2.

The Opioid Epidemic

Lily A. Upp, BS[a], Jennifer F. Waljee, MD, MPH[a,b],*

KEYWORDS

• Opioid • Narcotic • Pain • Surgery

KEY POINTS

- Opioid-related morbidity and mortality have dramatically increased in the United States over the last several decades.
- Opioid prescribing after surgery has often been in excess, in part owing to the absence of clear prescribing guidelines based on patient-reported pain and opioid-related outcomes.
- Disposal of excess pills after surgery remains low, and unused opioid pills are an important contributor to the opioid epidemic owing to diversion and misuse.

INTRODUCTION

By numerous measures, opioid-related harm in the United States has been increasing over the past 2 decades. Rates of opioid misuse and overdose have reached new highs in recent years, fueled by an abundance of prescription opioids and new spikes in heroin and synthetic opioid use.[1] Current estimates of the economic burden of the opioid crisis—including increased health care costs, productivity loss, and support from services such as law enforcement—top $100 billion per year.[2,3]

The human and financial tolls of this crisis have stimulated a variety of responses from clinicians, researchers, community workers, and policymakers, many of which focus on the role of clinical prescribing. At the center of such initiatives are questions weighting appropriate pain management against patient and public safety, and of the responsibilities of the prescriber. The purpose of this article is to review the current state of the epidemic in the context of surgical prescribing and explore methods within the purview of the plastic surgeon to mitigate opioid-related harm.

AN OVERVIEW OF THE OPIOID EPIDEMIC

In 2017, about 68% of all fatal drug overdoses involved an opioid.[1] This percentage represents 47,600 total opioid-related overdose deaths a year, or an average of 130 deaths per day. Opioid fatalities increased 12% between 2016 and 2017, reaching a number 6 times higher than in 1999, when opioid prescribing began to expand in response to concerted efforts to improve the treatment of pain[4,5] (**Fig. 1**A). Although the prevalence of prescription opioid misuse has significantly decreased since 2015, from 12.5 million to 11.1 million people, the number of people initiating misuse each year remains around 2 million (see **Fig. 1**B).[6,7]

Rates of nonfatal opioid overdose are somewhat inconsistent with those of opioid mortality, having decreased by 15% between 2017 and 2018 for states represented by The Centers for Disease Control and Prevention's Enhanced State Opioid Overdose Surveillance program. Still, several individual states still reported increases in nonfatal overdoses during the same time period, and rates again began to increase throughout the beginning of 2018 for all states.[8] Rates of opioid overdose throughout 2016 and 2017 varied almost 3-fold among US regions with the highest rates observed in the Northeast, followed by the West, Southeast, Midwest, and Southwest[9] (**Fig. 2**). In the same time period, the mortality rates in urban settings have remained stable, whereas those in rural areas

[a] Michigan Opioid Prescribing Engagement Network, Institute for Healthcare Policy and Innovation, University of Michigan, 2800 Plymouth Road, Building 16, Ann Arbor, MI 48109, USA; [b] Department of Plastic Surgery, University of Michigan Medical School, 2130 Taubman Center, 1500 East Medical Center Drive, Ann Arbor, MI 48109, USA
* Corresponding author. Section of Plastic Surgery, Michigan Medicine, 2130 Taubman Center, 1500 East Medical Center Drive, Ann Arbor, MI 48109.
E-mail address: filip@med.umich.edu

Clin Plastic Surg 47 (2020) 181–190
https://doi.org/10.1016/j.cps.2019.12.005
0094-1298/20/© 2020 Elsevier Inc. All rights reserved.

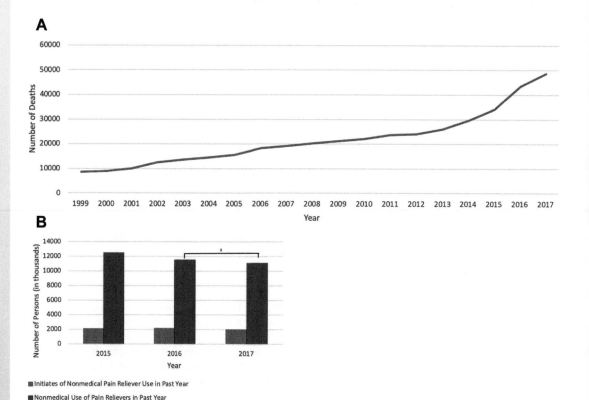

Fig. 1. (*A*) Opioid overdose death rates in the United States from 1999 to 2016. Deaths are classified using the *International Classification of Diseases, Tenth Revision* (ICD–10). Deaths are identified using underlying cause-of-death codes for drug-poisoning (X40–X44, X60–X64, X85, and Y10–Y14) and multiple cause of death codes for opioids (T40.0–T40.4). (*B*) Initiation of and past-year nonmedical use of prescription pain relievers among persons aged 12 or older from 2013 to 2017. [a] *P*<.05. (*Data from* Wide-ranging online data for epidemiologic research (WONDER). Atlanta, GA: CDC, National Center for Health Statistics; 2017. Available at http://wonder.cdc.gov; and the National Survey on Drug Use and Health. Available at https://nsduhweb.rti.org.)

have decreased, lessening the gap between the two.[8] Factors confounding urbanicity, such as economic distress, opioid supply, and race or ethnicity may be better predictors of geographic variation in some cases.[10] This variability suggests that smaller, regional analyses may be necessary to capture the sociodemographic nuances of this epidemic and offer opportunity to identify targets and processes for reduced morbidity.

THE ROLE OF PERIOPERATIVE OPIOID PRESCRIBING

Of the many opioid overdose deaths in 2017, 35% are attributed to prescription opioids specifically.[8] Moreover, use or misuse of prescription opioids remains the most common exposure to later heroin use.[11,12] These figures highlight the significant contribution of clinical prescribing to the opioid epidemic, and continuous review and revision of prescribing practices is critical to minimize risk to patients and the community.

Patterns of Opioid Prescribing

Historically, the rate of fatal opioid overdoses closely paralleled prescribing rates. Notably, in 2011, prescribing rates began to decrease,[13] owing to the combined effects of legislative regulation, clinical guidelines, financial controls, and increased national attention, which have encouraged or mandated changes in clinical practice, among other things.[14] However, overdoses continued to increase at a greater rate beyond 2011, fueled predominately by heroin and synthetic opioids, such as fentanyl and tramadol[1] (**Fig. 3**). The national rate of prescribing has continued to decrease through 2017.[15] From 2016 to 2017, the total opioid dosage filled saw a 12% decrease, the largest single-year decrease in 25 years.[13] However, more nuanced analyses have shown that prescribing in a handful of practices—including surgical, dental, and emergency care—has continued to increase from 2010 to 2016, despite the national downturn. Surgery in

Legend

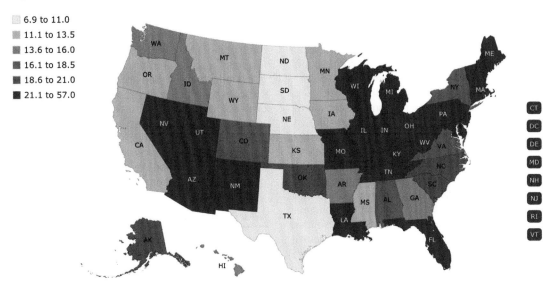

Fig. 2. Number and age-adjusted rates of drug overdose deaths by state in 2017. Deaths are classified using the *International Classification of Diseases, Tenth Revision* (ICD–10). Drug-poisoning deaths are identified using underlying cause-of-death codes X40–X44, X60–X64, X85, and Y10–Y14. Age-adjusted death rates were calculated as deaths per 100,000 population using the direct method and the 2000 standard population. (Courtesy of Center for Disease Control and Prevention. Available at https://www.cdc.gov/drugoverdose/data/statedeaths.html).

particular had an increase of nearly 70% in average total morphine milligram equivalents prescribed in this time period, and in 2016 surgery patients filled the most opioid prescriptions out of these 3 specialties.[16]

In addition to quantity, the types of opioid prescribed are also important to consider, given that increasing potency is correlated with a higher frequency of adverse events.[17] Hydrocodone and oxycodone, which are very commonly used for postoperative analgesia,[18] account for the majority (77%) of serious adverse events, including death.[17] Nevertheless, between 2013 and 2015, oxycodone prescribing dramatically increased,[19,20] translating

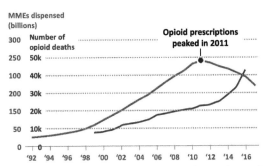

Fig. 3. Morphine milligram equivalents (MMEs) dispensed and opioid overdose deaths per year from 1992 to 2017. (Courtesy of Chad M. Brummett, MD, Ann Arbor, MI.)

into a greater number of patients exposed to this potent formulation. In the same period, 1 institution found that the frequency of tramadol prescriptions increased along with oxycodone after various procedures, a shift that coincided with the rescheduling of hydrocodone in 2014 prohibiting phoned prescriptions to pharmacies.[21] Notably, patients undergoing surgery are particularly more likely to receive oxycodone and hydrocodone as compared with dental or emergency care patients.[16]

Overprescription of Opioid Analgesics

Increasing rates of opioid prescribing within surgery are concerning, but more notable is the growing body of literature to suggest that opioids have been markedly overprescribed for postoperative pain management for decades. For example, Hill and colleagues[22] reported that more than 70% of opioids prescribed after common surgical procedures remain unused. In addition, in a systematic review of 6 studies on opioid prescribing and use, as many as 71% of opioid pills dispensed to surgical patients went unused, and as many as 92% of patients had pills leftover from their postoperative prescription.[23]

Other studies report median prescription sizes that are 2 (in outpatient plastic surgery procedures) to 5 (in abdominal procedures) times greater than patients actually use.[17,23–26] Prescribing is not only excessive, but also highly variable, even after the same procedure type,[25–27] perhaps indicating that prescribing is not consistently anchored by specific evidence. These findings suggest that both standardization and reduced prescribing are appropriate steps for surgical providers to reduce the amount of leftover opioids.

Although reduced postoperative opioid prescribing may raise concerns surrounding inadequate pain control or lower patient satisfaction, there is already growing evidence suggesting that these measures do not suffer when patients take fewer pills.[17,24,27] A recent study of outpatient plastic surgery procedures found that prescription size was not significantly correlated with patient satisfaction. Further, the top reason that patients reported not consuming the opioids prescribed to them, other than experiencing adverse events, was the ability to achieve adequate pain control without opioids.[23] Although the amount of opioid prescribed and consumed have both independently been correlated with pain scores,[24,26] Howard and colleagues[26] noted that one of the strongest predictors of the amount of opioid consumed among surgical patients is the prescription size provided after surgery. Recognizing that a larger prescription may influence patient behavior in taking opioids, and that appropriate pain control and patient satisfaction are achievable with limited use of opioids, it is critical that surgeons take a judicious approach to postoperative opioid prescribing.

Storage and Disposal of Leftover Opioids

Unused opioids leftover from prescriptions are available for misuse or diversion, especially if they are not stored or disposed of properly.[25] Despite these risks, rates of medication disposal are consistently low, and those that do dispose do not do so in alignment with guidelines from the US Food and Drug Administration.[23] Moreover, about three-quarters of patients report storing their opioids in unlocked locations, such as a cabinet or on a kitchen counter.[23] These poor practices may represent a gap in provider education surrounding safe storage and disposal practices. For example, in a poll of adults ages 50 to 80 years of age who had been prescribed an opioid in the last 2 years, just 37% recalled receiving disposal instructions from their surgeon or health care team,[28] and in another study only 18% of patients reported receiving such education.[25] Given the risk for diversion and misuse, it is important to not only match prescribing more closely to need, but also to educate patients on the proper storage and disposal of opioid medications.

Besides lack of appropriate counseling, barriers to disposal options outside the home (eg, law enforcement drop box, medication take back event) may also contribute to the failure of patients to dispose of leftover opioids. Brummett and colleagues[29] reports that providing patients with an activated charcoal bag for in-home medication disposal significantly increased the probability for disposal of unused medication, as compared with patients who received usual care or disposal education alone. Provision of materials for in-home disposal along with opioid prescriptions is a promising method to further promote safe disposal of medications.

New Persistent Use and Misuse after Surgery

New persistent use (NPU) is a significant risk of perioperative opioid prescribing. Although NPU has been defined in a variety of ways, this is commonly considered to be continued opioid fills after 3 months after the index procedure in the absence of additional surgical procedures among opioid naïve patients.[30] Estimates of the prevalence of NPU vary by procedure type and specialty. Various studies report the rate of NPU for opioid-naive patients to be anywhere from 4% to 15%,[31–36] including in pediatric general surgery procedures.[37] Studies on plastic surgery procedures in particular report rates at the higher end of that range, with 6.1% of patients undergoing body-contouring procedures,[35] 6.6% of patients having various plastic and reconstructive procedures,[38] and 13% of hand surgery patients[34,39] meeting criteria for NPU (**Fig. 4**). Additional studies suggest that rates of NPU vary between operating room and nonoperating room procedures,[30] as well as elective versus trauma surgeries.[39] Given that complications after most surgical procedures are relatively low, NPU is a common and important complication after surgical care.

Importantly, there are a number of factors that increase the risk of NPU among opioid-naive patients, including alcohol and substance abuse diagnoses, mental health disorders (anxiety, depression), tobacco use, and pain disorders.[38] For adolescents and young adults, long-term opioid use in a family member is associated with increased odds for persistent use after surgery.[40] Also, new persistent users are more likely to be younger, female, lower income, and have more comorbidities.[39] Attention to these patient-level factors is particularly warranted in light of the findings by Brummett and colleagues[36] that NPU is associated more strongly with patient-level predictors rather than the severity of a procedure.

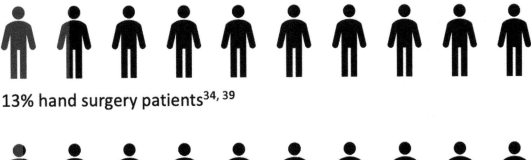

13% hand surgery patients[34, 39]

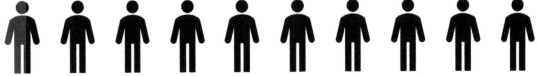

6.6% various plastic and reconstructive surgery patients[38]

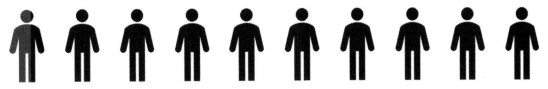

6.1% body-contouring patients[35]

Fig. 4. Rates of NPU in plastic surgery patients. Percentage of new persistent users after common plastic surgery procedures grouped by procedure type. (*Data from* Refs.[34,35,38,39])

There are also factors associated with higher rates of NPU that are at the discretion of the provider. Body-contouring patients that were exposed to high-risk prescribing practices (which include prescriptions of >100 oral morphine equivalents per day, of long-acting opioids, from >1 prescriber, or that overlap with benzodiazepine or other opioid prescriptions) were more likely to be new persistent users as compared with those patients who were not exposed to such practices.[35] These findings are consistent with other studies that have demonstrated that each refill and additional week of opioid use are associated with a higher adjusted rate of misuse,[41] that increasing total OMEs are associated with increased risk for NPU, and that long-acting opioids increase the risk for NPU compared with short-acting formulas.[33,41] Avoidance of these high-risk practices, and careful consideration of patient-level risk factors, should accompany perioperative opioid prescribing.

Transitions of Care After Surgery

In considering NPU, the question arises of who continues to provide opioid prescriptions long after the postoperative period. A retrospective study of national insurance claims found that although surgeons were responsible for the majority (69%) of prescriptions to opioid naive patients in the 3 months after surgery, they only accounted for 11% of prescriptions 9 to 12 months after surgery. In contrast, primary care providers prescribed 13% in the first 3 months then 53% in postoperative months 9 through 12, emergency medicine accounted for 2% then 5%, physical medicine and rehabilitation 1% then 6%, and all other specialties 15% then 25%.[32] These findings suggest that although NPU starts with a surgical prescription, primary care providers and other specialists are majorly responsible for the continuation of the provision of opioids. Surgeons should therefore take steps to better facilitate transitions of care for patients discharged with an opioid prescription, so as to monitor for misuse and NPU.

For opioid-exposed patients and those with chronic opioid use before surgery, facilitating transitions of care with other prescribers is an important step in minimizing exposures to high-risk prescribing practices. As reported by Lagisetty and colleagues,[42] 10% of such patients do not have a consistent prescriber before surgery and are thereby at increased risk for exposure to high-risk prescribing practices (eg, receiving prescriptions from multiple providers). Of the 90% that do have a usual opioid prescriber, return to that provider within 30 days postoperatively is associated with a decreased risk for multiple prescriptions.[42]

EFFORTS TOWARD SAFER PRESCRIBING AND USE OF OPIOIDS
The Legislative Response to the Opioid Epidemic

Policymakers at both state and national levels continue to pass regulatory measures to reduce opioid-related harm. Much of this effort has been reactive, focused on improving outcomes for those already struggling with opioid use disorders or experiencing overdose.[43] For example, the Federal Drug Administration is working to increase access to naloxone, an opioid antagonist that can reverse the effects of opioid overdose, in the hopes of reducing fatalities.[43] Access to Medication Assisted Treatment programs has improved with the passage of the Patient Protection and Affordable Care Act—which mandated that marketplace plans cover substance abuse treatment—by the expansion of coverage of these services for eligible Medicaid recipients, and increasingly by federal grants awarded to individual states to expand Medication Assisted Treatment services.[43] Experts believe these policies are responsible, at least in part, for the declining rate of overdose deaths by prescription opioids in recent years.[43]

Additional policy measures protect overdose victims and those who seek help on their behalf from legal repercussions, promote data collection on drug overdoses and fatalities, and discourage illegitimate prescribing of controlled medications.[44,45] More germane to surgical practice, there are several legal measures, which often vary by state, that directly impact providers' prescribing practice.

Preoperative counseling

Some recent mandates, such as Public Acts 246 and 248 of 2017 in Michigan,[45] and institutional policies[43] require that prescribers provide patient counseling before issuing a prescription for an opioid. Such education may communicate the risks of opioid use, expectations for pain, and alternative modalities for pain control.[22,45–47] A prospective study of carpal tunnel release patients (n = 40) suggests that this practice may have merit in decreasing postoperative opioid consumption. Patients randomized to a group receiving formal preoperative counseling reported taking significantly fewer pills than patients in the control group

who did not receive the counseling, despite receiving the same number of opioid pills. There was no difference in reported pain scores.[48] Based on these results, the authors recommended that surgeons incorporate preoperative counseling into routine practice,[48] an assertion supported by a number of other experts in the field.[22,46,47]

Prescription drug monitoring programs

As of 2017, prescription drug monitoring programs (PDMPs) have been authorized for creation and use in all 50 states and the District of Columbia.[43] PDMPs are valuable tools in identifying situations of potential opioid abuse, because they allow prescribers and pharmacists to view patients' prescription histories.[43] Owing to this central function, they have been leveraged in a handful of states to decrease inappropriate opioid prescribing. For example, New York and Tennessee experienced significant decreases in doctor shopping after a 2012 mandate required providers use the states' PDMPs.[43] Despite this and other evidence that PDMPs have the power to reduce high-risk prescribing and consumption patterns, their impact is limited by inconsistencies in use, the lack of connection between state systems, and prompt data updates.[43]

Prescribing limits

A number of states and individual organizations (eg, private health insurers, retail pharmacy, pharmacy benefit managers, health systems) have recently enacted opioid prescribing limits, generally capping prescriptions at a 3- to 7-day supply.[49,50] The goal is to curb excessive prescribing, which would limit opioid exposure for first-time users and minimize the amount of leftover prescriptions.[49] Skepticism remains, however, over the potential impact of this approach. Some critics have pointed out that a one-size-fits-all restriction will likely not be effective for a heterogeneous patient population, in which individuals have unique pain experiences and histories with opioid use.[50] The mandated limit may be too low for some patients, impeding adequate pain control,[49,50] while being too high for others, rendering the laws ineffectual in limiting prescribing to need.[50]

Additionally, broadly applicable limits must allow for a large number of exceptions to accommodate a variety of unique circumstances without introducing so much flexibility as to undermine the intention of the regulations, a balance that could be difficult to achieve.[49] Already there may be loopholes in these policies that allow physicians to circumvent the new limits. For example, a physician may prescribe higher doses within the daily limit, but direct patients to take fewer pills per dose over a longer duration, or they may forward-date an additional prescription to bypass restrictions on opioid refills.[50] Experts predict that detecting or mitigating this type of activity would be challenging.[50] Ultimately, these potential difficulties lead some to believe that sweeping prescribing limits will be ineffective in achieving their intended goal.[50]

Prescribing Guidelines and Best Practices

Regardless of legislation, it is ultimately incumbent upon the surgeon to use strategies that mitigate potential risks to patients and the community. To do this, providers may need to adopt additional precautionary practices outside of those mandated by law or by institutional policy. Besides the measures already discussed—including preoperative counseling, consistent use of PDMPs, and patient education on disposal methods—evidence and experts agree that prescribing guidelines and the use of nonopioid analgesics for postoperative pain may also be effective in curbing unnecessary prescribing[22,47] (**Fig. 5**).

Prescribing guidelines

Given the limitations of universally applied regulatory approaches, prescribing guidelines based on procedure-level and patient-level factors may be a more useful tool for matching prescribing to need.[47] Procedure-specific prescribing guidelines,[46,50–52] and recommendations based on inpatient opioid use in the 24 to 48 hours before discharge,[53] are available for many common surgeries and offer an evidence-based framework to guide clinician decision making. A study assessing the impact of such guidelines for elective laparoscopic cholecystectomy patients found that the recommendations significantly reduced prescribing with no change in refill requests or pain scores.[54] Notably, when patients were prescribed fewer opioids, as indicated by the guidelines, they reported taking fewer pills at home.[54] Thus, steps should be taken to continually revise guidelines, because consumption is likely to change along with prescription sizes.

A subsequent study found that the implementation of prescribing guidelines for laparoscopic cholecystectomy was associated with spillover effects, or reduced prescribing for other general surgery procedures (laparoscopic appendectomy, laparoscopic inguinal hernia repair, laparoscopic sleeve gastrectomy, and thyroidectomy/parathyroidectomy), again without substantial increases in refill requests. This evidence is important and suggests that the implementation of guidelines for 1 procedure results in an increased general awareness of safe and effective opioid prescribing and influences broader practice without compromising important patient-reported outcomes related to pain and opioids.[55]

There are several notable limitations of prescribing guidelines, the first of which is that may have variable application to patients who are exposed to opioids before surgery or with a history of or active opioid use disorders. In these cases, it is recommended that the surgeon use a patient-centered approach to devise the most appropriate prescription.[56] Caution should also be exercised in the development of guidelines to understand the reasons for which opioids are prescribed and consumed. For example, as part of study by Hill and colleagues[22] to inform guidelines for several general surgery procedures, researchers interviewed patients who consumed more opioid doses than suggested by guidelines. Many (53%) reported taking the medication for reasons unrelated to surgical pain, including for sleep, for nonsurgical pain, for indigestion or gastrointestinal discomfort, in anticipation of pain, or simply because they were provided the prescription, even if they were not experiencing pain.[53] Use motivated by extraneous factors may not always be distinguished in the data used to develop guidelines, thereby overestimating patient need

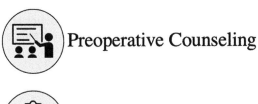
Preoperative Counseling

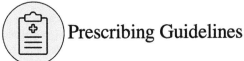
Prescribing Guidelines

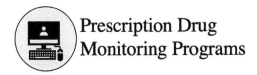
Prescription Drug Monitoring Programs

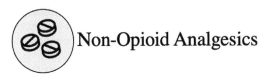
Non-Opioid Analgesics

Fig. 5. Evidence-based interventions for opioid reduction. A summary of 4 practices that have the potential to minimize opioid prescribing and consumption.

for opioids to treat surgical pain. Additionally, an expert panel of providers and patients, convened to devise appropriate prescribing guidelines, found that patients consistently advocated for smaller opioid prescriptions than did providers, indicating that even expert opinion may overrate patient need for opioids.[46]

Finally, guidelines specific to plastic surgery procedures are sparse in the literature, but evidence continues to emerge.[57,58] For example, guidelines set forth by Stanek and colleagues[51] address opioid prescribing for hand-related procedures (release of the first dorsal compartment, primary excision of wrist ganglion, open reduction internal fixation of a metacarpal fracture, and trigger finger release), whereas Fan and colleagues[28] and Rose and colleagues[24] describe prescription and consumption patterns for breast and aesthetic procedures. Further evaluation of prescribing and consumption patterns is necessary to develop guidelines appropriate for treating acute postoperative pain in plastic surgery.

Use of opioid alternatives for postoperative pain control

The use of nonopioid analgesics can decrease or eliminate the need for opioids after surgical procedures, thereby minimizing associated risks to the patient and community. A retrospective review of outpatient breast procedure patients (n = 560) found that 2 different oral multimodal analgesia regimens both significantly decreased the use of opioids in the postanesthesia care unit.[59] A prospective randomized controlled trial of patients undergoing elective soft tissue hand procedures (carpal tunnel release, trigger finger release, first dorsal compartment release, or ganglion cyst excision) reported similar results. Between patients who used ibuprofen and acetaminophen and those who used hydrocodone and acetaminophen, there were no significant differences in pain control, the number of patients needing rescue opioid prescription, or number of postoperative days until patients reported being pain free.[60] These results align with findings from nonopioid analgesic noninferiority studies of general surgical procedures[20] and expert panel recommendations to maximize use of acetaminophen and nonsteroidal anti-inflammatory drugs, where not contraindicated[46] to reduce opioid use.

SUMMARY

Although the growth of the opioid epidemic may be slowing in some ways,[13] prescription opioids remain a leading cause of morbidity and mortality in the United States.[1] Surgeons continue to contribute in large part to these consequences via postoperative opioid prescribing, which carries the risks of NPU, misuse, diversion, and adverse events. However, there are several strategies within the purview of the plastic surgeon for achieving adequate pain relief while mitigating opioid-related harm. Preoperative patient counseling, use of PDMPs, consultation of opioid prescribing guidelines, and maximized use of nonopioid analgesia all hold promise as tools for opioid reduction.

Future work should build on existing evidence demonstrating the adequacy of innovative, opioid-sparing pain management approaches. Further evidence is also needed to inform the development of prescribing guidelines for plastic surgery procedures, which are currently lacking. Finally, evaluation of the impact of public policy, with specific focus on the efficacy of legislative actions and inadvertent consequences, will also be pertinent as such regulatory measures continue to roll out across the nation.

DISCLOSURE

Dr J.F. Waljee receives funding from the National Institute on Drug Abuse (RO1 DA042859), NIAMS (P50 AR070600), and the Michigan Department of Health and Human Services (E20180672-00 Michigan DHHS - MA-2018 Master Agreement Program), as well as the Substance Abuse and Mental Health Administration (SAMHSA: E20180568-00 MA-2018 Master Agreement Program) and the Centers for Disease Control and Prevention (E20182818-00 MA-2018 Master Agreement Program).

REFERENCES

1. Opioid overdose: opioid overdose deaths. 2018. Available at: https://www.cdc.gov/drusgoverdose/epidemic/index.html. Accessed November 1, 2019.
2. Mallow PJ, Belk KW, Topmiller M, et al. Geographic variation in hospital costs, payments, and length of stay for opioid-related hospital visits in the USA. J Pain Res 2018;11:3079–88.
3. Rhyan CN. The potential societal benefit of eliminating opioid overdoses, deaths, and substance use disorders exceeds $95 billion per year executive summary. Senior Analyst, 1–2. 2017. Available at: https://altarum.org/sites/default/files/uploaded-publication-files/Research-Brief_Opioid-Epidemic-Economic-Burden.pdf. Accessed November 1, 2019.
4. Wide-ranging online data for epidemiologic research (WONDER). Atlanta (GA): CDC, National Center for Health Statistics; 2017. Available at: http://wonder.cdc.gov.

5. McGinty EE, Stuart EA, Caleb Alexander G, et al. Protocol: mixed-methods study to evaluate implementation, enforcement, and outcomes of U.S. state laws intended to curb high-risk opioid prescribing. Implement Sci 2018;13(1):37.

6. Substance Abuse and Mental Health Services Administration. Key substance use and mental health indicators in the United States: results from the 2017 National Survey on drug use and health. Department of Health and Human Services. (HHS publication No. SMA 17-5044, NSDUH series H-52), vol. 7, 2017 (1), 877–726.

7. McCance-Katz EF. The national Survey on drug Use and health: 2017 [PowerPoint Presentation]. 2018. Available at: https://www.samhsa.gov/data/sites/default/files/nsduh-ppt-09-2018.pdf. Accessed November 1, 2019.

8. Opioid overdose. 2018. Available at: https://www.cdc.gov/drugoverdose/data/nonfatal.html. Accessed November 1, 2019.

9. National Institute on Drug Abuse. Opioid overdose crisis. 2019. Available at: https://www.drugabuse.gov/drugs-abuse/opioids/opioid-overdose-crisis. Accessed November 1, 2019.

10. Monnat SM. The contributions of socioeconomic and opioid supply factors to U.S. drug mortality rates: urban-rural and within-rural differences. J Rural Stud 2019;68:319–35.

11. Compton WM, Jones CM, Baldwin GT. Relationship between nonmedical prescription-opioid use and heroin use. N Engl J Med 2016;374(2):154–63.

12. Cicero TJ, Ellis MS, Surratt HL, et al. The changing face of heroin use in the United States: a retrospective analysis of the past 50 years. JAMA Psychiatry 2014;71(7):821–6.

13. Brummett CM. The role of acute care prescribing in the opioid epidemic. Material presented at University of Michigan School of Dentistry. Ann Arbor, 2019.

14. Medicine use and spending in the U.S.. 2018. Available at: https://www.iqvia.com/institute/reports/medicine-use-and-spending-in-the-us-review-of-2017-outlook-to-2022. Accessed November 1, 2019.

15. Pezalla EJ, Rosen D, Erensen JG, et al. Secular trends in opioid prescribing in the USA. J Pain Res 2017;10:383–7.

16. Larach DB, Waljee JF, Hu H-M, et al. Patterns of initial opioid prescribing to opioid-naive patients. Ann Surg 2020;271(2):290–5.

17. Murphy DL, Lebin JA, Severtson SG, et al. Comparative rates of mortality and serious adverse effects among commonly prescribed opioid analgesics. Drug Saf 2018;41(8):787–95.

18. Tan WH, Yu J, Feaman S, et al. Opioid medication use in the surgical patient: an assessment of prescribing patterns and use. J Am Coll Surg 2018;227(2):203–11.

19. Tehrani AB, Henke RM, Ali MM, et al. Trends in average days' supply of opioid medications in Medicaid and commercial insurance. Addict Behav 2018;76:218–22.

20. Hartford LB, Van Koughnett JAM, Murphy PB, et al. Standardization of Outpatient Procedure (STOP) narcotics: a prospective non-inferiority study to reduce opioid use in outpatient general surgical procedures. J Am Coll Surg 2019;228(1):81–8.e1.

21. Tan WH, Feaman S, Milam L, et al. Postoperative opioid prescribing practices and the impact of the hydrocodone schedule change. Surgery 2018;164(4):879–86.

22. Hill MV, McMahon ML, Stucke RS, et al. Wide variation and excessive dosage of opioid prescriptions for common general surgical procedures. Ann Surg 2017;265:709–14.

23. Bicket MC, Long JJ, Pronovost PJ, et al. Prescription opioid analgesics commonly unused after surgery: a systematic review. JAMA Surg 2017;152(11):1066–71.

24. Rose KR, Christie BM, Block LM, et al. Opioid prescribing and consumption patterns following outpatient plastic surgery procedures. Plast Reconstr Surg 2019;143(3):929–38.

25. Fujii MH, Hodges AC, Russell RL, et al. Postdischarge opioid prescribing and use after common surgical procedure. J Am Coll Surg 2018;226(6):1004–12.

26. Howard R, Fry B, Gunaseelan V, et al. Association of opioid prescribing with opioid consumption after surgery in Michigan. JAMA Surg 2019;154(1):1–8.

27. Eid AI, DePesa C, Nordestgaard AT, et al. Variation of opioid prescribing patterns among patients undergoing similar surgery on the same acute care surgery service of the same institution: time for standardization? Surgery 2018;164(5):926–30.

28. Fan KL, Luvisa K, Black CK, et al. Gabapentin Decreases Narcotic Usage: Enhanced Recovery after Surgery Pathway in Free Autologous Breast Reconstruction. Plast Reconstr Surg Glob Open 2019;7(8):e2350.

29. Brummett CM, Steiger R, Englesbe M, et al. Effect of an activated charcoal bag on disposal of unused opioids after an outpatient surgical procedure: a randomized clinical trial. JAMA Surg 2019;154(6):558–61.

30. Bicket MC, Murimi IB, Mansour O, et al. Association of new opioid continuation with surgical specialty and type in the United States. Am J Surg 2019;218(5):818–27.

31. Sun EC, Darnall BD, Baker LC, et al. Incidence of and risk factors for chronic opioid use among opioid-naive patients in the postoperative period. JAMA Intern Med 2016;176(9):1286–93.

32. Klueh MP, Hu HM, Howard RA, et al. Transitions of care for postoperative opioid prescribing in previously opioid-naïve patients in the USA: a retrospective review. J Gen Intern Med 2018;33(10): 1685–91.

33. Deyo RA, Hallvik SE, Hildebran C, et al. Association between initial opioid prescribing patterns and subsequent long-term use among opioid-naïve patients: a statewide retrospective cohort study. J Gen Intern Med 2017;32(1):21–7.

34. Habermann EB. Are opioids overprescribed following elective surgery? Adv Surg 2018;52(1): 247–56.

35. Bennett KG, Kelley BP, Vick AD, et al. Persistent opioid use and high-risk prescribing in body contouring patients. Plast Reconstr Surg 2019;143(1): 87–96.

36. Brummett CM, Waljee JF, Goesling J, et al. New persistent opioid use after minor and major surgical procedures in us adults. JAMA Surg 2017;152(6): e170504.

37. Harbaugh CM, Lee JS, Hu HM, et al. Persistent opioid use among pediatric patients after surgery. Pediatrics 2018;141(1):e20172439.

38. Olds C, Spataro E, Li K, et al. Assessment of persistent and prolonged postoperative opioid use among patients undergoing plastic and reconstructive surgery. JAMA Facial Plast Surg 2019;94305:1–6.

39. Johnson SP, Chung KC, Zhong L, et al. Risk of prolonged opioid use among opioid-naïve patients following common hand surgery procedures. J Hand Surg 2016;41(10):947–57.e3.

40. Harbaugh CM, Lee JS, Chua K, et al. Association between long-term opioid use in family members and persistent opioid use after surgery among adolescents and young adults. JAMA Surg 2019;154(4): e185838.

41. Brat GA, Agniel D, Beam A, et al. Postsurgical prescriptions for opioid naive patients and association with overdose and misuse: retrospective cohort study. BMJ 2018;360:j5790.

42. Lagisetty P, Bohnert A, Goesling J, et al. Care coordination for patients on chronic opioid therapy following surgery. Ann Surg 2019. https://doi.org/10.1097/SLA.0000000000003235.

43. Barlas S. U.S. and states ramp up response to opioid crisis: regulatory, legislative, and legal tools brought to bear. P T 2017;42(9):569–92.

44. Phillips J. Prescription drug abuse: problem, policies, and implications. Nurs Outlook 2013;61(2): 78–84.

45. Legislation. 2019. Available at: https://michigan-open.org/legislation/. Accessed November 1, 2019.

46. Overton HN, Hanna MN, Bruhn WE, et al. Opioid-prescribing guidelines for common surgical procedures: an expert panel consensus. J Am Coll Surg 2018;227(4):411–8.

47. Kaafarani HMA, Weil E, Wakeman S, et al. The opioid epidemic and New Legislation in Massachusetts: time for a culture change in surgery? Ann Surg 2017;265:731–3.

48. Alter TH, Ilyas AM. A prospective randomized study analyzing preoperative opioid counseling in pain management after carpal tunnel release surgery. J Hand Surg 2017;42(10):810–5.

49. Bateman BT, Choudhry NK. Limiting the duration of opioid prescriptions: balancing excessive prescribing and the effective treatment of pain. JAMA Intern Med 2016;176(5):583–4.

50. Chua KP, Brummett CM, Waljee JF. Opioid prescribing limits for acute pain: potential problems with design and implementation. JAMA 2019;321(7): 643–4.

51. Stanek JJ, Renslow MA, Kalliainen LK. The effect of an educational program on opioid prescription patterns in hand surgery: a quality improvement program. J Hand Surg 2015;40(2):341–6.

52. Kim N, Matzon JL, Abboudi J. A prospective evaluation of opioid utilization after upper-extremity surgical procedures: identifying consumption patterns and determining prescribing guidelines. J Bone Joint Surg Am 2016;98(20):e89.

53. Hill MV, Stucke RS, Billmeier SE, et al. Guideline for discharge opioid prescriptions after inpatient general surgical procedures. J Am Coll Surg 2018; 226(6):996–1003.

54. Howard R, Waljee J, Brummett C, et al. Reduction in opioid prescribing through evidence-based prescribing guidelines. JAMA Surg 2018;153(3):284–5.

55. Howard R, Alameddine M, Klueh M, et al. Spillover effect of evidence-based postoperative opioid prescribing. J Am Coll Surg 2018;227(3):374–81.

56. Prescribing recommendations. 2019. Available at: https://michigan-open.org/prescribing-recommendations/. Accessed November 1, 2019.

57. Torabi R, Bourn L, Mundinger GS, et al. American Society of Plastic Surgeons member post-operative opioid prescribing patterns. Plast Reconstr Surg Glob Open 2019;7(3). https://doi.org/10.1097/gox. 0000000000002125.

58. Wang AMQ, Retrouvey H, Wanzel KR. Addressing the opioid epidemic: a review of the role of plastic surgery. Plast Reconstr Surg 2018;141(5):1295–301.

59. Barker JC, DiBartola K, Wee C, et al. Preoperative multimodal analgesia decreases postanesthesia care unit narcotic use and pain scores in outpatient breast surgery. Plast Reconstr Surg 2018;142(4): 443e–50e.

60. Weinheimer K, Michelotti B, Silver J, et al. A prospective, randomized, double-blinded controlled trial comparing ibuprofen and acetaminophen versus hydrocodone and acetaminophen for soft tissue hand procedures. J Hand Surg 2018; 44(5):387–93.

Pain Management in Plastic Surgery

Anna R. Schoenbrunner, MD, MAS[a], Jeffrey E. Janis, MD[b],*

KEYWORDS

- Pain management • Plastic surgery • Multimodal analgesia

KEY POINTS

- Poorly controlled postoperative pain is associated with worse clinical outcomes and negative patient experiences.
- Plastic surgeons must be well versed in multimodal analgesia (MMA) management strategies to optimize postoperative pain control and minimize narcotic use.
- MMA regimens are customized to the patient and procedure.
- Local anesthetics, regional blocks, and epidurals are powerful adjuncts in any MMA regimen.
- Plastic surgeons must be aware of dosing and contraindications for all medications used as part of an MMA regimen.

INTRODUCTION

Postoperative pain management in plastic surgery has become a topic of increasing interest. Pain is the perceived sensory and emotional reaction to actual or perceived tissue injury.[1] Nociceptive pain is caused by suprathreshold stimulation of peripheral pain receptors from damage to nonneural tissue.[2] Inflammatory pain results from peripheral pain sensitization caused by activation of the immune system via chemical mediators. Surgery causes tissue injury that leads to both nociceptive and inflammatory pain. Pathologic pain is caused by dysfunction of the nervous system without tissue damage; it is maladaptive in that it serves no biological function.[3]

Uncontrolled postsurgical pain has been associated with increased risk of poor pulmonary function, myocardial ischemia, ileus, thromboembolism, and impaired immune function.[4,5] It has been associated with increased postanesthesia care unit stays, prolonged admissions, and increased readmission rates, all of which may affect reimbursement and patient satisfaction.[6–11] Uncontrolled postsurgical pain has also been implicated in the development of persistent postsurgical pain (PPSP) caused by maladaptive neuronal plasticity.[12,13] PPSP is estimated to affect 20% to 25% of mastectomy patients, 50% to 85% of amputation patients, and 5% to 35% of hernia repair patients.[14,15]

In the era of the American opioid epidemic, surgeons play a crucial role in optimizing postoperative pain and minimizing narcotic use. Nonpharmacologic pain management strategies such as mindfulness, massage, and acupuncture have been found to be effective pain management strategies and should be used.[16] This article reviews pain management strategies available to plastic surgeons based on therapeutic class of medication and provides a framework for pain management based on Enhanced Recovery After Surgery (ERAS) protocols. Much of this content was previously covered in a *Plastic and Reconstructive Surgery* Pain Management Supplement

[a] Department of Plastic and Reconstructive Surgery, The Ohio State University, 915 Olentangy River Road, Columbus, OH 43212, USA; [b] Department of Plastic and Reconstructive Surgery, Ohio State University Wexner Medical Center, 915 Olentangy River Road, Columbus, OH 43212, USA
* Corresponding author.
E-mail address: jeffrey.janis@osumc.edu
Twitter: @aschoenbrunner (A.R.S.); @jjanismd (J.E.J.)

Clin Plastic Surg 47 (2020) 191–201
https://doi.org/10.1016/j.cps.2019.12.001
0094-1298/20/© 2019 Elsevier Inc. All rights reserved.

and the authors refer the reader to the supplement for a more in-depth discussion.[17]

OPIOIDS

Opioids are ubiquitous in the current health care system. This class of analgesics primarily act on mu opioid receptors in the central nervous system.[18] Opioids modify afferent pain signals by binding to opiate receptors and decrease the perception of pain. The mu opiate receptor not only has analgesic properties but also causes euphoria, sedation, anorexia, and respiratory depression; this accounts for the adverse effects associated with opiate use.[19] The addictive potential of opioids has been well established and cannot be overstated, with estimates of postoperative chronic opiate use in previously opiate-naive patients ranging from 5% to 13%.[20–22]

Opioids are generally administered parenterally or orally. Parenteral administration has predictable peak plasma concentration with rapid time to onset and offset. Parenteral formulations of opioids are an effective method of analgesia in patients without enteral absorptive capacity. Patient-controlled analgesia (PCA) devices allow repeated low doses of opioids to be administered by the patient. PCA has gained popularity because it decreases nursing burden; however, PCA has been shown to increase side effects such as nausea, vomiting, and pruritis.[23] Oral administration of opioids results in slower time of onset because of first-pass metabolism through the liver; however, the slower enteral absorption results in more steady and longer-lasting analgesic effects.[24]

Opioids should be used with caution in patients with obstructive sleep apnea, geriatric patients, and those with abuse history or potential. Caution must be used in prescribing opioids to patients who concurrently use other sedative medications, such as benzodiazepines, antihistamines, or sleep aids, because these can have additive effects and cause respiratory depression.[25] They should also be used with extreme caution in anyone with a history of alcohol consumption.

The authors recommend minimizing opiate use postoperatively by using a patient-specific and procedure-specific multimodal analgesia (MMA) approach for ambulatory or inpatient surgery patients. For patients who require opioids for acute postsurgical pain, we recommend the use of opioids without added acetaminophen (eg, tramadol or oxycodone alone) to decrease the risk of acetaminophen toxicity (maximum dose, 4000 mg in 24 hours).

ACETAMINOPHEN, NONSTEROIDAL ANTIINFLAMMATORY DRUGS, AND SELECTIVE CYCLOOXYGENASE-2 INHIBITORS
Acetaminophen

Acetaminophen's mechanism of action remains elusive but it is thought to inhibit cyclooxygenase-1 (COX-1) and COX-2 enzymes in the central nervous system.[26] This inhibition accounts for its analgesic and antipyretic effects.[27,28] Because acetaminophen does not affect peripheral COX enzymes, it does not have the same gastric ulceration and bleeding complications associated with nonsteroidal antiinflammatory drugs (NSAIDs). A Cochran Review found that a single dose of acetaminophen postoperatively achieves a 50% reduction in pain.[29] Acetaminophen is available in oral, rectal, and intravenous formulations. Intravenous acetaminophen is significantly more costly than oral acetaminophen and has not been shown to be more effective in reducing postoperative pain scores compared with oral acetaminophen.[30] Acetaminophen is metabolized by the liver and must be used with caution in patients with liver disease. The maximum dose of acetaminophen is 4000 mg in a 24-hour period.[31]

The authors recommend using acetaminophen in all postoperative patients who do not have contraindications to its use. Acetaminophen should be scheduled around the clock in the first 48 to 72 hours following surgery. Prescribers must exercise caution in patients who take medications at home containing acetaminophen, such as opioid combinations or cold medications.

Nonsteroidal Antiinflammatory Drugs

NSAIDs act by inhibiting peripheral COX-1 and COX-2 enzymes and inhibiting the synthesis of prostaglandin, a mediator of inflammation and vasodilation, and thromboxane, a mediator of vasoconstriction and platelet aggregation.[32] NSAIDs cause gastric ulceration, gastrointestinal (GI) bleeding, platelet dysfunction, asthma exacerbation, and renal impairment. Importantly, prescribers must be aware of the cardiovascular risks associated with NSAIDs and COX-2 inhibitors. These risks include myocardial infarction, stroke, heart failure, hypertension, atrial fibrillation, and venous thromboembolism in patients with and without known cardiovascular disease, elucidated largely through the landmark Vioxx gastrointestinal outcomes research (VIGOR) and Prospective Randomized Evaluation of Celecoxib Integrated Safety versus Ibuprofen or Naproxen (PRECISION) trials.[33,34] In 2015, the US Food and Drug Administration (FDA) strengthened its warning against NSAIDs, warning against the use of these medications because of increased risk of heart disease and stroke, both in patients with and without existing heart disease.[35]

Cyclooxygenase-2 Inhibitors

The COX-2 enzyme plays a role in inflammation.[36] Selective COX-2 inhibitors theoretically reduce the risk of GI bleeding. Several studies investigating the GI benefits of selective COX-2 inhibitors found they have decreased risk of GI bleeding compared with NSAIDs, but were still associated with higher bleeding risk compared with placebo.[33,37,38] A study investigating the effect of selective COX-2 inhibitors on platelet function found the drugs to have similar, undetectable effects on platelet function compared with placebo, whereas NSAIDs decreased platelet aggregation and increased bleeding time.[39] Selective COX-2 inhibitors have many of the same contraindications as NSAIDs with the exception that they have an improved GI risk profile. Importantly, they carry the same FDA warnings with regard to cardiovascular risks as NSAIDs.[40,41]

The authors recommend selective use of NSAIDs or COX-2 inhibitors in appropriately selected patients. These medications should not be used in patients with known cardiovascular disease, renal impairment, or GI bleeding risk factors. Duration should be minimized to the acute postoperative setting and the lowest effective dosage should be used. We prefer the use of celecoxib dosed 3 times per day.

ADJUVANT MULTIMODAL MEDICATIONS
Gabapentin

Gabapentin postsynaptically binds to dorsal horn neurons, blocking voltage-gated calcium channels, thereby decreasing neurotransmitter release.[42] The medication is orally administered. Gabapentin is not metabolized and is renally excreted via first-order kinetics; patients with renal impairment may require dose adjustment.[43,44] Gabapentin can cause somnolence, confusion, and dizziness and should be used cautiously in geriatric patients and those with obstructive sleep apnea.[45] High-dose gabapentin should be tapered, because abrupt cessation can cause withdrawal symptoms similar to those caused by alcohol and benzodiazepines.[46] A meta-analysis of postoperative gabapentin use found a 35% reduction in total opioid use within 24 hours following surgery and a significant reduction in postoperative pain.[47] However, a Cochrane Review on systemic medications for the prevention of chronic postoperative pain did not find a significant reduction of chronic postoperative pain with gabapentin.[48]

The authors recommend the use of gabapentin as an adjunctive multimodal medication for acute, postoperative pain in hospitalized patients. We advocate a loading dose the evening before surgery (usually 600 mg) as well as a preoperative dose before the operation (typically 300 mg). Postoperatively, in patients less than 65 years old, we favor 300 mg orally 3 times a day, whereas those more than 65 years old are dosed twice daily. Gabapentin must be dose adjusted for patients with renal impairment and used cautiously in geriatric patients and those with obstructive sleep apnea.

Muscle Relaxants

Cyclobenzaprine is a commonly prescribed muscle relaxant. Despite its classification, cyclobenzaprine does not act on skeletal muscle. It is a centrally acting medication that is thought to act at the brainstem level on the locus ceruleus, decreasing the activity of serotonergic descending neurons, thus decreasing muscle tone.[49,50] The effect on the locus ceruleus may help to explain the sedating qualities of the medication. Cyclobenzaprine, and most other muscle relaxants, are renally metabolized and require dose adjustments for patients with renal impairment. For patients unable to take oral medications, methocarbamol can be administered intravenously.

The authors recommend the use of muscle relaxants as adjuncts in an MMA regimen when a patient's pain is not controlled with a standard MMA regimen and when the operation involved a high likelihood of muscle spasm or tension. We use special caution in elderly patients because this class of medication can worsen fall risk and delirium.

Steroids

Steroids have potent and well-known antiinflammatory, immunomodulatory, and antiemetic effects. However, steroids also have innumerable side effects beyond the scope of this discussion. With regard to plastic surgery applications, steroids cause delayed wound healing, increased surgical site infections, and hyperglycemia.[51] A single dose of dexamethasone given preoperatively or intraoperatively has been found to decrease postoperative pain scores and narcotic usage.[52,53] Two retrospective studies, a meta-analysis, and a Cochrane Review have not found significant wound healing complications or surgical site infections within 30 days after a single perioperative dose of dexamethasone; however, long-term studies are lacking.[54–57]

There should be no concern or hesitation when the use of dexamethasone is warranted for its antiinflammatory or antiemetic effects. Typically, a single 8-mg intraoperative dose (Decadron) is recommended, and can be given at any time after induction. Clinicians should avoid preoperative administration because a known side effect is intense anal/perineal itching.

Topical Anesthetics

Topical anesthetics are the topical version of injectable local anesthetics. These classes of medications inactivate voltage-gated sodium channels, raising the threshold required to generate an action potential, rendering the area temporarily insensate.[58] Their structure consists of a lipophilic aromatic group attached to an amine group with a chain of either an amide or ester.[59] The amide or ester chain affects metabolism; amides are hepatically degraded, whereas esters are degraded by plasma cholinesterase. Esters form the metabolite para-aminobenzoic acid (PABA) and are more commonly implicated in allergic reactions.[60] Topical and local anesthetics preferentially affect type C nerve fibers (pain fibers) rather than type A nerve fibers (proprioception and pressure fibers); patients may therefore be entirely anesthetized in the injected area but continue to feel a pressure sensation.[61]

The most commonly used topical anesthetics include lidocaine patches; eutectic mixture of local anesthetics (EMLA) consisting of lidocaine and prilocaine; as well as a mixture of lidocaine, epinephrine, and tetracaine (LET). Time of onset, depth of penetration, and duration vary for each anesthetic based on the pKa, pH, solubility, and protein-binding potential.[58] Skin penetration can be increased by exfoliating skin and using alcohol to cleanse skin of sebaceous material. Efficacy of topical anesthetics depends on skin permeation and has a delayed onset of action compared with locally injected anesthetics. A Cochrane Review investigating the use of topical anesthetics during repair of dermal lacerations found that they can play an important role in analgesia before laceration repair.[62]

The concentrations of each local anesthetic vary and must be carefully calculated to avoid local anesthetic systemic toxicity (LAST) (**Table 1**).[63,64] Surgeons must be well versed in the management of LAST; guidelines are available from the American Society of Regional Anesthesia and Pain Medicine.[65]

The authors recommend the use of topical anesthetics applied at least 30 minutes before planned procedure for simple laceration repairs in pediatric patients.

Local Anesthetics

The importance of local anesthetics in plastic surgery practice cannot be overstated. The most commonly used local anesthetics include lidocaine, bupivacaine, and ropivacaine. These anesthetics are often combined with epinephrine to decrease intraoperative blood loss and allow better visualization. Lalonde has revolutionized wide-awake surgery with injection techniques that minimize discomfort and maximize efficacy.[66–72]

Local anesthetics not only allow painless wide-awake surgery but also improve postoperative pain. A meta-analysis found that local anesthetic injected before incision decreases somatic pain and decreases postoperative analgesic consumption and time to first rescue pain medication dose.[73] Joshi and colleagues[74] provide a framework for surgical site infiltration of local anesthetic for abdominal wall surgery based on a neuroanatomic approach; this framework is widely applicable.

Liposomal bupivacaine contains bupivacaine within a lipid-based vehicle that results in diffusion of the drug over time with initial peak at 0.25 to 2 hours and a second peak 12 to 24 hours after injection. Liposomal bupivacaine has been shown to provide pain relief over 48 to 72 hours.[75] Liposomal bupivacaine remains under patent and thus costs more than standard bupivacaine. A study by Little and colleagues[76] found decreased postoperative narcotic consumption, length of stay, direct and total costs, and 30-day readmission rate with liposomal bupivacaine compared with control patients undergoing abdominal wall, implant-based, and autologous breast reconstruction. However, a prospective, single-blinded, randomized controlled trial of a single surgeon using liposomal bupivacaine in addition to an enhanced recovery protocol including preoperative regional block failed to detect a clinical difference in total opioid consumption, pain score, or length of stay.[77] This finding suggests that the benefits of liposomal bupivacaine are clinically insignificant when combined with an enhanced recovery protocol that includes a regional or epidural analgesia.

The authors recommend the use of short-acting local anesthetics for bedside procedures and long-acting local anesthetics for postoperative pain control. We reserve the use of liposomal bupivacaine for patients at high risk of postoperative pain (such as those undergoing abdominal wall reconstruction who did not undergo preoperative epidural block), and usually administer it as a regional block for maximum effect.

Table 1
Local anesthetic dosing recommendations

Anesthetic	Onset (min)	Duration of Analgesia (h)	Maximum Dose Without Epinephrine (mg/kg)	Maximum Dose with Epinephrine (mg/kg)
Lidocaine	10–20	0.25–1	4.5	7
Mepivacaine	10–20	0.75–1.5	5	7
Ropivacaine	15–30	2–6	3	3.5
Bupivacaine	15–30	2–4	2.5	3

Data from Rosenberg, PH, Veering BT, Urmey WF. Maximum recommended doses of local anesthetics: a multi-factorial concept. Reg Anesth Pain Med. 2004; 29(6):564-75; discussion 524 and El-Boghdadly K, Pawa A, Chin KJ. Local anesthetic systemic toxicity: current perspectives. Local Reg Anesth. 2018; 11:35–44.

Tumescent Analgesia

Tumescent analgesia involves the use of dilute lidocaine or bupivacaine in large volumes of carrier fluid with or without epinephrine. This technique was popularized by Klein[78] in the late 1980s for use during liposuction. The practice has since been expanded to several surgical procedures, including body contouring, mastopexy, breast reduction, and mastectomy.[79] Because of the lipid solubility and distributive properties of local anesthetics, tumescent analgesia allows higher maximum concentrations of local anesthetics than traditional field blocks.[61] Klein[80] performed further studies measuring the maximum safe dose of lidocaine in wetting solution and found this to be 35 mg/kg, with more recent reports showing safety profiles up to 55 mg/kg.[80,81] The American Society of Plastic Surgeons Practice Advisory on Liposuction recommends limiting lidocaine to a maximum dose of 35 mg/kg; with adjustments for patients with metabolic conditions that may limit metabolism of local anesthetics.[82]

There is a dearth of evidence for the analgesic effects of tumescent techniques. However, 1 prospective, double-blinded, randomized controlled trial injecting wetting solution containing lidocaine into the side of a body site undergoing liposuction found a statistically significant decrease in postoperative pain at 18 hours after surgery.[83] However, this study did not account for the potential distributive effect of lidocaine or the systemic absorption of lidocaine, which, in itself, has been shown to decrease postoperative pain.[84]

The authors recommend the routine use of wetting solution in a superwet manner with lidocaine or bupivacaine, as described by Fodor,[85] within the safety profile of each respective local anesthetic for liposuction.[86]

Regional Anesthesia

Regional anesthesia is the technique whereby long-acting local anesthetic is injected or continuously infused into a targeted area surrounding peripheral nerves supplying specific dermatomes, thereby anesthetizing entire dermatomes. Regional anesthetics have been shown to decrease postoperative narcotic use, postoperative nausea/vomiting, and length of stay.[87–91] The most commonly used regional anesthetics in plastic surgery include the pectoralis nerve block (PECS) I and II block in breast surgery, transversus abdominis plane (TAP) block for abdominal wall surgery, and supraclavicular or infraclavicular blocks for wrist and hand surgery.

The PECS block is performed by injecting long-acting local anesthetic into the fascial plane between the pectoralis major and minor muscle (PECS I) and above the serratus anterior muscle at the level of the third rib (PECS II), blunting sensation from the pectoral, intercostobrachial, intercostal 3 to 6, and long thoracic nerves.[92–94] The TAP block is performed by injecting long-acting local anesthetic between the internal oblique and transversus abdominis fascial planes, blunting the afferent sensory fibers of the terminal branches of T10 to L1 sensory fibers.[95] The supraclavicular and infraclavicular blocks are performed by injecting local anesthetic around the trunks and divisions or cords of the brachial plexus, respectively.[96,97] Techniques vary but these blocks are typically performed with ultrasonography guidance; ultrasonography guidance decreases risk of pneumothorax.[98]

Because regional anesthesia uses local anesthetics, the same caution with regard to local anesthetic toxicity must be used. The authors recommend the use of regional anesthesia whenever possible. Certain regional anesthetics, such as the PECS and supraclavicular blocks, require skilled anesthetists; these capabilities may not be available in certain settings.

Table 2
Multimodal analgesia options

Medication/ Technique	Initiation	Dosage	Duration	Contraindications/ Caution
Epidural	Preoperatively	Per anesthesia acute pain team	3–5 d until patient able to tolerate PO MMA	Caution in patients with preexisting pulmonary disease, hypotension
Local and/or regional block	Preoperatively or intraoperatively	Attention to local anesthetic maximum dosage	—	—
Patient-controlled analgesia	Postoperatively as needed	Start at lowest dose without basal rate	Until patient able to tolerate CLD	Do not combine with epidural
Acetaminophen	Single preoperative dose; postoperatively when patient able to tolerate CLD	1000 mg pre-operative dose; 1000 mg q6 h post-operative	Continue 5 d after discharge	Liver disease
Celecoxib	Single preoperative dose; postoperatively when patient able to tolerate CLD	400 mg pre-operative dose; 200 mg TID post-operative	Continue 5 d after discharge	Cardiac or renal disease; caution in patients at risk for GI bleeding
Gabapentin	600-mg loading dose evening before surgery; single preoperative dose; postoperatively when patient able to tolerate CLD	900 mg pre-operative dose; 300 mg TID post-operative	Continue 5 d after discharge	OSA; caution in patients with renal impairment
Cyclobenzaprine	Postoperatively PRN when patient able to tolerate CLD	5–10 mg TID	Continue 5 d after discharge if initiated as inpatient	Caution in geriatric patients
Oxycodone	Single preoperative dose; postoperatively PRN when patient able to tolerate CLD	5 mg pre-operative; 5 mg q3–4 h PRN for breakthrough pain post-operative	Discontinue as soon as able	—
IV hydromorphone	Postoperatively PRN	0.5–1.0 mg hydromorphone q3 h PRN breakthrough pain	Discontinue as soon as able	—

Abbreviations: CLD, clear liquid diet; OSA, obstructive sleep apnea; PO, oral; PRN, as needed; q, every; TID, 3 times daily.

Epidural Anesthesia

Epidural anesthesia blocks the spinal nerve roots as they exit the spinal cord. This blocking is done by injecting or infusing local anesthetic and narcotic medications into the epidural space. At typical doses, epidurals do not cause motor weakness and thus allow early postoperative ambulation.[95] Epidurals are commonly used for abdominal wall reconstruction. They are typically placed preoperatively and continued for 3 to 5 days postoperatively until the patient is able to tolerate an oral MMA regimen.[99]

Outcomes data on epidural analgesia have been mixed, with few studies specifically assessing uses within plastic surgery. A 2016 Cochrane Review by Guay and colleagues[100] comparing epidurals with local anesthetics with opioids administered systemically or via epidural in abdominal surgery found that epidurals with opioids decrease postoperative pain and speed return of bowel function. A more recent Cochrane Review by Salicath and colleagues[101] comparing epidural analgesia with intravenous opiate PCAs in intra-abdominal surgery noted the decrease in postoperative pain to be clinically insignificant with higher chance of epidural failure caused by technical error and episodes of hypotension requiring intervention. Khansa and colleagues[99] studied the effect of preoperative epidural placement in an MMA regimen for abdominal wall reconstruction and found epidurals decreased postoperative narcotic requirements compared with patients who did not receive a preoperative epidural.

Epidurals have rare, but nontrivial, complications related to technique. These complications include epidural hematomas, abscesses, peripheral neuropathy, and spinal headaches. Their use is also associated with hypotension caused by efferent sympathetic blockade; this is seen in up to 33% of patients.[102] Epidurals can also cause respiratory complications in patients with preexisting pulmonary disease because the effect on intercostal and abdominal muscles can weaken forced exhalation.[95]

The authors recommend the use of epidural anesthesia in properly selected patients requiring inpatient reconstructive surgery, particularly abdominal wall reconstruction. We recommend the use of epidurals in combination with enhanced recovery protocols and MMA.

Putting it All Together: Multimodal Analgesia Regimen

In a time when the United States faces an opiate epidemic, surgeons must be ever mindful of their postoperative analgesic approach. The era of ERAS protocols, pioneered by Ljungqvist and colleagues[103,104] in the early 2000s, opened the surgical community's eyes to the benefits of preoperative nutritional and functional optimization, early postoperative liberalization of diet, and MMA.[103–105] The authors have adapted the lessons learned from the ERAS protocols as well as our own institutional experience to develop an MMA regimen to treat postsurgical pain.[99,106,107] **Table 2** summarizes our recommendations for MMA options that can be customized based on surgical procedure and patient characteristics.

DISCLOSURE

Dr J.E. Janis receives royalties from Thieme Publishing. Dr A.R. Schoenbrunner has no financial disclosures.

REFERENCES

1. IASP. Iasp Terminology. Available at: https://www.iasp-pain.org/Education/Content.aspx?ItemNumber=1698. Accessed Jan 23, 2020.
2. Fong A, Schug SA. Pathophysiology of pain: a practical primer. Plast Reconstr Surg 2014; 134(4 Suppl 2):8S–14S.
3. Cohen SP, Mao J. Neuropathic pain: mechanisms and their clinical implications. BMJ 2014;348: f7656.
4. Joshi GP, Ogunnaike BO. Consequences of inadequate postoperative pain relief and chronic persistent postoperative pain. Anesthesiol Clin North Am 2005;23(1):21–36.
5. Baratta JL, Schwenk ES, Viscusi ER. Clinical consequences of inadequate pain relief: barriers to optimal pain management. Plast Reconstr Surg 2014;134(4 Suppl 2):15S–21S.
6. Pavlin DJ, Chen C, Penaloza DA, et al. A survey of pain and other symptoms that affect the recovery process after discharge from an ambulatory surgery unit. J Clin Anesth 2004;16(3):200–6.
7. Herbst MO, Price MD, Soto RG. Pain related readmissions/revisits following same-day surgery: have they decreased over a decade? J Clin Anesth 2017;42:15.
8. Coley KC, Williams BA, DaPos SV, et al. Retrospective evaluation of unanticipated admissions and readmissions after same day surgery and associated costs. J Clin Anesth 2002;14(5):349–53.
9. Pavlin DJ, Chen C, Penaloza DA, et al. Pain as a factor complicating recovery and discharge after ambulatory surgery. Anesth Analg 2002;95(3): 627–34 [table of contents].
10. Pavlin DJ, Rapp SE, Polissar NL, et al. Factors affecting discharge time in adult outpatients. Anesth Analg 1998;87(4):816–26.

11. Wu CL, Naqibuddin M, Rowlingson AJ, et al. The effect of pain on health-related quality of life in the immediate postoperative period. Anesth Analg 2003;97(4):1078–85 [table of contents].

12. Kehlet H, Jensen TS, Woolf CJ. Persistent postsurgical pain: risk factors and prevention. Lancet 2006;367(9522):1618–25.

13. Beloeil H, Sulpice L. Peri-operative pain and its consequences. J Visc Surg 2016;153(6S):S15–8.

14. Niraj G, Rowbotham DJ. Persistent postoperative pain: where are we now? Br J Anaesth 2011; 107(1):25–9.

15. Stark N, Kerr S, Stevens J. Prevalence and predictors of persistent post-surgical opioid use: a prospective observational cohort study. Anaesth Intensive Care 2017;45(6):700–6.

16. Tick H, Nielsen A, Pelletier KR, et al. Evidence-based nonpharmacologic strategies for comprehensive pain care: the Consortium Pain Task Force White Paper. Explore (NY) 2018;14(3):177–211.

17. Janis JE, Joshi GP. Introduction to "current concepts in pain management in plastic surgery. Plast Reconstr Surg 2014;134(4 Suppl 2):6S–7S.

18. Pasternak GW. Opiate pharmacology and relief of pain. J Clin Oncol 2014;32(16):1655–61.

19. Trescot AM, Datta S, Lee M, et al. Opioid pharmacology. Pain Physician 2008;11(2 Suppl):S133–53.

20. Brummett CM, Waljee JF, Goesling J, et al. New persistent opioid use after minor and major surgical procedures in US adults. JAMA Surg 2017; 152(6):e170504.

21. Johnson SP, Chung KC, Zhong L, et al. Risk of prolonged opioid use among opioid-naive patients following common hand surgery procedures. J Hand Surg Am 2016;41(10):947–57.e3.

22. Jiang X, Orton M, Feng R, et al. Chronic opioid usage in surgical patients in a large Academic Center. Ann Surg 2017;265(4):722–7.

23. Roberts GW, Bekker TB, Carlsen HH, et al. Postoperative nausea and vomiting are strongly influenced by postoperative opioid use in a dose-related manner. Anesth Analg 2005;101(5):1343–8.

24. Glare PA, Walsh TD. Clinical pharmacokinetics of morphine. Ther Drug Monit 1991;13(1):1–23.

25. Funk RD, Hilliard P, Ramachandran SK. Perioperative opioid usage: avoiding adverse effects. Plast Reconstr Surg 2014;134(4 Suppl 2):32S–9S.

26. Ghanem CI, Perez MJ, Manautou JE, et al. Acetaminophen from liver to brain: new insights into drug pharmacological action and toxicity. Pharmacol Res 2016;109:119–31.

27. Flower RJ, Vane JR. Inhibition of prostaglandin synthetase in brain explains the anti-pyretic activity of paracetamol (4-acetamidophenol). Nature 1972; 240(5381):410–1.

28. Engstrom Ruud L, Wilhelms DB, Eskilsson A, et al. Acetaminophen reduces lipopolysaccharide-induced fever by inhibiting cyclooxygenase-2. Neuropharmacology 2013;71:124–9.

29. Toms L, McQuay HJ, Derry S, et al. Single dose oral paracetamol (acetaminophen) for postoperative pain in adults. Cochrane Database Syst Rev 2008;(4):CD004602.

30. Harricharan S, Frey N. Intravenous acetaminophen for the management of short-term post-operative pain: a review of clinical effectiveness and cost-effectiveness. Ottawa (Ontario): 2018.

31. Krenzelok EP, Royal MA. Confusion: acetaminophen dosing changes based on NO evidence in adults. Drugs R D 2012;12(2):45–8.

32. Cashman JN. The mechanisms of action of NSAIDs in analgesia. Drugs 1996;52(Suppl 5):13–23.

33. Bombardier C, Laine L, Reicin A, et al. Comparison of upper gastrointestinal toxicity of rofecoxib and naproxen in patients with rheumatoid arthritis. VIGOR Study Group. N Engl J Med 2000;343(21): 1520–8, 1522 p following 1528.

34. Nissen SE, Yeomans ND, Solomon DH, et al. Cardiovascular safety of celecoxib, naproxen, or ibuprofen for arthritis. N Engl J Med 2016; 375(26):2519–29.

35. [press release]FDA Drug Safety Communication: FDA strengthens warning that non-aspirin nonsteroidal anti-inflammatory drugs (NSAIDs) can cause heart attacks or strokes. Silver Spring, (MD): Food and Drug Administration (FDA); 2015.

36. Meade EA, Smith WL, DeWitt DL. Differential inhibition of prostaglandin endoperoxide synthase (cyclooxygenase) isozymes by aspirin and other non-steroidal anti-inflammatory drugs. J Biol Chem 1993;268(9):6610–4.

37. Simon LS, Weaver AL, Graham DY, et al. Anti-inflammatory and upper gastrointestinal effects of celecoxib in rheumatoid arthritis: a randomized controlled trial. JAMA 1999; 282(20):1921–8.

38. Emery P, Zeidler H, Kvien TK, et al. Celecoxib versus diclofenac in long-term management of rheumatoid arthritis: randomised double-blind comparison. Lancet 1999;354(9196):2106–11.

39. Leese PT, Hubbard RC, Karim A, et al. Effects of celecoxib, a novel cyclooxygenase-2 inhibitor, on platelet function in healthy adults: a randomized, controlled trial. J Clin Pharmacol 2000;40(2): 124–32.

40. Bresalier RS, Sandler RS, Quan H, et al. Cardiovascular events associated with rofecoxib in a colorectal adenoma chemoprevention trial. N Engl J Med 2005;352(11):1092–102.

41. Sibbald B. Rofecoxib (Vioxx) voluntarily withdrawn from market. CMAJ 2004;171(9):1027–8.

42. Chang CY, Challa CK, Shah J, et al. Gabapentin in acute postoperative pain management. Biomed Res Int 2014;2014:631756.

43. McLean MJ. Clinical pharmacokinetics of gabapentin. Neurology 1994;44(6 Suppl 5):S17–22 [discussion: S31–2].

44. Beydoun A, Uthman BM, Sackellares JC. Gabapentin: pharmacokinetics, efficacy, and safety. Clin Neuropharmacol 1995;18(6):469–81.

45. Mao J, Chen LL. Gabapentin in pain management. Anesth Analg 2000;91(3):680–7.

46. Norton JW. Gabapentin withdrawal syndrome. Clin Neuropharmacol 2001;24(4):245–6.

47. Peng PW, Wijeysundera DN, Li CC. Use of gabapentin for perioperative pain control – a meta-analysis. Pain Res Manag 2007;12(2):85–92.

48. Chaparro LE, Smith SA, Moore RA, et al. Pharmacotherapy for the prevention of chronic pain after surgery in adults. Cochrane Database Syst Rev 2013;(7):CD008307.

49. Kobayashi H, Hasegawa Y, Ono H. Cyclobenzaprine, a centrally acting muscle relaxant, acts on descending serotonergic systems. Eur J Pharmacol 1996;311(1):29–35.

50. Honda M, Nishida T, Ono H. Tricyclic analogs cyclobenzaprine, amitriptyline and cyproheptadine inhibit the spinal reflex transmission through 5-HT(2) receptors. Eur J Pharmacol 2003; 458(1–2):91–9.

51. Low YH, Gan TJ. NMDA receptor antagonists, gabapentinoids, alpha-2 agonists, and dexamethasone and other non-opioid adjuvants: do they have a role in plastic surgery? Plast Reconstr Surg 2014;134(4 Suppl 2):69S–82S.

52. Waldron NH, Jones CA, Gan TJ, et al. Impact of perioperative dexamethasone on postoperative analgesia and side-effects: systematic review and meta-analysis. Br J Anaesth 2013;110(2):191–200.

53. De Oliveira GS Jr, Almeida MD, Benzon HT, et al. Perioperative single dose systemic dexamethasone for postoperative pain: a meta-analysis of randomized controlled trials. Anesthesiology 2011; 115(3):575–88.

54. Thoren H, Snall J, Kormi E, et al. Does perioperative glucocorticosteroid treatment correlate with disturbance in surgical wound healing after treatment of facial fractures? A retrospective study. J Oral Maxillofac Surg 2009;67(9):1884–8.

55. Snall J, Kormi E, Lindqvist C, et al. Impairment of wound healing after operative treatment of mandibular fractures, and the influence of dexamethasone. Br J Oral Maxillofac Surg 2013;51(8):808–12.

56. Ali Khan S, McDonagh DL, Gan TJ. Wound complications with dexamethasone for postoperative nausea and vomiting prophylaxis: a moot point? Anesth Analg 2013;116(5):966–8.

57. Polderman JA, Farhang-Razi V, Van Dieren S, et al. Adverse side effects of dexamethasone in surgical patients. Cochrane Database Syst Rev 2018;(11): CD011940.

58. Kumar M, Chawla R, Goyal M. Topical anesthesia. J Anaesthesiol Clin Pharmacol 2015; 31(4):450–6.

59. Park KK, Sharon VR. A review of local anesthetics: minimizing risk and side effects in cutaneous surgery. Dermatol Surg 2017;43(2):173–87.

60. Becker DE, Reed KL. Essentials of local anesthetic pharmacology. Anesth Prog 2006;53(3):98–108 [quiz: 109–10].

61. Becker DE, Reed KL. Local anesthetics: review of pharmacological considerations. Anesth Prog 2012;59(2):90–101 [quiz: 102–3].

62. Tayeb BO, Eidelman A, Eidelman CL, et al. Topical anaesthetics for pain control during repair of dermal laceration. Cochrane Database Syst Rev 2017;(2):CD005364.

63. El-Boghdadly K, Pawa A, Chin KJ. Local anesthetic systemic toxicity: current perspectives. Local Reg Anesth 2018;11:35–44.

64. Clinical pharmacology of local anesthetics. 2019. Available at: https://www.nysora.com/foundations-of-regional-anesthesia/pharmacology/clinical-pharmacology-local-anesthetics/. Accessed July 22, 2019.

65. Neal JM, Woodward CM, Harrison TK. The American Society of Regional Anesthesia and Pain Medicine checklist for managing local anesthetic systemic toxicity: 2017 version. Reg Anesth Pain Med 2018;43(2):150–3.

66. Farhangkhoee H, Lalonde J, Lalonde DH. Teaching medical students and residents how to inject local anesthesia almost painlessly. Can J Plast Surg 2012;20(3):169–72.

67. Lalonde D, Martin A. Epinephrine in local anesthesia in finger and hand surgery: the case for wide-awake anesthesia. J Am Acad Orthop Surg 2013;21(8):443–7.

68. Lalonde DH, Wong A. Dosage of local anesthesia in wide awake hand surgery. J Hand Surg Am 2013;38(10):2025–8.

69. Lovely LM, Chishti YZ, Woodland JL, et al. How much volume of local anesthesia and how long should you wait after injection for an effective wrist median nerve block? Hand (N Y) 2018;13(3):281–4.

70. Strazar AR, Leynes PG, Lalonde DH. Minimizing the pain of local anesthesia injection. Plast Reconstr Surg 2013;132(3):675–84.

71. Lalonde D, Wong A. Local anesthetics: what's new in minimal pain injection and best evidence in pain control. Plast Reconstr Surg 2014;134(4 Suppl 2): 40S–9S.

72. Lalonde DH. Latest advances in wide awake hand surgery. Hand Clin 2019;35(1):1–6.

73. Ong CK, Lirk P, Seymour RA, et al. The efficacy of preemptive analgesia for acute postoperative pain management: a meta-analysis. Anesth Analg 2005; 100(3):757–73 [table of contents].

74. Joshi GP, Janis JE, Haas EM, et al. Surgical site infiltration for abdominal surgery: a novel neuroanatomical-based approach. Plast Reconstr Surg Glob Open 2016;4(12):e1181.

75. Chahar P, Cummings KC 3rd. Liposomal bupivacaine: a review of a new bupivacaine formulation. J Pain Res 2012;5:257–64.

76. Little A, Brower K, Keller D, et al. A cost-minimization analysis evaluating the use of liposomal bupivacaine in reconstructive plastic surgery procedures. Plast Reconstr Surg 2019;143(4):1269–74.

77. Ha AY, Keane G, Parikh R, et al. The analgesic effects of liposomal bupivacaine versus bupivacaine hydrochloride administered as a transversus abdominis plane block after abdominally based autologous microvascular breast reconstruction: a prospective, single-blind, randomized, controlled trial. Plast Reconstr Surg 2019;144(1):35–44.

78. Klein JA. Tumescent technique chronicles. Local anesthesia, liposuction, and beyond. Dermatol Surg 1995;21(5):449–57.

79. Gutowski KA. Tumescent analgesia in plastic surgery. Plast Reconstr Surg 2014;134(4 Suppl 2):50S–7S.

80. Klein JA. Tumescent technique for regional anesthesia permits lidocaine doses of 35 mg/kg for liposuction. J Dermatol Surg Oncol 1990;16(3):248–63.

81. Ostad A, Kageyama N, Moy RL. Tumescent anesthesia with a lidocaine dose of 55 mg/kg is safe for liposuction. Dermatol Surg 1996;22(11):921–7.

82. Iverson RE, Lynch DJ, ASPS Committee on Patient Safety. Practice Advisory on Liposuction. Plast Reconstr Surg 2004;113(5):1478–90.

83. Danilla S, Fontbona M, de Valdes VD, et al. Analgesic efficacy of lidocaine for suction-assisted lipectomy with tumescent technique under general anesthesia: a randomized, double-masked, controlled trial. Plast Reconstr Surg 2013;132(2):327–32.

84. Vigneault L, Turgeon AF, Cote D, et al. Perioperative intravenous lidocaine infusion for postoperative pain control: a meta-analysis of randomized controlled trials. Can J Anaesth 2011;58(1):22–37.

85. Fodor PB. Lipoplasty: A Personal, Conceptual, and Historical Perspective. Aesthetic Plast Surg 2007;31(4):313–6.

86. Rohrich RJ, Kenkel JM, Janis JE, et al. An update on the role of subcutaneous infiltration in suction-assisted lipoplasty. Plast Reconstr Surg 2003;111(2):926–7 [discussion: 928].

87. Schnabel A, Reichl SU, Kranke P, et al. Efficacy and safety of paravertebral blocks in breast surgery: a meta-analysis of randomized controlled trials. Br J Anaesth 2010;105(6):842–52.

88. Tahiri Y, Tran DQ, Bouteaud J, et al. General anaesthesia versus thoracic paravertebral block for breast surgery: a meta-analysis. J Plast Reconstr Aesthet Surg 2011;64(10):1261–9.

89. Rivedal DD, Nayar HS, Israel JS, et al. Paravertebral block associated with decreased opioid use and less nausea and vomiting after reduction mammaplasty. J Surg Res 2018;228:307–13.

90. Fayezizadeh M, Majumder A, Neupane R, et al. Efficacy of transversus abdominis plane block with liposomal bupivacaine during open abdominal wall reconstruction. Am J Surg 2016;212(3):399–405.

91. Rundgren J, Mellstrand Navarro C, Ponzer S, et al. Regional or general anesthesia in the surgical treatment of distal radial fractures: a randomized clinical trial. J Bone Joint Surg Am 2019;101(13):1168–76.

92. Blanco R. The 'pecs block': a novel technique for providing analgesia after breast surgery. Anaesthesia 2011;66(9):847–8.

93. Blanco R, Fajardo M, Parras Maldonado T. Ultrasound description of Pecs II (modified Pecs I): a novel approach to breast surgery. Rev Esp Anestesiol Reanim 2012;59(9):470–5.

94. Bashandy GM, Abbas DN. Pectoral nerves I and II blocks in multimodal analgesia for breast cancer surgery: a randomized clinical trial. Reg Anesth Pain Med 2015;40(1):68–74.

95. Momoh AO, Hilliard PE, Chung KC. Regional and neuraxial analgesia for plastic surgery: surgeon's and anesthesiologist's perspectives. Plast Reconstr Surg 2014;134(4 Suppl 2):58S–68S.

96. Ultrasound-guided infraclavicular brachial plexus block. 2019. Available at: https://www.nysora.com/regional-anesthesia-for-specific-surgical-procedures/upper-extremity-regional-anesthesia-for-specific-surgical-procedures/anesthesia-and-analgesia-for-elbow-and-forearm-procedures/ultrasound-guided-infraclavicular-brachial-plexus-block/. Accessed July 22, 2019.

97. Ultrasound-guided supraclavicular brachial plexus block. 2019. Available at: https://www.nysora.com/regional-anesthesia-for-specific-surgical-procedures/upper-extremity-regional-anesthesia-for-specific-surgical-procedures/anesthesia-and-analgesia-for-elbow-and-forearm-procedures/ultrasound-guided-supraclavicular-brachial-plexus-block/. Accessed July 22, 2019.

98. Lewis SR, Price A, Walker KJ, et al. Ultrasound guidance for upper and lower limb blocks. Cochrane Database Syst Rev 2015;(9):CD006459.

99. Khansa I, Koogler A, Richards J, et al. Pain management in abdominal wall reconstruction. Plast Reconstr Surg Glob Open 2017;5(6):e1400.

100. Guay J, Nishimori M, Kopp S. Epidural local anaesthetics versus opioid-based analgesic regimens for postoperative gastrointestinal paralysis, vomiting and pain after abdominal surgery. Cochrane Database Syst Rev 2016;(7):CD001893.

101. Salicath JH, Yeoh EC, Bennett MH. Epidural analgesia versus patient-controlled intravenous analgesia for pain following intra-abdominal surgery in adults. Cochrane Database Syst Rev 2018;(8): CD010434.

102. Carpenter RL, Caplan RA, Brown DL, et al. Incidence and risk factors for side effects of spinal anesthesia. Anesthesiology 1992;76(6): 906–16.

103. Ljungqvist O, Scott M, Fearon KC. Enhanced recovery after surgery: a review. JAMA Surg 2017; 152(3):292–8.

104. Ljungqvist O, Young-Fadok T, Demartines N. The history of enhanced recovery after surgery and the ERAS Society. J Laparoendosc Adv Surg Tech A 2017;27(9):860–2.

105. Temple-Oberle C, Shea-Budgell MA, Tan M, et al. Consensus review of optimal perioperative care in breast reconstruction: enhanced Recovery after Surgery (ERAS) Society recommendations. Plast Reconstr Surg 2017;139(5):1056e–71e.

106. Barker JC, DiBartola K, Wee C, et al. Preoperative multimodal analgesia decreases postanesthesia care unit narcotic use and pain scores in outpatient breast surgery. Plast Reconstr Surg 2018;142(4): 443e–50e.

107. Khansa I, Jefferson R, Khansa L, et al. Optimal pain control in abdominal wall reconstruction. Plast Reconstr Surg 2018;142(3 Suppl):142S–8S.

Fibromyalgia

Michael W. Neumeister, MD, FRCSC[a],*, Evyn L. Neumeister, MD, MPH[b]

KEYWORDS

- Fibromyalgia • Chronic pain • Pain • Pain disorders • Central sensitization

KEY POINTS

- Fibromyalgia is a complex systemic disorder characterized by generalized pain, specific sites of musculoskeletal tenderness, fatigue, sleep disturbance, headaches, and a myriad of other visceral and cognitive maladies.
- Diagnosis and treatment options are reviewed.

Pain syndromes seen by upper extremity surgeons have a variety of presentations. Compression neuropathies, neuromas, enthesopathies, tendinopathies, synovitis, arthritis, ischemia, trauma, and degenerative disorders may all play a role in the pain that afflicts our patients. Most conditions require either therapy exercises, immobilization, or anti-inflammatories. The history and physical examination become extremely important in helping the surgeon to differentiate surgical versus nonsurgical management in painful conditions and the upper extremity. Challenges arise, however, when the patient has multiple symptoms that do not seem to condense to a specific site or surgically manageable pathology. In fact, upper extremities surgeons often see patients with some distinct pathology, such as carpal metacarpal joint arthritis of the thumb or carpal tunnel syndrome, but the patient has complaints of chronic pain and tenderness in various areas in the upper extremity or the entire body. The patient may also complain of many conditions, such as a history of migraine headaches, irritable bowel syndrome, interstitial cystitis, myofascial pain syndrome, or restless leg syndrome. For the busy surgeon, this can be easily dismissed as they try to focus on one specific area that can be treated quickly and efficiently to render the patient pain free. The multiple symptoms outside of those to a specific area

in the upper extremity should alert the hand surgeon to other conditions such as fibromyalgia.

Fibromyalgia is a complex systemic disorder characterized by generalized pain, specific sites of musculoskeletal tenderness, fatigue, sleep disturbance, headaches, and a myriad of other visceral and cognitive maladies.[1,2] Fibromyalgia may be confused with other pain syndromes (**Box 1**). Previous fibromyalgia criteria used the term chronic wide spread pain defined as pain on the right or left side of the body, pain above or below the waist, or axial skeletal pain. Currently, regions of generalized pain are considered a more useful criteria.[3] Once termed fibrositis, fibromyalgia is now believed to be a part of the central sensitivity syndrome and not an inflammatory process.[4–6] With that being said, the triggers for the central sensitization are unclear. It is possible that inflammatory states or autoimmune conditions or physical trauma can be the initial trigger to fibromyalgia.[3] Ultimately, the condition is manifest by abnormal intense perception of pain with minimal stimuli. Abnormalities along the entire pain pathway, from the peripheral activation of nociceptors, to neurotransmitter changes, to the somatosensory cortical interpretation of the central nervous system, have been identified in patients with fibromyalgia.[3] Abnormalities in functional MRI provide objective evidence that

[a] Department of Surgery, Institute for Plastic Surgery, Southern Illinois University School of Medicine, 747 North Rutledge Suite 357, Baylis Building, Springfield, IL 62702, USA; [b] Institute for Plastic Surgery, Southern Illinois University School of Medicine, Springfield, IL, USA

* Corresponding author.

E-mail address: mneumeister@siumed.edu

Clin Plastic Surg 47 (2020) 203–213
https://doi.org/10.1016/j.cps.2019.12.007

Box 1
Characteristics of fibromyalgia and other centralized pain syndromes

Character and quality of pain

   Diffuse or multifocal, often waxes and wanes, and is frequently migratory in nature

   Often accompanied by dysethesia or parasthesias and described as more "neuropathic" (eg, with terms such as numbness, tingling, burning)

   Patients may note discomfort when they are touched or when wearing tight clothing

History of pain in other body regions earlier in life

Accompanying comorbid symptoms also of central nervous system origin

   Often fatigue, sleep disturbances, memory, and mood difficulties accompany centralized pain states such as fibromyalgia

   Several of these symptoms will typically improve along with pain when individuals are successfully treated with appropriate pharmacologic or nonpharmacological therapies

Symptoms suggesting more global sensory hyperresponsiveness

   Sensitivity to bright lights, loud noises, and odors and even many visceral symptoms may be in part due to a global sensory hyperresponsiveness seen in conditions such as fibromyalgia

   Often leads to a panpositive review of symptoms that has often mischaracterized these individuals as somatizers as the biology of somatization is increasingly recognized as that of sensory hyperresponsiveness[30]

From Clauw DJ. Fibromyalgia. A Clinical review. JAMA. 2014; 311(15):1574-55; with permission.

---

fibromyalgia has its foundation in an organic pathology.[2,3,6,7] Similarly, sustained higher levels of substance P and other pain-modulating neurotransmitters have been identified in the cerebral spinal fluid of patients with fibromyalgia.[2,3] Even more compelling is the recent finding by Albrecht and colleagues, demonstrating an increase in radioligands and uptake in specific brain regions through activated brain glia and neuroinflammation in patients with fibromyalgia.[7]

The prevalence of fibromyalgia is said to be in the range of 0.5% to 12.0% of the population with a female to male ratio 3 to 1.[3] Patients with fibromyalgia should be thought of as patients with a pain-prone phenotype, often experiencing episodes of chronic pain not only focused on the musculoskeletal system, but on all areas of the body.[1] Therefore, obtaining an extensive history defining the chronicity and regionality of the pain will direct management appropriately. Surgery and opioid use to relieve the pain is more often than not unresponsive in the pain-prone patient. Furthermore, the pain sensitivity is thought to be polygenic. Patients with fibromyalgia seem to have a familial preponderance of the condition with variable expression1.[3,6]

The diagnosis of fibromyalgia can be difficult, but is based predominantly on the patient's history. It often takes more than 2 years to confirm the diagnosis, with patients seeing an average of 3.7 physicians and or surgeons during this time.[8]

Many conditions may have similar clinical scenarios that mimic fibromyalgia; therefore, care should be taken into consideration during the workup of afflicted patients to try to identify ailments that will be treated differently. The differential diagnosis of fiber myalgia can be categorized into musculoskeletal, neurologic, psychiatric psychological, and drug-related disorders (**Box 2**).

Diagnostic dilemmas in the evaluation of a patient with chronic pain prompted the formation of the Analgesic, Anesthetic, and Addiction Clinical Trial Translations Innovation Opportunities and Networks public–private partnership with the US Food and Drug Administration and the American Pain Society initiation of the Analgesic, Anesthetic, and Addiction Clinical Trial Translations Innovation Opportunities and Networks–American Pain Society Pain Taxonomy group to develop a consistent diagnosis system for the various pain disorders.[9] As a result, the Analgesic, Anesthetic, and Addiction Clinical Trial Translations Innovation Opportunities and Networks–American Pain Society Pain Taxonomy identified 5 dimensions to differentiate diagnosis (**Box 3**).[3,8,9] Further clarifications were made through structured, focused fibromyalgia working groups to reach our current understanding of appropriate criteria for diagnosing fibromyalgia (**Box 4**).[3] Biomarkers do not exist for fibromyalgia, although increases in serum haptoglobin and fibrinogen levels offer some promise.[1] Systemic inflammation is not characteristic of

Box 2
A differential diagnosis for patients with fibromyalgia

Rheumatoid arthritis

Inflammatory spondyloarthritis

Systemic lupus erythematosus

Polymyalgia rheumatic

Myositis

Myofascial pain syndrome

Multiple sclerosis

Ehlers-Danlos syndrome

Neuropathy

Myopathies

Hypothyroidism

Depression

Lyme disease

Hepatitis C

Human immunodeficiency disease

Statins (secondary effects)

Aromatase inhibitors (secondary effects)

Bisphosphonates (secondary effects)

this condition. Recent evidence, however, suggests that profiles of microRNAs in saliva and cerebral spinal fluid may help to diagnose patients with fibromyalgia.[10–12] Proteomic analysis have shown increases in seotransferin, alpha-enolase,

Box 3
Fibromyalgia diagnostic dimensions from the Analgesic, Anesthetic, and Addiction Clinical Trial Translations Innovation Opportunities and Networks–American Pain Society Pain Taxonomy

Dimension 1: Core criteria

Pain in more than 6 of 9 regions

Sleep disturbance

Fatigue

Chronic pain, fatigue, sleep disturbance greater than 3 months

Dimension 2

Tenderness, generalized sensitivity of soft tissues or muscles

Dyscognition

Musculoskeletal stiffness

Hypervigilance (environmental hypersensitivity)

Dimension 3

Common medical and psychiatric comorbidities

Somatic pain disorders

Irritable bowel syndrome

Chronic pelvic pain

Interstitial cystitis

Chronic head and/or orofacial conditions

Rheumatic diseases

Psychiatric conditions

Major mood disorder

Anxiety disorders

Substance abuse disorder

Sleep disorders

Restless leg disorder

Sleep apnea

Obesity

Dimension 4

Neurobiological, psychological, and functional consequences

Disabilities

Greater health care costs

Poorer health status

Depression

Dimension 5

Putative neurobiological and psychosocial mechanisms, risk factors, and protective factors

Headaches

Dysmenorrhea

Temporomandibular joint disorder

Irritable bowel syndrome

Endometriosis

Other regional pain syndromes

Family history of fibromyalgia

Stressors as triggers, such as adverse life events

Data from Arnold LM, Bennett RM, Crofford LJ, Dean LE, Clauw DJ, Goldenberg DL, Fitzcharles M, Paiva ES, Staud R, Sarzi-Puttini P, Buskila D, MacFarlane GJ. Critical Reviews. AAPT Diagnostic Criteria for Fibromyalgia. J Pain, Vol 20, No 6 (June), 2019: pp 611-628.

phosphoglycerate-mutase-I, and trans-aldolase in patients with fibromyalgia relative to healthy, migraine, or rheumatoid arthritis patients.[13] Similarly, Ramirez-Tejero and colleagues[14] identified

Box 4
The 2019 Analgesic, Anesthetic, and Addiction Clinical Trial Translations Innovation Opportunities and Networks–American Pain Society Pain Taxonomy diagnostic criteria established for patients with fibromyalgia

1. Multisite pain, defined as pain in at least 6 sites of pain from a total of 9

2. Moderate to severe sleep problems OR fatigue

3. Multisite pain plus fatigue or sleep problems present for at least 3 months

From Arnold LM, Bennett RM, Crofford LJ, et al. AAPT Diagnostic Criteria for Fibromyalgia. J Pain. 2019; 20(6):611-628; with permission.

33 different proteins expressed in the plasma of patients with fibromyalgia and suggested that inflammation may have a role in the pathology. Metabolomic screening has recently differentiated

Box 5
General approach to pharmacologic therapy

All patients should receive

Education about nature of disorder

Counseling regarding role of exercise, cognitive–behavioral techniques

Pharmacologic therapy should be guided by predominant symptoms that accompany pain

All patients should have a good therapeutic trial of a low-dose tricyclic compound (eg, cyclobenzaprine, amitriptyline, nortriptyline)

Patients with comorbid depression or fatigue should next try a serotonin norepinephrine reuptake inhibitor

Patients with comorbid anxiety or sleep issues should next try a gabapentinoid

It is often necessary to use several of these classes of drugs together

Use of opioids is discouraged

Nonsteroidal anti-inflammatory drugs and acetaminophen can be used to treat comorbid peripheral pain generators

Therapies that have been less well-studied but show promise

Complementary and alternative therapies

Drugs including low-dose naltrexone, cannabinoids

Cortical electrostimulatory therapies

From Clauw DJ. Fibromyalgia. A Clinical review. JAMA. 2014; 311(15):1574-55; with permission.

patients with fibromyalgia from those patients with lupus and rheumatoid arthritis, identified through the analysis of vibrational spectra tyrosine residues in proteins, which highlighted possible roles of aromatic and carboxylic acid molecules, including tryptophan as potential biomarkers.[15]

Many patients with fibromyalgia often complain of areas of musculoskeletal pain, but may also described dysesthesias in the upper and lower extremities. Compression neuropathies may form a component of some of the physical complaints but recently small fiber neuropathies have been identified and a large number of patients with fibromyalgia. Biopsies indicating a reduction in the dermal unmylinated nerve fiber bundles may form a diagnostic tool for patients with fibromyalgia. Martinez-Lavin[16] described in vivo corneal confocal microscopy to identify small fiber pathology in patients with fibromyalgia. This option may be a plausible one for a noninvasive fibromyalgia diagnostic test.[16]

Neuroimmune activation has been suggested by Albrecht and colleagues[17] for a possible means to central sensitization in patients with fibromyalgia. The authors identified increased uptake of radioligands in specific areas of the brains in patients with fibromyalgia and implicated neuroinflammation as a possible target for biomarker identification.[17]

The treatment of patients with fibromyalgia requires a multidisciplinary approach.[1–3,7,17–21] Pharmacology alone will be fraught with failure. Education, behavioral changes, and exercise regimens are the mainstay of treating patients with fibromyalgia with pharmacology assisting in the management of pain and associated conditions (**Box 5**).[1,3,18] Patients with questionable diagnoses should be sent to a rheumatologist to identify other possible inflammatory or autoimmune conditions that may explain the patient's symptoms. The psychological support may involve basic body awareness therapy, cognitive–behavioral therapy, group music and imagery intervention, and virtual reality.[19–24] Other nonpharmacologic therapies have included yoga, Tai Chi, acupuncture, heat application, and dietary modulation.[25,26]

There are a variety of medications that have been used to treat the chronic pain of fibromyalgia.[1,3,7,27–29] The extent of this polypharmacy is beyond the scope of this article but the pharmacology should be guided toward not only the pain but the symptoms and comorbidities that accompany the pain (**Table 1**).[1,3]

Attempts to elucidate the treatment options in patients with fibromyalgia many investigators to study the role of the gut-brain axis, microbiome, and nutrition in the pathophysiology of this

Table 1
Summary of treatment guidelines

Treatment	Cost	Details	Evidence Level	Adverse Effects	Clinical Pearls
General recommendations					
Patient education[35]	Low	Incorporate principles of self-management including a multimodal approach	1A		Following initial diagnosis, spend several visits (or use separate educational sessions) to explain the conditions and set treatment expectations
Nonpharmacologic therapies					
Graded exercise[36]	Low	Aerobic exercise has been best studied but strengthening and stretching have also been shown to be of value	1A	Worsening of symptoms when program is begun too rapidly	Counsel patients to "start low, go slow" For many patients, focusing first on increasing daily "activity" is helpful before actually starting exercise
CBT[37]	Low	Pain-based CBT programs have been shown to be effective in one-on-one settings, small groups, and via the Internet	1A	No significant adverse effects of CBT per se but patient acceptance is often poor when viewed as a "psychological" intervention	Internet-based programs are gaining acceptance and are more convenient for working patients
CAM therapies[38]	Variable	Most CAM therapies have not been rigorously studied	1A	Generally safe	Evidence emerging that CAM treatments such as tai chi, yoga, balneotherapy, and acupuncture may be effective Allowing patients to choose which CAM therapies to incorporate into an active treatment program can increase self-efficacy

(continued on next page)

Table 1
(continued)

Treatment	Cost	Details	Evidence Level	Adverse Effects	Clinical Pearls
CNS neurostimulatory therapies[39]		Several types of CNS neurostimulatory therapies have been effective in fibromyalgia and other chronic pain states		Headache	These treatments continue to be refined as optimal stimulation targets, "dosing," etc, become understood
Pharmacologic therapies		Therapies best chosen based on predominant symptoms and initiated in low doses with slow dose escalation	5, Consensus		Prescribing patients a drug regimen that helps improve symptoms before initiating nonpharmacologic therapies can help to improve adherence
Tricyclic compounds[40,41]		Amitriptyline, 10–70 mg once daily before bedtime Cyclobenzaprine, 5–20 mg once daily before bedtime	1A	Dry mouth, weight gain, constipations, groggy, or drugged feeling	When effective, can improve a wide range of symptoms including pain, sleep, bowel, and bladder symptoms Taking several hours before bedtime improves adverse effect profile
Serotonin norepinephrine reuptake inhibitors[40]	Duloxetine is generic; milnacipran is not	Duloxetine, 30–120 mg/d Milnacipran, 100–200 mg/d	1A	Nausea, palpitations, headache, fatigue, tachycardia, hypertension	Warning patients about transient nausea, taking with food, and slowly increasing dose can increase tolerability Milnacipran might be slightly more noradrenergic than duloxetine and thus potentially more helpful for fatigue and memory problems but also more likely to cause hypertension

Gabapentinoids[42]	Gabapentin is generic, pregabalin not	Gabapentin, 800–2400 mg/d in divided doses; Pregabalin, up to 600 mg/d in divided doses	1A	Sedation, weight gain, dizziness	Giving most or all of the dose at bedtime can increase tolerability
γ-Hydroxybutyrate[43]	For treating narcolepsy/cataplexy	4.5–6.0 g per night in divided doses	1A	Sedation, respiratory depression, and death	Shown as efficacious but not approved by the US Food and Drug Administration because of safety concerns
Low-dose naltrexone[44]	Low	4.5 mg/d	Two small single-center randomized trials[a]		
Cannabanoids[45]	NA	Nabilone, 0.5 mg orally at bedtime to 1.0 twice daily	1A[a]	Sedation, dizziness, dry mouth	No synthetic cannabinoid has US approval for treatment of pain
SSRIs[40]	SSRIs that should be used in fibromyalgia are all generic	Fluoxetine, sertraline, paroxetine	1A	Nausea, sexual dysfunction, weight gain, sleep disturbance	Older, less selective SSRIs may have some efficacy in improving pain, especially at higher doses that have more prominent noradrenergic effects; Newer SSRIs (citalopram, escitalopram, desvenlafaxine) are less effective or ineffective as analgesics
Nonsteroidal anti-inflammatory drugs		No evidence of efficacy; can be helpful for comorbid peripheral pain generators	5D	Gastrointestinal, renal, and cardiac adverse effects	Use the lowest dose for the shortest period of time to reduce adverse effects

(continued on next page)

Table 1
(continued)

Treatment	Cost	Details	Evidence Level	Adverse Effects	Clinical Pearls
Opioids		Tramadol with or without acetaminophen, 50–100 mg every 6 h No evidence of efficacy for stronger opioids	5D	Sedations, addictions, tolerance, opioid-induced hyperalgesia	Increasing evidence suggests that opioids are less effective for treating chronic pain than previously thought and their risk-benefit profile is worse than other classes of analgesics

Abbreviations: CAM, complementary and alternative medicine; CNS, central nervous system; SSRI, selective serotonin reuptake inhibitors.
[a] Evidence rated by author; not rated by Canadian National Fibromyalgia Guideline Advisory Panel.
Data from Clauw DJ. Fibromyalgia. A Clinical review. JAMA, April, 2014; 311(15): 1547-1555 and Arnold LM, Bennett RM, Crofford LJ, et al. AAPT Diagnostic Criteria for Fibromyalgia. J Pain. 2019; 20(6):611-628.

syndrome and as a target for treatment. There is a high incidence of comorbidity between fibromyalgia, chronic fatigue syndrome, depression, and irritable bowel syndrome, and some have postulated that the gut–brain axis could be the common denominator.[30] Communication between the gut and the central nervous system may be through the vagus nerve, enteric nervous system, endocrine system, and/or the immune system.[31] Research into the gut microbiome and its vast impact on every aspect of human health is in its infancy, but recent studies have implicated the gut microbiome in metabolism, weight management, cardiovascular health, psychiatric illness, cancers, inflammatory diseases such as rheumatoid arthritis, and other inflammatory syndromes, including fibromyalgia, chronic fatigue syndrome, and irritable bowel syndrome through the gut–brain axis.[32] In fact, several studies have shown promising results regarding the connection between fibromyalgia, the gut microbiome, and dysbiosis.[30–32] Dysbiosis refers to relative abundance or depletion of certain microbes that lead to overgrowth of pathogenic microbes. This affects the gastrointestinal, metabolic, and immunologic health and function, and several studies have shown dysbiosis particularly within patients with fibromyalgia.[30–32] In patients with fibromyalgia, 1 study showed a relative depletion of species of bacteria that are known to have anti-inflammatory and antinociceptive effects.[32]

The idea that the microbiome may play a role in fibromyalgia has led to interest in probiotics and diet as potential therapies for fibromyalgia. Probiotics are live bacteria that can be consumed and, at appropriate, levels may help to combat intestinal dysbiosis by competing with pathogenic bacteria in the gastrointestinal system, enhancing the epithelial barrier, increasing immune function within the gastrointestinal system, and enhancing secretory IgA production.[31] Probiotics have been shown to improve symptoms of irritable bowel syndrome, chronic fatigue syndrome, and depression, and they have also been shown to decrease inflammatory markers in patients with rheumatoid arthritis,[31] but further studies need to be performed to determine whether or not probiotics are a viable option for fibromyalgia treatment.

The types of foods eaten as well as the timing of meals affect not only the endocrine system, weight management, and energy, but also the gut microbiome. The effects of several diets on fibromyalgia symptoms have yielded some significant results, but there is as yet no consensus on the most effective diet for fibromyalgia. Vegan and vegetarian diets have been studied and haven't been shown to significantly reduce the amount of FM symptoms; others have found no association between vegetarian diets and improvement in FM symptoms.[33] Patients with FM have been found to have higher levels of proinflammatory cytokines compared with controls. Anti-inflammatory diets, which include high numbers of fruits and vegetables with moderate low-fat proteins and low amounts of breads and grains, especially refined grains, have shown to be effective in reducing hypersensitivity in patients with fibromyalgia.[33] Additionally, low-calorie diets, with and without bariatric surgery, have been shown to improve symptoms.[34]

Malnutrition may also play a role in the development of fibromyalgia. Patients with fibromyalgia have been shown to have lower levels of essential amino acids including valine, leucine, isoleucine, and phenylalanine when compared with people without the diagnosis. These amino acids cannot be produced by the body and thus must be acquired from the diet. These are essential for protein synthesis and muscle energy. Zinc, magnesium, iron, selenium, and vitamin D deficiencies have been associated with fibromyalgia; no results are conclusive regarding micronutrient deficiencies and fibromyalgia at this time.[34]

Although the microbiome's and diet's impact on fibromyalgia pathophysiology and treatment remains largely unknown, it is reasonable to consider that a healthy diet rich in vegetables and nutrients may be a useful treatment or preventative option patients with fibromyalgia based on the evidence that we do have to date. Many patients with fibromyalgia have tried several medical and perhaps even surgical treatment options with minimal improvement. Referrals to a dietician for these patients is, therefore, a reasonable option.

SUMMARY

Fibromyalgia is a complex generalized pain disorder that affects a significant proportion of our population. The epidemiology is not well-elucidated and the diagnoses and management can be difficult. Extremity surgeons see patients with a variety of pain ailments, but surgery may not be the most appropriate management of some of these pain conditions like fibromyalgia. It may even be more difficult to discern some surgical conditions from points of heightened sensitivity in the fibromyalgia patient. Close attention to the current and past medical history in such patients should aid the surgeon in his attempt to rid the patient of painful conditions through surgery.

DISCLOSURE

Nothing to disclose.

REFERENCES

1. Clauw D. Fibromyalgia: a clinical review. JAMA 2014;311(15):1547–55.
2. Hawkins R. Fibromyalgia: a clinical update. J Am Osteopath Assoc 2013;113(9):680–9.
3. Arnold LM, Bennett RM, Crofford LJ, et al. Critical reviews. AAPT diagnostic criteria for fibromyalgia. J Pain 2019;20(6):611–28.
4. Phillips K, Clauw D. Central pain mechanisms in chronic pain states – Maybe it is all in their head. Best Pract Res Clin Rheumatol 2011;25:141–54.
5. Bennett RM. Fibrositis a misnomer for a common rheumatic disorder. The West J Med 1981;134:405–13.
6. Yunus M. Fibromyalgia and overlapping disorders: the unifying concept of central sensitivity syndromes. Semin Arthritis Rheum 2007;36(6):339–56.
7. Atzeni F, Talotta R, Masala IF, et al. One year in review 2019: fibromyalgia. Clin Exp Rheumatol 2019;37(Suppl. 116):S3–10.
8. Choy E, Perrot S, Leon T, et al. A patient survey of the impact of fibromyalgia and the journey to diagnosis. BMC Health Serv Res 2010;10:102.
9. Fillingim RB, Bruehl S, Dworkin RH, et al. The ACTTION-American Pain Society Pain Taxonomy (AAPT): an evidence-based and multidimensional approach to classifying chronic pain conditions. J Pain 2014;15:241–9.
10. Davis F, Gostin M, Roberts B, et al. Characterizing classes of fibromyalgia within the continuum of central sensitization syndrome. J Pain Res 2018;11:2551–60.
11. Masotti A, Baldassarre A, Guzzo MP, et al. Circulating microRNA profiles as liquid biopsies for the characterization and diagnosis of fibromyalgia syndrome. Mol Neurobiol 2017;54:7129–36.
12. Bjersing JL, Lundborg C, Bokarewa MI, et al. Profile of cerebrospinal microRNAs in fibromyalgia. PLoS One 2013;8:e78762.
13. Ciregia F, Giacomelli C, Giusti L, et al. Putative salivary biomarkers useful to differentiate patients with fibromyalgia. J Proteomics 2019;190:44–54.
14. Ramirez-Tejero JA, Martinez-Lara E, Rus A, et al. Insight into the biological pathways underlying fibromyalgia by a proteomic approach. J Proteomics 2018;186:47–55.
15. Hackshaw KV, Aykas DP, Sigurdson GT, et al. Metabolic fingerprinting for diagnosis of fibromyalgia and other rheumatologic dis- orders. J Biol Chem 2019;294(7):2555–68.
16. Martinez-Lavin M. Fibromyalgia and small fiber neuropathy: the plot thickens! Clin Rheumatol 2018;37:3167–71.
17. Albrecht DS, Forsberg A, Sandstrom A, et al. Brain glial activation in fibromyalgia – a multi-site positron emission tomography investigation. Brain Behav Immun 2019;75:72–83.
18. MacFarlane GJ, Kronisch C, Dean LE, et al. EULAR revised recommendations for the management of fibromyalgia. Ann Rheum Dis 2017;76:318–28.
19. Bravo C, Skjaerven LH, Espart A, et al. Basic Body Awareness Therapy in patients suffering from fibromyalgia: a randomized clinical trial. Physiother Theor Pract 2019;35(10):919–29.
20. Kashikar-Zuck S, Black WR, Pfeiffer M, et al. Pilot randomized trial of integrated cognitive-behavioral therapy and neuro- muscular training for juvenile fibromyalgia: the FIT Teens Program. J Pain 2018;19:1049–62.
21. McCrae CS, Mundt JM, Curtis AF, et al. Gray matter changes following cognitive behavioral therapy for patients with comorbid fibromyalgia and insomnia: a pilot Study. J Clin Sleep Med 2018;14:1595–603.
22. Torres E, Pedersen IN, Perez-Fernan-Dez JI. Randomized trial of a group music and imagery method (GrpMI) for women with fibromyalgia. J Music Ther 2018;55:186–220.
23. Hedman-Lagerlof M, Hedman-Lagerlof E, Axelsson E, et al. Internet-delivered exposure therapy for fibromyalgia: a randomized controlled trial. Clin J Pain 2018;34:532–42.
24. Hedman-Lagerlof M, Hedman-Lagerlof E, Ljotsson B, et al. Cost-effectiveness and cost utility of internet-delivered exposure therapy for fibromyalgia: results from a randomized controlled study. J Pain 2019;20:47–59.
25. Ostrovsky DA. Tai Chi may be more effective for improving fibromyalgia symptoms than aerobic exercise. Explore 2018;14:391–2.
26. Merriwether BAEN, Frey-Law LA, Rakel BA, et al. Physical activity is related to function and fatigue but not pain in women with fibromyalgia: baseline analysis from the Fibromyalgia Active Study with TENS (FAST). Arthritis Res Ther 2018;20:199.
27. Thorpe J, Shum B, Moore RA, et al. Combination pharmacotherapy for the treatment of fibromyalgia in adults. Cochrane Database Syst Rev 2018;(2):CD010585.
28. Goldenberg DL, Clauw DJ, Palmer RE, et al. Opioid use in fibromyalgia: a cautionary tale. Mayo Clin Proc 2016;91:640–8.
29. Stockings E, Campbell G, Hall WD, et al. Cannabis and cannabinoids for the treatment of people with chronic non-cancer pain conditions: a systematic review and meta- analysis of controlled and observational studies. Pain 2018;159:1932–54.
30. Malatji BG, Mason S, Mienie LJ, et al. The GC-MS metabolomics signature in patients with fibromyalgia syndrome directs to dysbiosis as an aspect contributing factor of FMS pathophysiology. Metabolomics 2019;15(4):54.

31. Roman P, Carrillo-Trabalón F, Sánchez-Labraca N, et al. Are probiotic treatments useful on fibromyalgia syndrome or chronic fatigue syndrome patients? A systematic review. Benef Microbes 2018;9(4): 603–11.

32. Minerbi A, Gonzalez E, Brereton NJB, et al. Altered microbiome composition in individuals with fibromyalgia. Pain 2019;160(11):2589–602.

33. Correa-Rodríguez M, Casas-Barragán A, González-Jiménez E, et al. Dietary inflammatory index scores are associated with pressure pain hypersensitivity in women with fibromyalgia. Pain Med 2019. https://doi.org/10.1093/pm/pnz238.

34. Rossi A, Di Lollo AC, Guzzo MP, et al. Fibromyalgia and nutrition: what news? Clin Exp Rheumatol 2015; 33(1 Suppl 88):S117–25.

Pediatric Pain Management in Plastic Surgery

Kory D. Blank, MD[a],*, Norman Y. Otsuka, MSc, MD, FRCSC[b]

KEYWORDS

- Pediatrics • Pain management • Plastic surgery

KEY POINTS

- Pediatric pain is often undermanaged because of concerns of overmedicating children.
- Pain assessment in the pediatric population is difficult and requires different strategies than in adults.
- There are a variety of pharmacologic and nonpharmacologic techniques to manage pediatric pain.
- Compartment syndrome in pediatric patients may present in a different fashion than in adult patients.

INTRODUCTION

Pain management in the pediatric population can be a daunting task for treating physicians. Although this is an important responsibility, it has been reported that a large percentage of children's pain goes undertreated.[1] This untreated pain can be a significant cause of morbidity and mortality, especially in the postoperative period. Acute pain, from injury, illness, or medical and surgical procedures, is the most common type of pain experienced by the pediatric population.

Over the last 2 decades, pediatric pain management has progressed greatly. In the 1970s, pediatric procedural and postoperative pain was almost completely disregarded. It soon became evident that inadequate pain control had negative short-term and long-term effects on these patients.[2] New pediatric pain assessment tools have been developed and validated. In the past, proper treatment of pediatric pain was lacking compared with adult pain, mainly because of a deficiency of clinical knowledge, inadequate research in the realm of pediatric pain, and a fear of using opioid analgesia. However, most major children's hospitals in the United States have a dedicated department focusing on the evaluation and treatment of pediatric pain.[3] A multimodal approach using pharmacologic measures, opioid and nonopioid analgesics, local and regional anesthesia, as well as nonpharmacologic measures is being used to adequately treat pain.

ASSESSMENT OF PAIN

The accurate assessment of pain is vital when managing pain in any population, but may be especially difficult in the pediatric population. In general, pediatric patients experience more fear and anxiety surrounding painful situations, including postoperative pain. Young children and infants pose a challenge in the assessment of pain, especially if they are nonverbal or minimally communicative because of age or developmental disabilities. Self-reporting of pain has been considered the gold standard for accurate pain assessment (**Table 1**). However, this is only practical in older children that have the capabilities to rate their pain on a scale.

Observing behavioral changes in the pediatric population may be useful to help quantify pain. A behavioral checklist can be performed, and, based

[a] Southern Illinois University School of Medicine, Springfield, IL, USA; [b] Division of Orthopaedic Surgery, Southern Illinois University School of Medicine, 747 North Rutledge Street, 5th Floor, Springfield, IL 62702, USA
* Corresponding author. 520 South Second Street Apartment 1110, Springfield, IL 62701.
E-mail address: koryblankmd@gmail.com

Clin Plastic Surg 47 (2020) 215–219
https://doi.org/10.1016/j.cps.2020.01.001

Table 1
Types of pain scales used in the pediatric population

Types of Scale	Name of Tool	First Author, Year	Age Range (y)
Numerical rating scale	Visual analogue scale	Atiken, 1969	>6
Faces scales	Wong-Baker Faces Pain Scale Faces Pain Scale–Revised Faces Pain Scale Oucher pain scale	Wong, 1998 Hicks, 2001 Bieri, 1990 Beyer, 1992	>3 — — —
Adjective scales	Verbal Rating Scale	Tesler, 1991	>9
Pieces of hurt	Pieces of hurt, poker chip tools	Hester, 1979	>3
Color scales	Colored analogue scale	McGrath, 1996	>4
Universal pain scale	Universal pain assessment tool	Department of Anesthesiology and Reanimation, California University, 2005	All ages

From Shindova M, Belcheva, A. Pain Assessment Methods Among Pediatric Patients in Medical and Dental Research. International Scientific On-Line Journal Science & Technologies. Medical Biology Studies, Clinical Studies, Social Medicine and Health Care. 6(1): 16-23; with permission.

on the behaviors present, a numerical score can be given. An estimate can then be made of the level of pain of the patient. These pain checklists may be a reliable resource to aid in the assessment of pain in noncommunicative or developmentally disabled children.[3]

MODALITIES OF PAIN CONTROL

It is imperative to provide both the patient as well as the family with education on the various pharmacologic and nonpharmacologic analgesia options. This education should include effectiveness of the treatment plan as well as the potential side effects and adverse reactions associated with the various medications.

The ideal method of providing perioperative analgesia to the pediatric population is through a multimodal approach. For example, preoperative regional anesthesia, postoperative local anesthetic use, and a variety of intravenous and oral analgesics postoperatively can be used to create a synergistic or additive effect that allows appropriate analgesia in the perioperative setting. Analgesics can work at the peripheral level. These analgesics include modalities such as local anesthesia, regional nerve block, and nonopioid and opioid pain medications. Analgesia can also be achieved at the level of the brain, and include such modalities as local anesthetics, opioids, and alpha-2 agonists.[3]

NONPHARMACOLOGIC

As discussed previously, the pediatric population is unique in that generally there is increased fear and anxiety associated with painful situations and procedures. The unique neurodevelopmental stages of newborns, infants, and children dictate the way this population perceives and copes with pain. Interventions should be individualized to patients based on the age and developmental stage of the patient.

In instances of traumatic situations, first aid maneuvers should be used. Immobilization through splints can stabilize fractures and dislocations, which can reduce pain. Cryotherapy decreases swelling and may provide localized topical pain relief in the setting of a traumatic injury.[4]

The role of child life specialists has been shown in the acute setting to reduce children's pain and anxiety.[5] The presence of the children's parents may also play a beneficial role, with the caveat that parental anxiety can increase pain. For this reason, physicians should counsel parents before any procedures and instruct them on different coping strategies specific to the child's current neurodevelopmental stage.

Distraction techniques may be a useful adjunct to treat pain in preschool and school-aged children. Toddlers showed improved pain tolerance when distraction techniques, such as playing peek-a-boo, blowing bubbles, and looking at books, were used. In older children, distraction via video games, cartoons, or other forms of TV entertainment were effective in lessening self-reported anxiety.[4]

In the neonatal and infant population, oral stimulation and physical touch has shown effectiveness in both anxiety reduction as well as pain control. Skin-to-skin care occurs when the infant is placed directly on the parent's chest for 30 minutes before and during the procedure.[6] A sucrose solution has been recommended in neonates less than 30 days old for certain painful procedures. It is easy to administer, accessible, cost-effective, and has a very low risk of adverse events.[7]

Acupuncture has also been proposed as a modality to treat pain in pediatric patients. Up to 30% of the pediatric pain centers reported acupuncture services. One study reported on 243 children treated with acupuncture for 6 weeks for various pain complaints. The visual analogue scale score decreased significantly from 8.3 at the beginning of the study to 3.3 after the final treatment. The safety of acupuncture has been shown in several studies, but it is recommended that only experienced and qualified individuals perform these services.[8]

NONOPIOID ANALGESICS

Medications such as acetaminophen, aspirin, nonsteroidal antiinflammatory drugs (NSAIDs), and selective cyclooxygenase (COX) 2 inhibitors make up the broad category of nonopioid analgesics. COX enzymes are implicated in the pain and inflammation pathway by converting arachidonic acid to prostanoid products. There are different subtypes of COX enzymes that are differentially found in the peripheral tissues and vary in function. COX-1 is found in platelets. Both NSAIDs and aspirin inhibit the action of COX-1, but aspirin ingestion results in an irreversible inhibition. Of note, aspirin and NSAIDs inhibit a broad spectrum of COX enzymes. COX-2 is found primarily in leukocytes and other inflammatory cells. COX-2 inhibitors such as celecoxib are designed specifically to inhibit this subtype of COX enzyme. COX-3 is found in the central nervous system and is inhibited by acetaminophen.[9]

Acetaminophen is probably the most widely used analgesic in the pediatric population. Unlike the other nonopioid analgesics, it has minimal effect in the periphery. It also acts as an antipyretic, which further increases its popularity among the pediatric population.[9] Acetaminophen is primarily metabolized by the liver. Toxicity caused by acute and chronic overdose can result in hepatic injury. To avoid hepatic toxicity, the daily dose should not exceed 4 g/d. Acetaminophen is available in both oral and rectal formulations in the United States.[10]

NSAIDs reversibly inhibit the COX enzyme, resulting in peripheral antiinflammatory and analgesic effects. They are commonly used for mild to moderate pain and are often used in conjunction with opioids to serve as an adjuvant. Unlike opioids, NSAIDs are not associated with respiratory depression, sedation, tolerance, or urinary retention. However, NSAIDs are associated with unique risks. These risks include, but are not limited to, nephropathy, gastropathy, and bleeding caused by reversible inhibition of platelets.

One area of controversy surrounding NSAID use revolves around bone healing in children with fractures or in pediatric patients who have undergone certain types of procedures that require bone formation, such as a posterior spinal instrumented fusion for scoliosis. Prostanoids play a key role in osteoblast activation and new bone formation. Animal models have raised theoretic concerns of potential nonunion complications with NSAID use. Some researchers have suggested that judicious use of NSAIDs is likely to have minimal to no effect on fracture healing or fusion formation.

Ketorolac is the most popular intravenous NSAID used in the United States, with an analgesic efficacy similar to most opioids. It may be particularly useful in patients that cannot tolerate opioids for any reason or in procedures that have a high affinity to cause nausea or vomiting. At present, oral ketorolac is not available for pediatric use.[9,10]

A 2014 randomized trial in Canada studied the use of morphine versus ibuprofen in acute postfracture pain in the pediatric population. Children that presented to the emergency department with a nonoperative fracture within the previous 24 hours were blindly randomized to either a morphine group or ibuprofen group. No statistically significant difference was found in analgesic efficacy between the two groups. However, morphine was associated with significantly more adverse effects.[11]

COX-2 inhibitors provide similar analgesia and antiinflammatory effects to other NSAIDs, with the theoretic benefit of lower incidence of gastric issues. However, there does not seem to be a difference in renal toxicity compared with traditional NSAIDs. In the adult population, there have been reports of cardiovascular complications seen in patients with limited use. It is still unknown whether this risk is conferred to the pediatric population.[9]

Ketamine is used as an adjuvant analgesic in perioperative pain management. It has recently been more widely used for procedural sedation and analgesia in a variety of settings, including the emergency department. It is widely recommended to administer ketamine along with an anticholinergic agent and benzodiazepine to reduce sialorrhea and hallucinations, respectively. When used, it is vital to have appropriate monitoring and resuscitation equipment available in the event of respiratory distress.[10]

OPIOID ANALGESICS

The fear of patient opioid use, opiophobia, is present in all patient populations but is especially present in the pediatric population. An initial concern for addiction was diminished when a *New England Journal of Medicine* article cited that only 4 of 11,000 patients with a legitimate medical condition that are prescribed oral opioids for pain control develop addiction.[12] To address the long-standing history of undertreatment of pediatric pain, opioid prescriptions doubled between 1990 and 2010. However, with this increase in opioid prescriptions, new areas of concerns began to appear: accidental opioid overdose in young children and illegal and/or recreational use by teenagers.[2] A 2009 report by a poison control center cited more than 9000 accidental exposures to opioids in children younger than 6 years. These 9000 exposures resulted in multiple hospitalizations and 8 recorded deaths.[13] Despite these considerations and valid concerns, opioids can play a key role in relief of acute pain and remain underused in the pediatric population.[2]

Recent literature has been directed toward the use of opioid analgesics, tramadol and codeine, in the pediatric population. Both of these analgesics are metabolized via the cytochrome P450 2D6 enzyme into active compounds. There have been several case reports of children being rapid metabolizers of these specific opioid analgesics because of an overactive cytochrome P450 2D6 enzyme. This condition could lead to oversedation, respiratory distress, and potentially death. As of 2017, the US Food and Drug Administration updated the warnings regarding codeine and tramadol use in pediatric patients. It is now contraindicated in patients 12 years of age and younger.[14]

INTRAVENOUS PATIENT-CONTROLLED AND NURSE-CONTROLLED ANALGESIA

Patient-controlled analgesia (PCA) institutes a delivery system with small doses of opioid that are preset before administration. A button can be pressed by the patient or the nursing staff to deliver the opioid intravenously. PCA usage seems to be more effective in children older than 7 years of age because of greater understanding of the cause-and-effect concept of pushing and button and receiving medication and pain relief.

Nurse-controlled analgesia is used in the younger pediatric population. This population is more likely to be physically or cognitively unable to control the PCA appropriately. Evidence supports that nurse-controlled analgesia is a safe way to titrate opioids in the younger patient population.[9]

SUMMARY

Adequate pain management in the pediatric population is a difficult undertaking for treating physicians. Pain management in the pediatric population has evolved greatly in the last 2 decades. Proper assessment of a child's pain is the first step to adequately controlling pain. There are different modalities that can be used to treat pain in this population, including both pharmacologic and nonpharmacologic methods. Common pharmacologic methods include, but are not limited to, nonopioid medications such as nonsteroidal antiinflammatories, opioids, and ketamine. Regional anesthesia is also becoming increasingly popular. Nonpharmacologic methods include cryotherapy, distraction techniques, and, in some cases, acupuncture. A child life specialist can be a great asset with these nonpharmacologic pain control modalities.

DISCLOSURE

The authors have nothing to disclose.

REFERENCES

1. Schechter NL, Berde CB, Yaster M. Pain in infants, children, and adolescents: an overview. In: Schechter NL, Berde CB, Yaster M, editors. Pain in infants, children, and adolescents. Baltimore (MD): Williams & Wilkins; 1993. p. 3–9.
2. Schechter NL. Pediatric pain management and opioids: the baby and the bathwater. JAMA Pediatr 2014;168(11):987–8.
3. Verghese ST, Hannallah RS. Acute pain management in children. J Pain Res 2010;3:105–23.
4. Gaglani A, Gross T. Pediatric pain management. Emerg Med Clin North Am 2018;36(2):323–34.
5. Corwin DJ, Kessler DO, Auerbach M, et al. An intervention to improve pain management in the pediatric emergency department. Pediatr Emerg Care 2012; 28:524–8.
6. Johnston C, Campbell-Yeo M, Disher T, et al. Skin-to-skin care for procedural pain in neonates. Cochrane Database Syst Rev 2017;(2):CD008435.
7. Zempsky WT, Cravero JP. The committee on pediatric emergency medicine and section on anesthesiology and pain medicine: relief of pain and anxiety in pediatric patients in emergency medical systems. Pediatrics 2004;114:1248–354.
8. Kundu A, Berman B. Acupuncture for pediatric pain and symptom management. Pediatr Clin North Am 2007;(54):885–99.
9. Greco C, Berde C. Pain management for the hospitalized pediatric patient. Pediatr Clin North Am 2005; 52(4):995–1027. vii-viii.

10. Landsman IS, Hayes SR, Karsenac CJ, et al. Pediatric surgery. Chapter 13. p. 201–222.
11. Poonai N, Bhullar G, Lin K, et al. Oral administration of morphine versus ibuprofen to manage postfracture pain in children: a randomized trial. CMAJ 2014;186(18):1358–63.
12. Porter J, Jick H. Addiction rare in patients treated with narcotics. N Engl J Med 1980;302(2):123.
13. Bailey JE, Campagna E, Dart RC, RADARS System Poison Center Investigators. The underrecognized toll of prescription opioid abuse on young children. Ann Emerg Med 2009;53(4):419–24.
14. Fortenberry M, Crowder J, So T. The use of codeine and tramadol in the pediatric population—what is the verdict now? J Pediatr Health Care 2019;33(1):117–33.

Enhanced Recovery After Surgery Pathways in Breast Reconstruction

Sarah Persing, MD, MPH, Michele Manahan, MD, Gedge Rosson, MD*

KEYWORDS

- Enhanced recovery after surgery • Breast reconstruction • Microsurgery • Fast track surgery
- Surgery pathways

KEY POINTS

- The Enhanced Recovery After Surgery (ERAS) protocol is a multidisciplinary, multimodal, and evidence-based approach to perioperative management.
- ERAS protocols help to streamline perioperative care based on evidence-based review and consensus across all multidisciplinary aspects of care in breast reconstruction.
- In plastic surgery procedures, ERAS pathways have been shown to reduce hospital length of stay and opioid consumption, which may have cost-saving implications down the line. They also enhance the patient experience by improving postoperative analgesia, nausea, and vomiting.

BACKGROUND

The Enhanced Recovery After Surgery (ERAS) protocol is a multidisciplinary, multimodal, and evidence-based approach to perioperative management.[1] This concept was first introduced in 1997 by a group of general surgeons from Europe, led by Henrik Kehlet,[2,3] with a background experience in colorectal "fast-track surgery." A formal research group, called the ERAS Study Group, was then formed by a group of surgeons from several academic hospitals in Europe in 2001, with the aim of exploring an improved care pathway for patients undergoing open colorectal procedures, with the specific goals of improving care, reducing cost, and reducing length of hospital stay. The ERAS pathway has since been applied to numerous major surgical procedures throughout various specialties and has shown very promising results, namely reduced postoperative morbidity, reduced opioid use, and shortened hospital length of stay.[1,4,5] The ERAS Society was subsequently established in 2003 with the aim of further developing formal perioperative care pathways to improve recovery through evidence-based practices.

Breast cancer is the most common malignancy in women worldwide according to the World Health Organization, contributing more than 25% to new cancer diagnoses in 2012 (excluding nonmelanoma skin cancer).[6] In the United States, there has been a gradual increase in immediate and delayed reconstruction over the past few decades (**Fig. 1**).[7] In 2017, there were 106,000 breast reconstructions in the United States, which represents a 35% increase from 2000.[8]

In the current health care climate, there has been a growing focus on optimizing the quality of care for patients and reducing the overall cost burden of health care. More attention has thus been given to ERAS pathways as a quality improvement initiative in breast reconstruction. Several studies have examined the efficacy and safety of ERAS pathways in patients undergoing

Department of Plastic and Reconstructive Surgery, Johns Hopkins Hospital, 601 North Caroline Street, 2nd Floor JHOC Building, Baltimore, MD 21287, USA
* Corresponding author.
E-mail address: gedge@jhmi.edu

Clin Plastic Surg 47 (2020) 221–243
https://doi.org/10.1016/j.cps.2019.12.002

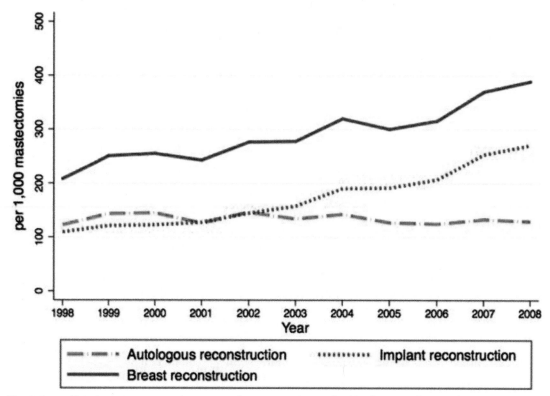

Fig. 1. Immediate breast reconstruction rate and reconstructive method in the United States from 1998 to 2008. (*Adapted from* Alboronz CR, Bach PB, Mehrara BJ, et al. A paradigm shift in U.S. breast reconstruction: increasing implant rates. Plast Reconstr Surg. 2013;131(1):15-23; with permission.)

breast reconstruction.[9–11] In this article, the authors review the ERAS pathways for breast reconstruction procedures.

ENHANCED RECOVERY AFTER SURGERY SOCIETY RECOMMENDATIONS IN BREAST RECONSTRUCTION

In 2017, a consensus report developed by the ERAS Society provides guidelines specific for breast reconstruction (**Table 1**).[12] These guidelines describe 18 care elements in the preoperative, intraoperative, and postoperative periods for breast reconstruction. These care elements will be reviewed based on the following consensus data[12]:

1. Preadmission information, education, counseling
2. Preadmission optimization
3. Perforator flap planning
4. Perioperative fasting
5. Preoperative carbohydrate loading
6. Venous thromboembolism prophylaxis
7. Antimicrobial prophylaxis
8. Postoperative nausea and vomiting prophylaxis
9. Perioperative and intraoperative analgesia
10. Standard anesthetic protocol
11. Preventing intraoperative hypothermia
12. Perioperative intravenous fluid management
13. Postoperative analgesia
14. Early feeding
15. Postoperative flap monitoring
16. Postoperative wound management
17. Early mobilization
18. Postdischarge home support and physiotherapy

Preadmission Information, Education, and Counseling

Recommendation
Patients should receive detailed preoperative counseling.

Discussion of the surgical and anesthetic plans with the patient helps manage their expectations and concerns about the procedure. Offering patients preoperative education enables them to be a part of the decision-making process about breast reconstruction. This discussion has been shown to reduce anxiety and improve patient satisfaction independent of the reconstruction type.[13,14]

Table 1
Enhanced Recovery after Surgery Society enhanced recovery after surgery recommendations for perioperative care in breast reconstruction

Item	Recommendation	Evidence Level	Recommendation Grade
1. Preadimission information, education, and counseling	Patients should receive detailed preoperative counseling	Moderate	Strong
2. Preadimission optimization	For daily smokers, 1 mo of abstinence before surgery is beneficial. For patients who are obese, weight reduction to achieve a BMI $\leq$30 kg/m^2 before surgery is beneficial. For alcohol abusers, 1 mo of abstinence before surgery is beneficial. For appropriate groups, referral should be made to resources for these behavior changes	Moderate (smoking) High (obesity) Low (alcohol)	Strong Strong Strong
3. Perforator flap planning	If preoperative perforator mapping is required, CTA is recommended	Moderate	Strong
4. Perioperative fasting	Preoperative fasting should be minimized, and patients should be allowed to drink clear fluids up to 2 h before surgery	Moderate	Strong
5. Preoperative carbohydrate loading	Preoperative maltodextrin-based drinks should be given to patients 2 h before surgery	Low	Strong
6. Venous thromboembolism prophylaxis	Patients should be assessed for venous thromboembolism risk. Unless contraindicated, and balanced by the risk of bleeding, patients at a higher risk should receive low-molecular-weight heparin or unfractionated heparin until ambulatory or discharged. Mechanical methods should be added	Moderate	Strong

(continued on next page)

Table 1
(continued)

Item	Recommendation	Evidence Level	Recommendation Grade
7. Antimicrobial prophylaxis	Chlorhexidine skin preparation should be performed, and intravenous antibiotics covering common skin organisms should be given within 1 h of incision	Moderate	Strong
8. Postoperative nausea and vomiting prophylaxis	Women should receive preoperative and intraoperative medications to mitigate postoperative nausea and vomiting	Moderate	Strong
9. Preoperative and intraoperative analgesia	Women should receive multimodal analgesia to mitigate pain	Moderate	Strong
10. Standard anesthetic protocol	General anesthesia with TIVA is recommended	Moderate	Strong
11. Preventing intraoperative hypothermia	Preoperative and intraoperative measures, such as forced air, to prevent hypothermia should be instituted. Temperature monitoring is required to ensure the patient's body temperature is maintained higher than 36°C	Moderate	Strong
12. Perioperative intravenous fluid management	Overresuscitation or underresuscitation of fluids should be avoided, and water and electrolyte balance should be maintained. Goal-directed therapy is a useful method of achieving these goals. Balanced crystalloid solutions, rather than saline, are recommended. Vasopressors are recommended to support fluid management and do not negatively affect free flaps	Moderate	Strong

(continued on next page)

Table 1
(continued)

Item	Recommendation	Evidence Level	Recommendation Grade
13. Postoperative analgesia	Multimodel postoperative pain management regimens are opioid sparing and should be used	High	Strong
14. Early feeding	Patients should be encouraged to take fluids and food orally as soon as possible, preferably within 24 h after surgery	Moderate	Strong
15. Postoperative flap monitoring	Flap monitoring within the first 72 h should occur frequently. Clinical evaluation is sufficient for monitoring, with implantable Doppler devices recommended in cases of buried flaps	Moderate	Strong
16. Postoperative wound management	For incisional closure, conventional sutures are recommended. Complex wounds following skin necrosis are treatable with debridement and negative-pressure wound therapy	High (sutures), moderate (NPWT)	Strong
17. Early mobilization	Patients should be mobilized within the first 24 h after surgery	Moderate	Strong
18. Postdischarge home support and physiotherapy	Early physiotherapy, supervised exercise programs, and other supportive care initiatives should be instituted after discharge	Moderate	Strong

Abbreviations: BMI, body mass index; NPWT, negative-pressure wound therapy; TIVA, total intravenous anesthesia.
   Adapted from Temple-Oberle C, Shea-Budgell M, Tan M, et al. Consensus review of optimal perioperative care in breast reconstruction: Enhanced recovery after surgery (ERAS) society recommendations. Plast Reconstr Surg. 2017;135(5):1056e-1071e; with permission.

Preadmission Optimization

Recommendation

For daily smokers, 1 month of abstinence before surgery is beneficial.

For patients who are obese, weight reduction to achieve a body mass index less than or equal to 30 kg/m^2 before surgery is beneficial. For alcohol abusers, 1 month of abstinence before surgery is beneficial. For appropriate groups, referral should be made to resources for these behavior changes.

Variables, such as smoking, alcohol consumption, poor nutrition, diabetes, and obesity, are some factors that are known to have an adverse effect on postoperative outcomes in breast reconstruction surgery. Patients with an active smoking history have more mastectomy flap necrosis, reconstructive failure, and higher rates of infection compared with nonsmokers.[15,16] Heavy alcohol consumption (defined as 5 or more drinks on each of 5 or more days in the past 30 days) has also been shown to increase the risk of surgical site infections.[17] It is therefore recommended that patients stop smoking and drinking alcohol for at least 1 month before surgery.

Obesity (>30 kg/m²) is associated with flap loss and donor-site morbidity as well as increases the risk of surgical site infection and venous thromboembolism.[18–23] Patients are encouraged to lose weight before surgery. In obese patients, muscle-preserving flaps (ie, deep inferior epigastric perforator [(DIEP] flap) reduce the risk abdominal wall complications, such as hernia, compared with non-muscle-sparing flaps (ie, free or pedicled transverse rectus abdominis musculocutaneous [TRAM] flap).[21,24]

With respect to diabetes, the National Surgical Quality Improvement Program (NSQIP) data on 29,736 women with breast reconstruction showed an increased risk of overall surgical complications (Operating room, 1.85).[25] Poor glycemic control is associated with worse outcomes in primary closure of surgical wounds in these high-risk patients.[26] Although not formally included in the consensus report, it has been shown that glucose levels greater than 200 mg/dL are associated with worse outcomes in terms of wound healing.[27] Current guidelines outlined by the Society for Healthcare Epidemiology of America recommend maintaining postoperative blood glucose of 180 mg/dL or lower.[28]

Perforator Flap Planning

Recommendation
If preoperative perforator mapping is required, computed tomographic angiography (CTA) is recommended.

Despite risks of contrast allergy, nephrotoxicity, and exposure to radiation,[29] modern CTA scanning protocols have been able to reduce the amount of radiation patients are exposed to.[30] Prior metaanalysis has shown the benefits of CTA with respect to reducing operative time, postoperative flap-related complications, and donor-site morbidity compared with Doppler ultrasonography.[31]

Preoperative Fasting

Recommendation
Preoperative fasting should be minimized, and patients should be allowed to drink clear fluids up to 2 hours before surgery.

A 2003 Cochrane Review of 22 randomized controlled trials showed that drinking clear fluids 2 hours before surgery is safe and does not increase the risk regurgitation and aspiration.[32] The ERAS guidelines for gastrointestinal surgery recommend a 6-hour preoperative fasting for solid foods and 2-hour fasting for clear liquids before general anesthesia.[33] The guidelines note that the recommendations have not been applied to patients at increased risk of gastric emptying.

Preoperative Carbohydrate Loading

Recommendation
Preoperative maltodextrin-based drinks should be given to patients 2 hours before surgery.

Studies have shown that maltodextrin-based drinks (400 mL) taken 2 hours before surgery have positive metabolic effects, such as increasing insulin sensitivity and reducing preoperative thirst and anxiety.[34–36] The effect of carbohydrate loading preoperatively reduces the catabolic effects of surgery, including loss of nitrogen and protein, lean body mass, and muscle strength,[37–39] resulting in a reduced length of hospital stay.[40] Furthermore, for patients with well-controlled type 2 diabetes, a carbohydrate drink given up to 3 hours before surgery (instead of 2 hours) along with their normal medication does not delay gastric emptying and allows glucose concentrations to return to baseline.[41]

Prophylaxis Against Venous Thromboembolism

Recommendation
Patients should be assessed for venous thromboembolism risk. Unless contraindicated, and balanced by risk of bleeding, patients at higher risk should receive low-molecular-weight heparin or unfractionated heparin until they are ambulatory or discharged. Mechanical methods (as with intermittent pneumatic compression) should be added.

Patients undergoing breast reconstruction procedures are at greater risk for venous thromboembolism. NSQIP data on 68,285 patients have shown an almost 2-fold increased risk of venous thromboembolism compared with lumpectomy or mastectomy alone (0.41% vs 0.13% and 0.29%, respectively; $P<.0001$).[22] According to the American Society of Plastic Surgeons Executive Committee–approved Caprini Risk Assessment Module, patients undergoing immediate reconstruction after mastectomy meet criteria for "higher" risk of venous thromboembolism and are "highest" risk if they are obese or elderly.[42,43] For this population, pharmacologic anticoagulation with or without mechanical methods (ie, intermittent pneumatic compression) is recommended.[43,44] The ERAS guidelines recommend that prophylaxis be initiated before surgery and continue for at least 7 to 10 days.[45] Although low-molecular-weight heparin has been shown not to increase bleeding risk in some studies,[46,47] other studies have shown low-molecular-weight heparin may have a higher bleeding risk than unfractionated heparin in breast surgery procedures.[48,49]

Antimicrobial Prophylaxis

Recommendation
Chlorhexidine skin preparation and intravenous antibiotics covering common skin organisms should be given within 1 hour of incision.

The risk of infection following mastectomy is higher than other clean surgeries (3%–15% vs 2%).[50,51] This risk is further increased with the addition of a flap or prosthesis.[52–54] Prophylactic antibiotics have been shown to decrease the risk of surgical-site infections.[55] Antibiotics against common skin organisms (ie, cephalosporins) should be administered 1 hour before incision.[56,57] Despite the common practice of continued use of postoperative antibiotics while surgical drains are in place, prolonged use of antibiotics in breast reconstruction beyond 24 hours has not been proven beneficial in implant- and flap-based surgeries.[52,58–60] Chlorhexidine-based antiseptic skin preparations applied before surgery have been shown to decrease surgical site infections.[61,62]

Preoperative and Intraoperative Prophylaxis Against Postoperative Nausea and Vomiting

Recommendation
Women should receive preoperative and intraoperative multimodal medications to mitigate postoperative nausea and vomiting.

Metaanalysis has demonstrated the efficacy of 5-hydroxytryptamine-3 receptor antagonists over placebo in reducing postoperative nausea and vomiting in breast surgery.[63] Steroids alone have been shown to reduce postoperative nausea, vomiting, and pain.[64] When combined, steroids and 5-hydroxytryptamine-3 receptor antagonists have superior effects than either alone.[65] Preoperative neurokinin-1 receptor antagonists provide even further reduction in postoperative nausea and vomiting compared with 5-hydroxytryptamine-3 receptor antagonists.[66–68]

Preoperative and Intraoperative Analgesia

Recommendation
Women should receive multimodal analgesia to mitigate pain.

Gabapentin has been shown to reduce analgesic requirements and pain in women undergoing mastectomy.[69,70] Nonsteroidal anti-inflammatory drugs (NSAIDs) and cyclooxygenase-2 inhibitor medications are effective preoperatively or intraoperatively in reducing pain without increasing bleeding complications.[71–73] Bupivacaine infiltrated into the area of planned surgical incision for mastectomy is also shown to decrease pain and opiate demand postoperatively.[74] In addition, adenosine,[75] systemic magnesium,[76] venlafaxine,[77] and clonidine[78] are also effective analgesics when administered preoperatively.

Standard Anesthetic Protocol

Recommendation
General anesthesia with total intravenous anesthesia is recommended for breast reconstruction procedures.

There are 3 common modalities for maintenance of anesthesia during breast surgery: general anesthesia with total intravenous anesthesia, general anesthesia with a volatile anesthetic, and regional anesthesia. Regional anesthesia, with paravertebral or transversus abdominis plane (TAP) blocks, is shown to decrease postoperative narcotic use,[79–81] but does not decrease pain, nausea, sedation, time to ambulation, or length of hospital stay.[80] General anesthesia with total intravenous anesthesia decreases postoperative nausea and vomiting compared with a volatile anesthetic in breast surgery.[82,83]

Preventing Intraoperative Hypothermia

Recommendation
Preoperative and intraoperative measures, such as forced air, to prevent hypothermia should be instituted. Temperature monitoring is required to ensure the patient's body temperature is maintained higher than 36°C.

The Surgical Care Improvement Project found an association with hypothermia and impaired wound healing, prolonged hospitalization, and a 3-fold higher wound infection risk.[84] Maintaining patient temperature higher than 36°C reduces multiple complications, including cardiac conditions, altered drug metabolism, as well as decreased wound infections.[85] Preoperative patient-warming strategies affect intraoperative warming strategies,[86] so warming an operating room will not be sufficient to prevent hypothermia.[87] In a systematic review of multiple randomized controlled trials, forced-air warming is safe and effective in preventing hypothermia.[88] Warmed intravenous fluid reduces hypothermia for short procedures,[89] but in longer surgeries, it is insufficient.[90]

Perioperative Intravenous Fluid Management

Recommendation

Overresuscitation or underresuscitation of fluids should be avoided, and water and electrolyte balance should be maintained. Goal-directed therapy is a useful method to achieve these goals. Balanced crystalloid solutions rather than saline is recommended. Vasopressors are recommended to support fluid management and do not negatively affect free-flap breast reconstruction.

Overresuscitation can affect cardiopulmonary events and wound infection and can increase wound-healing problems and length of hospital stay.[91,92] Both overresuscitation and underresuscitation have been shown to increase the risk of anastomosis thrombosis in free-flap breast reconstruction.[93,94] Historically, vasopressors used to maintain blood pressure have been avoided in flap patients, but studies have shown that they are safe to use in normovolemic patients.[95–97] Balanced crystalloid solutions are shown to be superior to 0.9% saline for maintaining electrolyte balance.[94]

Postoperative Analgesia

Recommendation

Multimodal postoperative pain management regimens that are opioid sparing should be used with the goal of facilitating early mobilization.

Consideration to reducing opioid use after surgery can help alleviate some of the effects of postoperative nausea and vomiting, as well as constipation. According to Cochrane data from randomized controlled trials, the combination of acetaminophen and NSAIDs is more effective than either alone.[98] Multiple randomized controlled trials further demonstrate that NSAIDs reduce the need for narcotics with minimal surgical site bleeding risk.[99–101] A metaanalysis of randomized controlled trials showed that ketorolac does not increase perioperative bleeding.[102] Gabapentin administered preoperatively or postoperatively is effective for pain control and also demonstrates reduced narcotic requirements.[103,104]

The use of regional or local blocks can help minimize pain, narcotic use, and sedation. Paravertebral blocks with continuous bupivacaine infusion catheters have been shown to reduce opioid requirements,[105,106] and TAP blocks have been effective in decreasing abdominal donor site pain in flap patients.[80]

Early Feeding

Recommendation

Patients should be encouraged to take fluids and food orally as soon as possible, preferably within 24 hours after surgery.

Early refeeding within 24 hours after surgery is safe and associated with improved healing, reduced infection, and reduced hospital stay.[107] The decision of when to resume a diet after surgery should be weighed against the risk of a possible urgent return to the operating room, for example, in patients who develop a microvascular thrombosis in their free-flap reconstruction.[108,109] Rapid-sequence intubation can help mitigate the risk of aspiration in the event of an urgent return to the operating room.[110]

Postoperative Flap Monitoring

Recommendation

Flap monitoring within the first 72 hours should occur frequently. Clinical evaluation is sufficient for monitoring, with implantable Doppler recommended in cases of buried flaps.

Microvascular thrombosis of the free flap occurs in 2% to 5% of cases and typically within the first 72 hours.[108,109,111] In most cases (60%–74%), thrombosis occurred in the venous system.[109,112] Studies have shown that the outcomes are improved in earlier salvage interventions in a compromised free flap.[112,113] Monitoring of flaps includes clinical observation for color, temperature, and capillary refill, as well as the use of monitoring devices. The hand-held Doppler is a noninvasive adjunct to clinical observation and is shown to be highly effective in monitoring free flaps.[114] The typical protocol is 1-hour monitoring in the first 24 hours, every 2 hours for the next 24 hours, and then every 3 to 4 hours for the next 24 hours.

Implantable Doppler devices have excellent sensitivity in detecting flap compromise, but may detach and result in a higher false-positive rate than clinical observation.[115] Clinical observation with or without implantable Doppler monitors has equivocal rates of flap salvage.[116,117] In the case of buried flaps, implantable Doppler is the only objective measure.[114] Alternative flap monitoring devices include a venous coupler with an embedded implantable Doppler device, laser Doppler monitoring, infrared spectroscopy, tissue oximetry, and microdialysis.[118–120]

Postoperative Wound Management

Recommendation

For incisional closure, conventional sutures are typically recommended. Complex wounds following skin necrosis are treatable with debridement and negative pressure wound therapy.

Typically, breast and abdominal incisions following breast reconstruction are closed with layered intradermal absorbable sutures.[121] Skin adhesive octyl-2-cyanoacrylate is widely used in breast surgery and shows patient preference but no objective difference in cosmesis or complications.[122] The length of time for a dressing to stay in place is variable. A clinical trial comparing dressing removal at day 1 versus dressing removal at day 6 is ongoing. Preliminary results may support standard recommendations of dressing removal after breast reconstruction in 24 to 48 hours.[123]

Regarding complex wounds associated with mastectomy flap, DIEP flap and abdominal skin necrosis are known possible complications of breast reconstruction.[124,125] Surgical debridement and negative-pressure wound therapy is an effective adjunct in wound management, with studies showing complete healing in 97% of breast wounds.[126]

Early Mobilization

Recommendation

Patients should be mobilized within the first 24 hours after surgery.

Prolonged inactivity combined with a catabolic state (ie, postoperative stress) exacerbates muscle atrophy.[127] Early mobilization of patients improves muscle strength and reduces risk of pulmonary embolism, pneumonia, and decubitus ulcers.[128] In addition, early mobilization decreases length of hospital stay and improves overall psychological well-being.[129–131]

Postdischarge Home Support and Physiotherapy

Recommendation

Early physiotherapy, supervised exercise programs, and other supportive care initiatives should be instituted after discharge.

For patients undergoing mastectomy and axillary dissection, early physical rehabilitation has been shown to improve physical and emotional recovery.[132,133] Physical rehabilitation programs in the postoperative period improve mobility, decrease pain, and enhance quality of life for patients with breast cancer.[134] Visiting nurses also provide an important role in delivering physical care and education, as well as psychosocial support following TRAM flap reconstruction.[135]

The Johns Hopkins Enhanced Recovery After Surgery Protocol for Microsurgical Breast Reconstruction

The Johns Hopkins breast reconstruction team developed a protocol for microsurgical breast reconstruction that details the care elements based on the ERAS Society consensus report for microsurgical breast reconstruction (**Table 2**). During the development of the protocol, multidisciplinary "buy-in" was first addressed through discussion with all members involved in the care of breast reconstruction patients at this institution, and all members came to a consensus based on evidence-based review of the literature. To highlight several specifications or modifications of the ERAS consensus report to the Johns Hopkins ERAS protocol, the preoperative analgesic regimen includes a combination of celecoxib, gabapentin, and oral acetaminophen. For antiemetic therapy, patients have a scopolamine patch applied in the preoperative holding area and may receive any combination of dexamethasone, ondansetron, or dimenhydrinate. Routine administration of 5000 units of subcutaneous heparin is given to patients in the preoperative holding area. Intraoperatively, TAP blocks are performed by the anesthesia team while the microanastomosis is being performed. Postoperatively, the diet is advanced in the morning after surgery to balance early feeding protocol and possible urgent return to the operating room in the event of flap failure.[136]

The Johns Hopkins Enhanced Recovery After Surgery Protocol for Alloplastic Breast Reconstruction

There are few ERAS protocols developed for alloplastic breast reconstruction. The Johns Hopkins breast reconstruction team developed a protocol for patients undergoing implant-based breast reconstruction following multidisciplinary consensus input from the care teams involved, as shown in **Table 3**. Similar to the microsurgical ERAS protocols, this protocol is divided into 4 phases: before surgery, day of surgery, intraoperative, and postoperative phases.

Before surgery, patients are counseled and provided with educational materials about the procedure. They undergo the same preadmission fasting and optimization. They are also instructed to use chlorhexidine gluconate wipes before surgery to help reduce the risk of infection.

On the day of surgery, patients receive multimodal analgesia and antiemetic therapy. Patients may drink up to 20 ounces of noncarbonated sports drink up to 2 hours before surgery. Subcutaneous heparin is not given preoperatively.

Intraoperatively, patients receive appropriate prophylactic antibiotics, anesthesia, analgesia, and intravenous fluid therapy according to prior ERAS guidelines for breast reconstruction.

Table 2
Enhanced Recovery after Surgery protocol for microsurgical breast reconstruction as implemented at the Department of Plastic and Reconstructive Surgery at The Johns Hopkins Hospital

	Before Surgery	Day of Surgery–Preoperative Holding Area	Intraoperative	Postoperative Day 0 (T)	Postoperative Day 1 (T + 1)	Postoperative Day 2 (T + 2)	Postoperative Day 3 (T + 3)	Discharge
Laboratory tests	Normal preoperative workup		As needed	As needed				
Medications		Antiemetics: Scopolamine patch (do not give with narrow/closed angle glaucoma) Analgesics: Acetaminophen 1 g po (do not give with liver failure/elevated liver enzymes) Celecoxib 400 mg po (do not give with poor renal function) Gabapentin 600 mg po (do not give with poor renal function) Anticoagulation: Heparin 5000 units SC in preoperative holding area	Antiemetics (PRN): Dexamethasone 4 mg IV after induction of anesthesia Ondansetron 4-8 mg IV 30 min before end of case Promethazine (Phenergan) 6 mg IV Analgesics: Fentanyl or hydromorphone IV PRN Antibiotics: Cefazolin 2 g IV before incision, redose every 3 h and 59 min or sooner Clindamycin 600 mg for penicillin allergy redose	Antiemetics: Ondansetron (Zofran) 4 mg IV/po q8h Promethazine (Phenergan) 5–12.5 mg IV (administer 15 min after ondansetron dose if patient has persistent nausea) Analgesics: Acetaminophen 1 g po q8h Gabapentin 100 mg po tid Celecoxib 200 mg po bid Analgesics (IV PRN): Fentanyl 50 µg IV q3h PRN for severe pain (pain scale rating 7–10 out of 10) Hydromorphone 0.5 mg IV q3h PRN for severe pain (pain scale rating 7–10 out of 10) Analgesics (po PRN):	Antiemetics: Ondansetron (Zofran) 4 mg IV/po q8h Analgesia: As before Anticoagulation: Heparin 5000 units SC q8h Stool softener: Docusate sodium (Colace) 100 mg po bid Senna (Senekot) 8.6-mg tablets, take 2 tablets qhs PRN Glycerin suppository rectally once PRN	Antiemetics: As before Analgesics: As before Anticoagulation: Continue DVTp Stool softener: As before	Antiemetics: As before Analgesics: As before Anticoagulation: Continue DVTp Stool softener: As before	Discharge patient with the following prescriptions: Analgesics: Acetaminophen 650 mg po q6h PRN for 7 d Ibuprofen 600 mg q6h PRN for 7 d Tramadol 50 mg po q4h PRN OR Oxycodone 5 mg q4h PRN (30 tablets maximum) Gabapentin 100 mg po tid for 1 wk (if tolerating well) Anticoagulation:

	(Preoperative)	(Intraoperative)	(Postoperative)				(Discharge)
		every 7 h 59 min or sooner Fluids: Crystalloid IV 20–30 mL/kg minimum during case, avoid overload Anesthesia: Avoid nitrous oxide Avoid inhalational agents Total IV anesthesia if possible Circuit humidified low oxygen (>21/min) TAP blocks performed with ultrasound guidance	Oxycodone 5 mg po q4h PRN for moderate pain (pain scale rating 4–6 out of 10) Tramadol 50 mg po q4h PRN for mild pain (pain scale rating 1–3 out of 10) Antibiotics: Cefadroxil 1 g IV q8h × 24 h, administer after last intraoperative dose Clindamycin 600 mg q8h IV for penicillin allergy, administer 12 h after last intraoperative dose Fluids: Crystalloid IV at maintenance, discontinue when taking good po Anticoagulation: Heparin 5000 units SC q8h to start in PM				± Enoxaparin (Lovenox) 30 mg SC q12h for extended DVTp if high risk Stool softener: Docusate sodium (Colace) 100 bid for 7 d
Nursing and treatments	Warming blanket IV start	Anesthesia head-turning guidelines for patients undergoing prolonged surgery Foley catheter Warming blanket	Flap checks q1h × 24 h, then q2h × 24 h, then q4h onward while in hospital SCD to be worn when patient	As before Foley out by 16:00 (nurses to activate order if appropriate)	As before	As before	Remove marking suture and Viotix probe before discharge

(continued on next page)

Table 2
(*continued*)

	Before Surgery	Day of Surgery—Preoperative Holding Area	Intraoperative	Postoperative Day 0 (T)	Postoperative Day 1 (T + 1)	Postoperative Day 2 (T + 2)	Postoperative Day 3 (T + 3)	Discharge
			SCDs to lower extremities Padding to protect all prominent surfaces Pillow behind knees	is in bed or chair, remove when ambulating Record in and outs, including drain Prime and empty drain PRN 3–4 drains, right and left abdomen plus right and/or left breast Inspect IV, drain, and surgical sites as per nursing protocol				
Activity				Hip flexion—continuous Bedrest overnight	Provide total assistance, transfer to chair in morning Ambulate with 1 person assist until ambulating independently	Ambulate 3 times per day, progress as tolerated	As before	As before
Nutrition		Drink up to 20 noncarbonated sports drink up to 2 h before surgery		Sips of water	Advance diet as tolerated, regular diet	Regular diet	Regular diet	Regular diet
Consults	Preoperative anesthesia consultation				Physiotherapy			Physiotherapy outpatient referral

Teaching	ERAS free-flap education booklet provided to patient, which includes risks, benefits, and alternatives to surgery, expected length of stay, and postoperative course	No bra Drain care teaching Verify postoperative follow-up appointment, scheduled within 7 d of discharge

Abbreviations: bid, twice per day; DVTp, deep vein thrombosis prophylaxis; IV, intravenous; po, by mouth; PRN, when necessary; SC, subcutaneous; SCD, sequential compression devices; tid, 3 times per day; qhs, Every night at bedtime.

Adapted from Stone J, Siotos C, Sarmiento S, et al. Implementing our microsurgical breast reconstruction enhanced recovery after surgery pathway: Consensus obstacles and recommendations. *Plast Reconstr Surg Glob Open.* 2019;7(1):e1855.

Table 3
Enhanced Recovery after Surgery protocol for alloplastic breast reconstruction as implemented at the Department of Plastic and Reconstructive Surgery at The Johns Hopkins Hospital

	Before Surgery	Day of Surgery–Preoperative Area	Intraoperative	Postoperative Day 0 (T)	Postoperative Day 1 (T + 1)	Postoperative Day 2 (T + 2)	Postoperative Day 3 (T + 3)	Discharge
Laboratory tests	Normal preoperative workup							
Medications and pain control		Antiemetics: Scopolamine patch (do not give with narrow/closed angle glaucoma) Analgesia: Gabapentin 600 mg po (do not give with poor renal function) Acetaminophen 1 g po (do not give with liver failure/elevated liver enzymes) Celecoxib 400 mg po (do not give with allergic type reactions to sulfonamides)	As needed	Antiemetics (PRN): Dexamethasone 4 mg IV after induction of anesthesia Ondansetron 4-8 mg IV 30 min before end of case Promethazine (Phenergan) 6 mg IV Analgesics: Fentanyl or hydromorphone IV PRN Antibiotics: Cefazolin 2 g IV before incision, redose every 3 h and 59 min or sooner Clindamycin 600 mg for penicillin allergy redose every 7 h 59 min or sooner Fluids: Crystalloid IV 20–30 mL/kg minimum during case, avoid overload	Antiemetics: Zofran 4 mg IV q6h po until discharge Antiemetics (PRN): Promothazine (Phenergan) 5–12.5 mg IV ×1 Antihistamine: H1 receptor antagonist Metoclopramide (Reglan) 10 mg IV ×1 Haloperidol (Haldol) 1 mg IV ×1 Analgesics: Acetaminophen 1 g IV Tylenol ×2 q6h then follow with po q6h Gabapentin 100 mg po tid Celebrex 200 mg po bid Valium 5 mg q8h for 24 h Analgesics (IV PRN): Fentanyl 50 μg IV q3h PRN for severe pain	Antiemetics: Continue scopolamine patch (DC on day 3) Continue Zofran 4 mg IV q6h po until discharge Analgesics: As before Stool softener: Docusate sodium (Colace) 100 mg po bid Antibiotics: Duricef 500 mg bid Clindamycin 300 mg q6h for penicillin allergy Fluids: Discontinue IV fluids if taking adequate po Anticoagulation: Heparin 5000 units SC q8h prophylaxis	Antiemetics: As before Analgesics: As before Stool softener: As before Antibiotics: As before Anticoagulation: As before	Antiemetics: As before Analgesics: As before Stool softener: As before Antibiotics: As before Anticoagulation: As before	Discharge patient with following prescriptions: Antiemetics: Patient to remove Scopolamine patch on postoperative day 3 Analgesics: Tramadol 50 mg po q4h PRN OR Oxycodone 5 mg q4h PRN Acetaminophen 650 mg po q6h PRN Ibuprofen 600 mg q6h PRN for 7 d Gabapentin 100 mg po tid Valium 5 mg

Nursing and treatments	Provide chlorhexidine wipes to be applied to	Warming blanket Chlorhexidine wipes applied before	Anesthesia: Avoid nitrous oxide Avoid inhalational agents Minimize opioids Circuit humidified low oxygen (>21/min) Total IV anesthesia if possible: propofol drip as needed; midazolam 2–5 g IV, titrate to BIS of 40–60 IV lidocaine drip (if tumescent solution is used, consider omitting lidocaine drip) 1.5 mg/kg bolus on induction + 1.5 mg mg/kg/h; stop when surgeon starts to close	(pain scale rating 7–10 out of 10) Hydromorphone 0.5 mg IV q3h PRN for severe pain (pain scale rating 7–10 out of 10) Analgesics (po PRN): Oxycodone 5 mg po q4h PRN for moderate pain (pain scale rating 4–6 out of 10) Tramadol 50 mg po q4h PRN for mild pain (pain scale rating 1–3 out of 10) Fluids: D5 1/2 NS +20 KCl @ 84 mL/h, discontinue when po >500 mL Anticoagulation: Heparin 5000 units SC q8h prophylaxis to start in PM	Consider placement of OG tube Anesthesia head-	SCD to be worn when patient is in bed or	Order surgical bra as needed SCD to be worn when patient	q8h for 24 h Stool softener: Docusate sodium (Colace) 100 bid for 7 d Antibiotics: Duricef 500 mg bid If penicillin allergy, give Clindamycin 300 mg q6h for 14 d

(continued on next page)

Table 3
(continued)

	Before Surgery	Day of Surgery—Preoperative Area	Intraoperative	Postoperative Day 0 (T)	Postoperative Day 1 (T + 1)	Postoperative Day 2 (T + 2)	Postoperative Day 3 (T + 3)	Discharge
	surgical sites before surgical marking	surgical marking If not done already, nurse will help patient with chlorhexidine application	turning guidelines for patients undergoing prolonged surgery Foley catheter (avoid Foley in cases <3 h), discontinue Foley at end of case Warming blanket SCDs to lower extremities Padding to protect all prominent surfaces Pillow behind knees Check IV sites every 2 h Biopatch on drain sites	chair, remove when ambulating	is in bed or chair, remove when ambulating			
Activity				Ambulate with 1 person assist until ambulating	Ambulate 3 times per day, progress as tolerated	Ambulate 3 times per day, progress as tolerated	Ambulate 3 times per day, progress as tolerated	
Nutrition		Drink up to 20 ounces of noncarbonated sports drink up to 2 h before surgery		Advance diet as tolerated	Regular diet	Regular diet	Regular diet	

Consults			
Teaching	Education materials (booklet) provided discussing risks and benefits of surgery and length of stay Online modules Consents completed	Drain teaching Leave dressing on until clinic visit or POD 7. Remove if dressing becomes saturated	Drains to stay in place until follow-up visit Biopatches around drains Wound care Patient has postoperative follow-up appointment scheduled within 7 d of discharge

Abbreviations: BIS, bispectral index; DC, discharge; OG, oral gastric.

Biopatches are used around the drain sites, and a surgical bra is applied at the end of the procedure.

Postoperatively, patients again receive multimodal analgesia and antiemetic therapy as well as subcutaneous heparin prophylaxis. Most patients are discharged on postoperative day 1 with a course of Duricef 500 mg twice daily (or Clindamycin 300 mg 4 times daily if penicillin allergic) for a duration of 14 days. Pain control is multimodal with tramadol, acetaminophen, Celebrex, gabapentin, valium, and oxycodone. Patients remove the scopolamine patch on postoperative day 3. Wound and drain care teaching is provided on day of discharge, and patients typically follow up 1 week after discharge.

OUTCOMES OF ENHANCED RECOVERY AFTER SURGERY PROTOCOLS

ERAS pathways are widely used in many specialties; however, the concept is relatively new to plastic surgery. There are several studies demonstrating the safety and efficacy of ERAS protocols in plastic surgery.[9,11,134,136,137] ERAS protocols have been shown to reduce postoperative opioid use and reduce length of hospital stay in microvascular breast reconstruction.[138] They also improve postoperative analgesia for patients and reduce the risk of nausea and vomiting.[139] A recent large metaanalysis of retrospective and prospective studies again demonstrated overall shortened length of hospital stay and no increase in postoperative morbidity for patients undergoing autologous breast reconstruction.[140]

There are few ERAS protocols described for patients undergoing mastectomy with alloplastic breast reconstruction. Dumestre and colleagues[141] were the first to develop and implement an ERAS protocol for mastectomy with implant-based reconstruction based on multidisciplinary consensus input. They demonstrated that their ERAS protocol was safe, with improved patient satisfaction, and patients were able to be discharged on the same day without an increase in complications.

SUMMARY

ERAS protocols help to streamline perioperative care based on evidence-based review and consensus across all multidisciplinary aspects of care in breast reconstruction. Although ERAS protocols are not yet considered standard of care, they are likely the future of postoperative care delivery in plastic surgery. In plastic surgery, ERAS pathways have been shown to reduce hospital length of stay and opioid consumption, which may have cost-saving implications down the line. They also enhance the patient experience by improving postoperative analgesia, nausea, and vomiting. As consensus is achieved regarding best practices within plastic surgery based on the available evidence, it is likely that ERAS protocols will become standard throughout health care institutions.

REFERENCES

1. Offodile A, Boukovalas S, Coroneos C, et al. Enhanced recovery after surgery (ERAS) pathways in breast reconstruction: systematic review and meta-analysis of the literature. Breast Cancer Res Treat 2019;173:65–77.
2. Kehlet H. Multimodal approach to control postoperative pathophysiology and rehabilitation. Br J Anaesth 1997;78:606–17.
3. Kehlet H, Wilmore D. Multimodal strategies to improve surgical outcome. Am J Surg 2002;183:630–41.
4. Gustafsson U, Hausel J, Thorell A, et al. Adherence to enhanced recovery after surgery protocol and outcomes after colorectal cancer surgery. JAMA 2011;146(5):571–7.
5. Greco M, Capretti G, Beretta L, et al. Enhanced recovery program in colorectal surgery: a meta-analysis of randomized controlled trials. World J Surg 2014;38(6):1531–41.
6. Ferlay J, Soerjomataram I, Dikshit R, et al. Cancer incidence and mortality worldwide: sources, methods, and major patterns in GLOBOCAN 2012. Int J Cancer 2015;136:E359–86.
7. Panchal H, Matros E. Current trends in postmastectomy breast reconstruction. Plast Reconstr Surg 2017;150(5):7S–13S.
8. American Society of Plastic Surgeons. Plastic surgery statistics report. 2017. Available at: http://www.plasticsurgery.org/documents/News/Statistics/2017/plastic-surgery-statistics-report-2017.pdf. Accessed August 25, 2019.
9. Batdorf N, Lemaine V, Lovely J, et al. Enhanced recovery after surgery in microvascular breast reconstruction. J Plast Reconstr Aesthet Surg 2015;68:395–402.
10. Astanehe A, Temple-Oberle C, Nielsen M, et al. An enhanced recovery after surgery pathway for microvascular breast reconstruction is safe and effective. Plast Reconstr Surg Glob Open 2018;6(1):e1634.
11. Bonde C, Khorasani H, Eriksen K, et al. Introducing fast track surgery principles can reduce length of stay after autologous breast reconstruction using free flaps: a case-control study. J Plast Surg Hand Surg 2015;49(6):367–71.
12. Temple-Oberle C, Shea-Budgell M, Tan M, et al. Consensus review of optimal perioperative care in

breast reconstruction: Enhanced Recovery After Surgery (ERAS) Society recommendations. Plast Reconstr Surg 2017;135(5):1056e–71e.

13. Temple-Oberle C, Ayeni O, Webb C, et al. Shared decision-making: applying a person-centered approach to tailored breast reconstruction information provides high satisfaction across a variety of breast reconstruction operations. J Surg Oncol 2014;110:796–800.

14. Kiecolt-Glaser J, Page G, Marucha P, et al. Psychological influences on surgical recovery: perspectives from psychoneuroimmunology. Am Psychol 1998;53:1209–18.

15. Goodwin S, McCarthy C, Pusic A, et al. Complications in smokers after postmastectomy tissue expander/implant breast reconstruction. Ann Plast Surg 2005;55(1):16–9.

16. Chang D, Reece G, Wang B, et al. Effect of smoking on complications in patients undergoing free TRAM flap breast reconstruction. Plast Reconstr Surg 2000;105(7):2374–80.

17. Nguyen T, Costa M, Vidar E, et al. Effect of immediate reconstruction on postmastectomy surgical site infection. Ann Surg 2012;256(2):326–33.

18. Fischer J, Nelson J, Kovach S, et al. Impact of obesity on outcomes in breast reconstruction: analysis of 15,937 patients from the ACS-NSQIP datasets. J Am Coll Surg 2013;217:656–64.

19. Schaverien M, Mcculley S. Effect of obesity on outcomes of free autologous breast reconstruction: a meta-analysis. Microsurgery 2014;34:484–97.

20. Fischer J, Nelson J, Sieber B, et al. Free tissue transfer in the obese patient: an outcome and cost analysis in 1258 consecutive abdominally based reconstructions. Plast Reconstr Surg 2013;131(5):681e–92e.

21. Lee K, Mun G. Effects of obesity on postoperative complications after breast reconstruction using free muscle-sparing transversus rectus abdominis myocutaneous, deep inferior epigastric artery perforator, and superficial inferior epigastric artery flap: a systematic review and meta-analysis. Ann Plast Surg 2016;76:576–84.

22. Nwaogu I, Yan Y, Margenthaler J, et al. Venous thromboembolism after breast reconstruction in patients undergoing breast surgery: an American College of Surgeons NSQIP analysis. J Am Coll Surg 2015;220:886–93.

23. Chung C, Wink J, Nelson J, et al. Surgical site infections after free flap breast reconstruction: an analysis of 2,899 patients from the ACS-NSQIP datasets. J Reconstr Microsurg 2015;31:434–41.

24. Mennie J, Mohanna P, O'Donoghue J, et al. Donor-site hernia repair in abdominal flap breast reconstruction: a population-based cohort study of 7,929 patients. Plast Reconstr Surg 2015;136:1–9.

25. Qin C, Vaca E, Lovecchio F, et al. Differential impact of non-insulin-dependent diabetes mellitus and insulin-dependent diabetes mellitus on breast reconstruction outcomes. Breast Cancer Res Treat 2014;146:429–38.

26. Endara M, Masden D, Goldstein J, et al. The role of chronic and perioperative glucose management in high-risk surgical closures: a case for tighter glycemic control. Plast Reconstr Surg 2013;132:996–1004.

27. Coursin D, Connery L, Ketzler J. Perioperative diabetic and hyperglycemic management issues. Crit Care Med 2004;32(4 Suppl):S116–25.

28. Anderson D, Podgorny K, Berrios-Torres S, et al. Strategies to prevent surgical site infections in acute care hospitals: 2014 update. Infect Control Hosp Epidemiol 2014;35(6):605–27.

29. Symonette C, Gan B. Computed tomography-based preoperative vascular imaging in autologous breast reconstruction: a Canadian perspective. Can J Plast Surg 2013;21:11–4.

30. Phillips T, Stella D, Rozen W, et al. Abdominal wall CT angiography: a detailed account of a newly established preoperative imaging technique. Radiology 2008;249:32–44.

31. Ohkuma R, Mohan R, Baltodano P, et al. Abdominally based free flap planning in breast reconstruction with computed tomographic angiography: systematic review and meta-analysis. Plast Reconstr Surg 2014;133(3):483–94.

32. Brady M, Kinn S, Stuart P. Preoperative fasting for adults to prevent perioperative complications. Cochrane Database Syst Rev 2003;(4):CD004423.

33. Feldheiser A, Aziz O, Baldini G, et al. Enhanced recovery after surgery (ERAS) for gastrointestinal surgery, part 2: consensus statement for anesthesia practice. Acta Anaesthesiol Scand 2016;60(3):289–334.

34. Bilku D, Dennison A, Hall T, et al. Role of preoperative carbohydrate loading: a systematic review. Ann R Coll Surg Engl 2014;96:15–22.

35. Hausel J, Nygren J, Lagerkranser M, et al. A carbohydrate-rich drink reduces preoperative discomfort in elective surgery patients. Anesth Analg 2001;93(5):1344–50.

36. Nygren J, Soop M, Thorell A, et al. Preoperative oral carbohydrate administration reduces postoperative insulin resistance. Clin Nutr 1998;17:65–71.

37. Crowe P, Dennison A, Royle G. The effect of preoperative glucose loading on postoperative nitrogen metabolism. Br J Surg 1984;71:635–7.

38. Yuill K, Richardson R, Davidson H, et al. The administration of an oral carbohydrate-containing fluid prior to major elective upper gastro-intestinal surgery preserves skeletal muscle mass postoperatively: a randomised clinical trial. Clin Nutr 2005;24:32–7.

39. Henriksen M, Hessov I, Dela F, et al. Effects of preoperative oral carbohydrates and peptides on

postoperative endocrine response, mobilization, nutrition, and muscle function in abdominal surgery. Acta Anaesthesiol Scand 2003;47:191–9.

40. Nygren J, Thorell A, Ljungqvist O. Preoperative oral carbohydrate nutrition: an update. Curr Opin Clin Nutr Metab Care 2001;4:255–9.

41. Gustafsson U, Nygren J, Thorell A, et al. Pre-operative carbohydrate loading may be used in type 2 diabetes patients. Acta Anaesthesiol Scand 2008; 52(7):946–51.

42. Murphy R, Alderman A, Gutowski K, et al. Evidence-based practices for thromboembolism prevention: summary of the ASPS venous thromboembolism task force report. Plast Reconstr Surg 2012;130(1):168e–75e.

43. Caprini J. Thrombosis risk assessment as a guide to quality patient care. Dis Mon 2005;51:70–8.

44. patiar S, Kirwan C, McDowell G, et al. Prevention of venous thromboembolism in surgical patients with breast cancer. Br J Surg 2007;94:412–20.

45. Rasmussen M, Jorgensen L, Wille-Jorgensen P. Prolonged thromboprophylaxis with low molecular weight heparin for abdominal or pelvic surgery. Cochrane Database Syst Rev 2009;(1):CD004318.

46. Pannucci C, Wachtman C, Dreszer G, et al. The effect of postoperative enoxaparin on right of reoperative hematoma. Plast Reconstr Surg 2012;129(1):160–8.

47. Kim E, Eom J, Ahn S, et al. The efficacy of prophylactic low-molecular-weight heparin to prevent pulmonary thromboembolism in immediate breast reconstruction using the TRAM flap. Plast Reconstr Surg 2009;123:9–12.

48. Lapid O, Pietersen L, Horst CV. Reoperation for haematoma after breast reduction with preoperative administration of low-molecular-weight heparin: experience in 720 patients. J Plast Reconstr Aesthet Surg 2012;65:1513–7.

49. Hardy R, Williams L, Dixon J. Use of enoxaparin results in more haemorrhagic complications after breast surgery than unfractionated heparin. Br J Surg 2008;95:834–6.

50. Cruse P, Foord R. The epidemiology of wound infection: a 10-year prospective study of 62,939 wounds. Surg Clin North Am 1980;60:27–40.

51. Sanguinetti A, Rosato L, Cirocchi R, et al. Antibiotic prophylaxis in breast surgery. Preliminary results of a multicenter randomized study on 1400 cases. Ann Ital Chir 2009;80(4):275–9.

52. Phillips B, Bishawi M, Dagum A, et al. A systematic review of infection rates and associated antibiotic duration in acellular dermal matrix in breast reconstruction. Eplasty 2014;14:e42.

53. Sajid M, Hutson K, Akhter N, et al. An updated meta-analysis on the effectiveness of preoperative prophylactic antibiotics in patients undergoing breast surgical procedures. Breast J 2012;18: 312–7.

54. Olsen M, Nickel K, Fox I, et al. Incidence of surgical site infection following mastectomy with and without immediate reconstruction using private insurer claims data. Infect Control Hosp Epidemiol 2015;36(8):907–14.

55. Jones D, Bunn F, Bell-Syer S. Prophylactic antibiotics to prevent surgical site infection after breast cancer surgery. Cochrane Database Syst Rev 2014;(3):CD005360.

56. Huang N, Liu M, Yu P, et al. Antibiotic prophylaxis in prosthesis-based mammoplasty: a systematic review. Int J Surg 2015;15:31–7.

57. Hardwicke J, Bechar J, Skillman J. Are systemic antibiotics indicated in aesthetic breast surgery? A systematic review of the literature. Plast Reconstr Surg 2013;131:1395–403.

58. Collins J, Verheyden C, Mahabir R. Core measures: implications for plastic surgery. Plast Reconstr Surg 2013;131:1266–71.

59. Thomas R, Alvino P, Cortino G, et al. Long-acting versus short-acting cephalosporins for preoperative prophylaxis in breast surgery: a randomized double-blind trial involving 1,766 patients. Chemotherapy 1999;45(3):217–23.

60. Drury K, Lanier S, Khavanin N, et al. Impact of postoperative antibiotic prophylaxis duration on surgical site infections in autologous breast reconstruction. Ann Plast Surg 2016;76(2):174–9.

61. Craft R, Damjanovic B, Colwell A. Evidence-based protocol for infection control in immediate implant-based breast reconstruction. Ann Plast Surg 2012; 69:446–50.

62. Dumville J, McFarlane E, Edwards P, et al. Preoperative skin antiseptics for preventing surgical wound infections after clean surgery. Cochrane Database Syst Rev 2015;(4):CD003949.

63. Singhal A, Kannan S, Gota V. 5HT3 antagonists for prophylaxis of postoperative nausea and vomiting in breast surgery: a meta-analysis. J Postgrad Med 2012;58:23–31.

64. Olanders K, Lundgren G, Johansson A. Betamethasone in prevention of postoperative nausea and vomiting following breast surgery. J Clin Anesth 2014;26:461–5.

65. Gupta P, Jain S. Postoperative nausea and vomiting prophylaxis: a comparative study of ondansetron, granisetron and granisetron and dexamethasone combinations after radical mastectomy. Saudi J Anaesth 2014;8(Suppl 1):S67–71.

66. Diemunsch P, Gan T, Philip B, et al. Single-dose aprepitant vs ondansetron for the prevention of postoperative nausea and vomiting: a randomized, double-blind phase III trial in patients undergoing open abdominal surgery. Br J Anaesth 2007; 99(2):202–11.

67. Vallejo M, Phelps A, Ibinson J, et al. Aprepitant plus ondansetron compared with ondansetron alone in

reducing postoperative nausea and vomiting in ambulatory patients undergoing plastic surgery. Plast Reconstr Surg 2012;129(2):519–26.

68. Habib A, Keifer J, Borel C, et al. A comparison of the combination of aprepitant and dexamethasone versus the combination of ondansetron and dexamethasone for the prevention of postoperative nausea and vomiting in patients undergoing craniotomy. Anesth Analg 2011;112:813–8.

69. Dirks J, Fredensborg B, Christensen D, et al. A randomized study of the effects of single-dose gabapentin versus placebo on postoperative pain and morphine consumption after mastectomy. Anesthesiology 2002;97:560–4.

70. Kim S, Song J, Park B, et al. Pregabalin reduces post-operative pain after mastectomy: a double-blind, randomized, placebo-controlled study. Acta Anaesthesiol Scand 2001;55:290–6.

71. Priya V, Divatia J, Sareen R, et al. Efficacy of intravenous ketoprofen for pre-emptive analgesia. J Postgrad Med 2002;48:109–12.

72. Sun M, Liao Q, Wen L, et al. Effect of perioperative intravenous flurbiprofen axetil on chronic mastectomy pain. Zhong Nan Da Xue Xue Bao Yi Xue Ban 2013;38:653–60.

73. Riest G, Peters J, Weiss M, et al. Does perioperative administration of rofecoxib improve analgesia after spine, breast and orthopaedic surgery? Eur J Anaesthesiol 2006;23(3):219–26.

74. Zielinksi J, Jaworski R, Smietanska I, et al. A randomized, double-blind, placebo-controlled trial of preemptive analgesia with bupivacaine in patients undergoing mastectomy for carcinoma of the breast. Med Sci Monit 2011;17:CR589–97.

75. Segerdahl M, Ekblom A, Sandelin K, et al. Preoperative adenosine infusion reduces the requirements for isoflurane and postoperative analgesics. Anesth Analg 1995;80:1145–9.

76. Oliveria GD, Bialek J, Fitzgerald P, et al. Systemic magnesium to improve quality of post-surgical recovery in outpatient segmental mastectomy: a randomized, double-blind, placebo-controlled trial. Magnes Res 2013;26:156–64.

77. Amr Y, Yousef A. Evaluation of efficacy of the perioperative administration of Venlafaxine fo gabapentin on acute and chronic postmastectomy pain. Clin J Pain 2010;26:381–5.

78. Imai Y, Mammoto T, Murakami K, et al. The effects of preanesthetic oral clonidine on total requirement of propofol for general anesthesia. J Clin Anesth 1998;10(8):660–5.

79. Glissmeyer C, Johnson W, Sherman B, et al. Effect of paravertebral nerve blocks on narcotic use after mastectomy with reconstruction. Am J Surg 2015; 209:881–3.

80. Zhong T, Ojha M, Bagher S, et al. Transversus abdominis plane block reduces morphine consumption in the early postoperative period following microsurgical abdominal tissue breast reconstruction: a double-blind, placebo-controlled, randomized trial. Plast Reconstr Surg 2014;134(5): 870–8.

81. Karmakar M, Samy W, Li J, et al. Thoracic paravertebral block and its effects on chronic pain and health-related quality of life after modified radical mastectomy. Reg Anesth Pain Med 2014;39(4): 289–98.

82. Hong J, Kang Y, Kil H. Anaesthesia for day case excisional breast biopsy: propofol-remifentanil compared with sevoflurane-nitrous oxide. Eur J Anaesthesiol 2008;25:460–7.

83. Chen H, Hsu Y, Hua K, et al. Comparison of sevoflurane versus propofol under auditory evoked potential monitoring in female patients undergoing breast surgery. Biomed J 2013;36: 125–31.

84. Kurz A, Sessler D, Lenhardt R. Perioperative normothermia to reduce the incidence of surgical-wound infection and shorten hospitalization. Study of Wound Infection and Temperature Group. N Engl J Med 1996;334:1209–15.

85. National Institute for Health and Care Excellence. Clinical practice guideline: the management of inadvertent perioperative hypothermia in adults. National Collaborating Centre for Nursing and Supportive care commissioned by National Institute for Health and Care Excellence (NICE). London: Royal College of Nursing; 2008. Available at: http://guidance.nice.org.uk/CG65. Accessed August 25, 2019.

86. Roberson M, Dieckmann L, Rodriguez R, et al. A review of the evidence for active preoperative warming in adults undergoing general anesthesia. AANA J 2013;81:351–6.

87. Deren M, Machan J, DiGiovanni C, et al. Prewarming operating rooms for prevention of intraoperative hypothermia during total knee and hip arthroplasties. J Arthroplasty 2011;26:1380–6.

88. Munday J, Hines S, Wallace K, et al. A systematic review of effectiveness of warming interventions for women undergoing cesarean section. Worldviews Evid Based Nurs 2014;11:383–93.

89. Andrzejowski J, Turnbull D, Nandakumar A, et al. A randomised single blinded study of the administration of pre-warmed fluid vs active fluid warming on the incidence of peri-operative hypothermia in short surgical procedures. Anaesthesia 2010;65: 942–5.

90. Campbell G, Alderson P, Smith A, et al. Warming of intravenous and irrigation fluids for preventing inadvertent perioperative hypothermia. Cochrane Database Syst Rev 2015;(13):CD009891.

91. Giglio M, Marucci M, Testini M, et al. Goal-directed haemodynamic therapy and gastrointestinal

complications in major surgery: a meta-analysis of randomized controlled trials. Br J Anaesth 2009; 103:637–46.

92. Nisanevich V, Felsenstein I, Almogy G, et al. Effect of intraoperative fluid management on outcome after intraabdominal surgery. Anesthesiology 2005; 103:25–32.

93. Booi D. Perioperative fluid overload increases anastomosis thrombosis in the free TRAM flap used for breast reconstruction. Eur J Plast Surg 2011;34:81–6.

94. Nelson J, Fischer J, Grover R, et al. Intraoperative perfusion management impacts postoperative outcomes: an analysis of 682 autologous breast reconstruction patients. J Plast Reconstr Aesthet Surg 2015;68(2):175–83.

95. Chen C, Nguyen M, Bar-Meir E, et al. Effects of vasopressor administration on the outcomes of microsurgical breast reconstruction. Ann Plast Surg 2010;65(1):28–31.

96. Kelly D, Reynolds M, Crantford C, et al. Impact of intraoperative vasopressor use in free tissue transfer for head, neck, and extremity reconstruction. Ann Plast Surg 2014;72:S135–8.

97. Harris L, Goldstein D, Hofer S, et al. Impact of vasopressors on outcomes in head and neck free tissue transfer. Microsurgery 2012;32:15–9.

98. Derry C, Derry S, Moore R. Single dose oral ibuprofen plus paracetamol (acetaminophen) for acute postoperative pain. Cochrane Database Syst Rev 2013;(6):CD010210.

99. Hall P, Derry S, Moore R, et al. Single dose oral lornoxicam for acute postoperative pain in adults. Cochrane Database Syst Rev 2009;(7):CD007441.

100. Barden J, Derry S, McQuay H, et al. Single dose oral ketoprofen and dexketoprofen for acute postoperative pain in adults. Cochrane Database Syst Rev 2009;(4):CD007355.

101. Legeby M, Sandelin K, Wickman M, et al. Analgesic efficacy of diclofenac in combination with morphine and paracetamol after mastectomy and immediate breast reconstruction. Acta Anaesthesiol Scand 2005;49:1360–6.

102. Gobble R, Hoang H, Kachniarz B, et al. Ketorolac does not increase perioperative bleeding: a meta-analysis of randomized controlled trials. Plast Reconstr Surg 2014;133:741–55.

103. Seon R, Paul K. Preoperative gabapentin for postoperative analgesia: a meta-analysis. Can J Anaesth 2006;53:461–9.

104. Engelman E, Cateloy F. Efficacy and safety of perioperative pregabalin for post-operative pain: a meta-analysis of randomized-controlled trials. Acta Anaesthesiol Scand 2011;55:927–43.

105. Heller L, Kowalski A, Wei C, et al. Prospective, randomized, double-blind trial of local anesthetic infusion and intravenous narcotic patient-controlled anesthesia pump for pain management after free TRAM flap breast reconstruction. Plast Reconstr Surg 2008;122:1010–8.

106. Boehmler J, Venturi M, Nahabedian M. Decreased narcotic use with an implantable local anesthetic catheter after deep inferior epigastric perforator flap breast reconstruction. Ann Plast Surg 2009; 62:618–20.

107. Lambert E, Carey S. Practice guideline recommendations on perioperative fasting: a systematic review. JPEN J Parenter Enteral Nutr 2016;40: 1158–65.

108. Bui D, Cordeiro P, Hu Q, et al. Free flap reexploration: indications, treatment, and outcomes in 1193 free flaps. Plast Reconstr Surg 2007;119: 2092–100.

109. Chang E, Carlsen B, Festekjian J, et al. Salvage rates of compromised free flap breast reconstruction after recurrent thrombosis. Ann Plast Surg 2013;71:68–71.

110. Stollings J, Diedrich D, Oyen L, et al. Rapid-sequence intubation: a review of the process and considerations when choosing medications. Ann Pharmacother 2014;48:62–76.

111. Masoomi H, Clark E, Paydar K, et al. Predictive risk factors of free flap thrombosis in breast reconstruction surgery. Microsurgery 2014;34(8):589–94.

112. Nahabedian M, Momen B, Manson P. Factors associated with anastomotic failure after microvascular reconstruction of the breast. Plast Reconstr Surg 2004;114:74–82.

113. Mirzabeigi M, Wang T, Kovach S, et al. Free flap take-back following postoperative microvascular compromise: predicting salvage versus failure. Plast Reconstr Surg 2012;130:579–89.

114. Disa J, Cordeiro P, Hidalgo D. Efficacy of conventional monitoring techniques in free tissue transfer: an 11-year experience in 750 consecutive cases. Plast Reconstr Surg 1999;104(1):97–101.

115. Schmulder A, Gur E, Zaretski A. Eight-year experience of the Cook-Swartz Doppler in free flap operations: microsurgical and reexploration results with regard to a wide spectrum of surgeries. Microsurgery 2011;31:1–6.

116. Whitaker I, Rozen W, Chubb D, et al. Postoperative monitoring of free flaps in autologous breast reconstruction: a multicenter comparison of 398 flaps using clinical monitoring, microdialysis, and the implantable Doppler probe. J Reconstr Microsurg 2010;26(6):409–16.

117. Smit J, Werker P, Liss A, et al. Introduction of the implantable Doppler system did not lead to an increased salvage rate of compromised flaps: a multivariate analysis. Plast Reconstr Surg 2010; 125(6):1710–7.

118. Um G, Chang J, Louie O, et al. Implantable Cook-Swartz Doppler probe versus Synovis Flow Coupler

for the post-operative monitoring of free flap breast reconstruction. J Plast Reconstr Aesthet Surg 2014;67(7):960–6.

119. Pelletier A, Tseng C, Agarwal S, et al. Cost analysis of near-infrared spectroscopy tissue oximetry for monitoring autologous free tissue breast reconstruction. J Reconstr Microsurg 2011;27:487–94.

120. Lin S, Nguyen M, Chen C, et al. Tissue oximetry monitoring in microsurgical breast reconstruction decreases flap loss and improves rate of flap salvage. Plast Reconstr Surg 2011;127(3):1080–5.

121. Duteille F, Rouif M, Alfandari B, et al. Reduction of skin closure time without loss of healing quality: a multicenter prospective study in 100 patients comparing the use of Insorb absorbable staples with absorbable thread for dermal suture. Surg Innov 2013;20(1):70–3.

122. Nipshagen M, Hage J, Beekman W. Use of 2-octyl-cyanoacrylate skin adhesive (Dermabond) for wound closure following reduction mammaplasty: a prospective, randomized intervention study. Plast Reconstr Surg 2008;122:10–8.

123. Veiga D, Veiga-Filho J, Damasceno C, et al. Dressing wear time after breast reconstruction: study protocol for a randomized controlled trial. Trials 2013;14:58.

124. Nahabedian M. Achieving ideal donor site aesthetics with autologous breast reconstruction. Gland Surg 2015;4:145–53.

125. Kim J, Davila A, Persing S, et al. A meta-analysis of human acellular dermis and submuscular tissue expander breast reconstruction. Plast Reconstr Surg 2012;129(1):28–41.

126. Kostaras E, Tansarli G, Falagas M. Use of negative-pressure wound therapy in breast tissues: evaluation of the literature. Surg Infect (Larchmt) 2014; 15:679–85.

127. Paddon-Jones D, Sheffield-Moore M, Cree M, et al. Atrophy and impaired muscle protein synthesis during prolonged inactivity and stress. J Clin Endocrinol Metab 2006;91(12):4836–41.

128. Henriksen M, Jensen M, Hansen H, et al. Enforced mobilization, early oral feeding, and balanced analgesia improve convalescence after colorectal surgery. Nutrition 2002;18:147–52.

129. Brower R. Consequences of bed rest. Crit Care Med 2009;37(Suppl):S422–8.

130. Jones C, Kelliher L, Dickenson M, et al. Randomized clinical trial on enhanced recovery versus standard care following open liver resection. Br J Surg 2013;100(8):1015–24.

131. Bartolo M, Zycchella C, Pace A, et al. Early rehabilitation after surgery improves functional outcome in inpatients with brain tumours. J Neurooncol 2012; 107(3):537–44.

132. Testa A, Iannace C, Libero LD. Strengths of early physical rehabilitation programs in surgical breast cancer patients: results of a randomized controlled study. Eur J Phys Rehabil Med 2014;50:275–84.

133. Scaffidi M, Vulpiani M, Vetrano M, et al. Early rehabilitation reduces the onset of complications in the upper limb following breast cancer surgery. Eur J Phys Rehabil Med 2012;48(4):601–11.

134. Davidge K, Brown M, Morgan P, et al. Processes of care in autogenous breast reconstruction with pedicled TRAM flaps: expediting postoperative discharge in an ambulatory setting. Plast Reconstr Surg 2013;132:339e–44e.

135. Holtzmann J, Timm H. The experiences of and the nursing care for breast cancer patients undergoing immediate breast reconstruction. Eur J Cancer Care (Engl) 2005;14:310–8.

136. Stone J, Siotos C, Sarmiento S, et al. Implementing our microsurgical breast reconstruction enhanced recovery after surgery pathway: consensus obstacles and recommendations. Plast Reconstr Surg Glob Open 2019;7(1):e1855.

137. Afonso A, Oskar S, Tan K, et al. Is enhanced recovery the new standard of care in microsurgical breast reconstruction? Plast Reconstr Surg 2017; 139(5):1053–61.

138. Sharif-Askary B, Hompe E, Broadwater G, et al. The effect of enhanced recovery after surgery pathway implementation on abdominal-based microvascular breast reconstruction. J Surg Res 2019;242:276–85.

139. Chiu C, Aleshi P, Esserman J, et al. Improved analgesia and reduced post-operative nausea and vomiting after implementation of an enhanced recovery after surgery (ERAS) pathway for total mastectomy. BMC Anesthesiol 2018;18:1–9.

140. Sebai M, Siotos C, Payne R, et al. Enhanced recovery after surgery pathway for microsurgical breast reconstruction: a systematic review and meta-analysis. Plast Reconstr Surg 2019;143(3):655–66.

141. Dumestre D, Webb C, Temple-Oberle C. Improved recovery experience achieved for women undergoing implant-based breast reconstruction using an enhanced recovery after surgery model. Plast Reconstr Surg 2016;139(3):550–9.

Imaging of Damaged Nerves

David A. Purger, MD, PhD[a], Sarada Sakamuri, MD[b], Nicholas F. Hug, BA[a], Sandip Biswal, MD[c], Thomas J. Wilson, MD[d],*

KEYWORDS

- Diffusion tensor imaging • MRI • Magnetic resonance neurography • Nerve injury • Peripheral nerve
- Ultrasound

KEY POINTS

- The history and physical examination are the cornerstones of evaluation for patients presenting with peripheral nerve pathology. Imaging is an important adjunct, but not a replacement for a thorough and skillful history and physical examination.
- Magnetic resonance neurography (MRN) and ultrasound are the most commonly utilized modalities for evaluating peripheral nerves. Each has its advantages and disadvantages.
- Important parameters to assess on imaging studies of peripheral nerves include the caliber of the nerve, changes in signal intensity (whether magnetic resonance signal or echogenicity), course of the nerve, fascicular structure, continuity/discontinuity of the nerve, and the presence of mass lesions.
- Fat-saturated images and gadolinium contrast enhancement are valuable in gleaning information from magnetic resonance neurography studies.
- Emerging techniques for evaluating peripheral nerves include 7 T MRN, ultrasound elastography, and positron emission tomography using novel radiotracers.

INTRODUCTION

Nerve damage occurs in various ways. One commonly thinks about traumatic nerve injuries and nerve entrapments, but a variety of other conditions can damage nerves, including inflammatory and autoimmune conditions, primary nerve tumors, and perineural spread of malignancy. Regardless of the cause, damage to the nerve can cause weakness, numbness, paresthesias, neuropathic pain, and/or autonomic dysfunction. The mainstays in diagnosis are the history and physical examination. As an extension of the physical examination, electrodiagnostics can be helpful in localizing the injury, characterizing the injury,

and in some cases, suggesting the pathology responsible for the injury. Although never a replacement for the history and physical examination, imaging also is increasingly playing an important role in the evaluation of damaged nerves. Again, imaging studies can not only help localize the nerve injury but can also play an important role in diagnosing the pathology responsible for nerve injury.

Improved imaging of damaged nerves has the power to transform clinical care and the way clinicians approach nerve injuries. For example, after closed traumatic nerve injuries, the typical approach is to wait 3 to 6 months to see if there

Funding: None.
[a] Department of Neurosurgery, Stanford University, 300 Pasteur Drive, Stanford, CA 94305, USA; [b] Department of Neurology and Neurological Sciences, 213 Quarry Road, MC 5979, Palo Alto, CA 94304, USA; [c] Department of Radiology, Stanford University, 300 Pasteur Drive, S-068B, Stanford, CA 94305, USA; [d] Department of Neurosurgery, Stanford University, 300 Pasteur Drive, R293, Stanford, CA 94305, USA
* Corresponding author.
E-mail address: wilsontj@stanford.edu

Clin Plastic Surg 47 (2020) 245–259
https://doi.org/10.1016/j.cps.2019.12.003

will be evidence of spontaneous recovery before deciding whether surgery is appropriate. Imagine how this would change if one could image the damaged nerve and predict which nerves will go on to spontaneous recovery and which will not. As imaging improves, this may become a reality. Although new techniques are emerging, old techniques and the improvements that have already occurred are still an important part of the evaluation of nerve injuries and nerve pain and are already reshaping the way one thinks about nerve pathology. As an example, the literature would suggest that complex regional pain syndrome (CRPS) type 1 is more common than CRPS type 2.[1] However, the authors have found at their institution that using a combination of a multidisciplinary approach and magnetic resonance neurography (MRN), many times a nerve injury can be identified in patients diagnosed with CRPS type 1, converting the diagnosis to CRPS type 2 and changing the approach to care. The authors observed that CRPS type 2 is more common than type 1 using this approach (Johnson, unpublished data, 2020).

The focus of this article is imaging of damaged nerves, focusing on nerve injuries and entrapment neuropathies. It discusses the currently available imaging techniques and some emerging techniques that may take a more prominent role in the future.

MAGNETIC RESONANCE NEUROGRAPHY
Introduction

With the advent of widespread MRI technology in the 1980s, the technique has been applied to imaging of a variety of specific anatomic structures. MRN is nothing more than MRI of peripheral nerves. This technique continues to evolve, allowing better depiction of peripheral nerves, their anatomic structure, and their pathologic states. Initial applications included anatomic imaging of the carpal tunnel, where the median nerve was identified as a structure with slightly higher signal intensity compared with surrounding tendons.[2] One of the first demonstrations of peripheral nerve pathology via MRN was the finding that in carpal tunnel syndrome, the median nerve demonstrates T2-hyperintensity and an increased caliber.[3] As MRN technology has developed, its indications have continued to expand.[4–11]

Magnetic Resonance Neurography Technique

The mainstay of MRN is the identification of peripheral nerve anatomy and pathology using T1-weighted and T2-weighted fluid-sensitive (eg, short tau inversion recovery [STIR]) sequences, which are analyzed to understand nerve signal intensity, size and caliber, course, fascicular pattern, perineural tissues, and nerve-associated mass lesions.[12] Imaging is generally performed on scanners with 1.5- or 3-T (T) magnets using phased-array surface coils shaped around the area of interest to increase signal-to-noise ratio and parallel imaging that allows for precise localization of the magnetic resonance signal.[13] Normal nerves display an intermediate signal intensity similar to muscle on T1-weighted images and intermediate to slightly increased intensity on T2-weighted images, depending on the amount of background fat suppression and the presence of endoneurial fluid.[14] Obtaining fat-saturated images is extremely important when trying to image nerves (**Fig. 1**). Healthy peripheral nerves do not normally enhance with gadolinium contrast because of the presence of the blood-nerve barrier.[15] Contrast administration may assist in cases where there is suspicion for infection, inflammation, diffuse lesions, or tumors, or in physical injury, where nearby denervated muscles may also demonstrate contrast enhancement.[12] Thus, in the authors' opinion, contrast should be given for all MRN studies, unless there is a specific contraindication. In abnormal nerves, the most common and easily identifiable change is an increase in the signal intensity of the nerve on T2-weighted images, approaching the intensity of adjacent blood vessels.[16]

During the first 2 decades of MRN imaging, clinicians were limited to 2-dimensional sections in standard anatomic planes (ie, axial, coronal, and sagittal), which are adequate for anatomy that is aligned with the axis of an MRI magnetic field, such as an upper extremity lying flat against an examination table. Although advances in magnetic resonance sequences, such as T1-weighted spin echo (SE) and T2-weighted SPAIR (spectrally adiabatic inversion recovery) allowed for more homogeneous fat suppression, helping to show a nerve's fascicular microstructure in greater detail. Anatomic structures obliquely situated within the body, such as the brachial plexus, were not easily depicted with even the most advanced 2-dimensional sequences.[12] The development of 3-dimensional magnetic resonance sequences, such as curved multiplanar reconstructions (MPRs), allowed for the visualization of nervous structures with tortuous courses or oblique orientations.[17] Newer sequences such as 3-dimensional STIR SPACE (Sampling Perfection with Application optimized Contrasts using different flip angle Evolutions) combine modern fat suppression techniques with MPR and maximal intensity projection (MIP) technology to optimize the

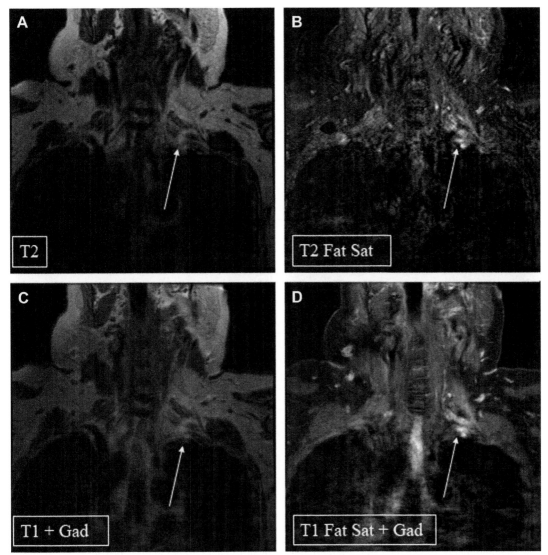

Fig. 1. Coronal sequences from an MRN of the brachial plexus, including (*A*) T2, (*B*) T2 with fat saturation, (*C*) T1 with gadolinium, and (*D*) T1 with gadolinium and fat saturation, showing enlargement, T2-hyperintensity, and contrast-enhancement in the left C7, C8, and T1 nerve roots (*arrow*). The T2-hyperintensity and contrast enhancement are much more difficult to appreciate on the nonfat saturated images (Panels *A* and *C*).

visualization of the brachial plexus and other anatomically complex structures.[18] Evaluating small, distal nerves situated next to blood vessels may be difficult. At their institution, the authors have found one of the most useful sequences to be the double-echo steady-state (DESS) sequence, which is sensitive to motion and helps differentiate blood vessels from nerves, particularly when attempting to image small nerves (**Fig. 2**). For intradural applications, such as imaging nerve root avulsions, heavily T2-weighted myelography sequences, such as FIESTA, DRIVE, and CISS are preferred to compensate for cerebrospinal fluid flow.[19,20]

Magnetic Resonance Neuropathy for Traumatic Nerve Injuries

MRN allows for the identification of nerve transection and helps distinguish injury patterns in nontransected nerves by visualizing details of nerve architecture. The resulting detailed characterization of nerve injury is important for management and prognostication.[15,21] Seddon's classification system for nerve injuries defined 3 types of injuries: neurapraxia, axonotmesis, and neurotmesis, each associated with different pathologic features and clinical outcomes.[22] Sunderland expanded the original Seddon classification based on the degree

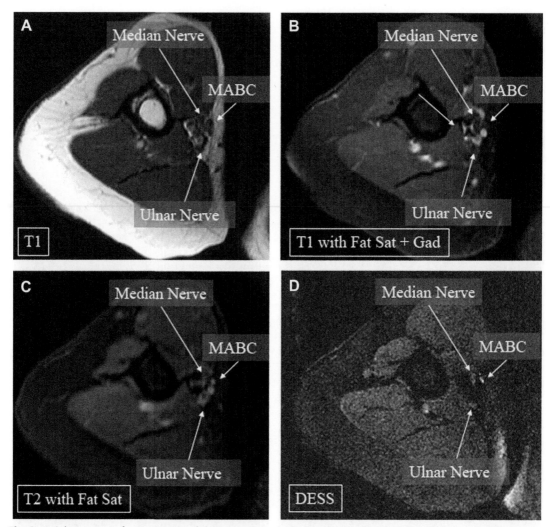

Fig. 2. Axial sequences from an MRN of the upper arm, including (*A*) T1, (*B*) T1 with gadolinium and fat saturation, (*C*) T2 with fat saturation, and (*D*) DESS, showing enlargement and T2-hyperintensity of the medial antebrachial cutaneous nerve. DESS allows the differentiation of small T2-hyperintense nerves, such as the MABC in this case, from nearby blood vessels.

of injury to the axons and surrounding connective tissue.[23] The increase in routine use of MRN has established findings suggestive of each of these levels of nerve injury. Although these findings can be suggestive, MRN cannot always reliably differentiate between different injury types or grades.

Neurapraxic, or Sunderland grade 1, injuries result in damage to the myelin sheath, with preservation of the axon and surrounding connective tissues.[22,23] The most characteristic sign on MRN is nerve enlargement and hyperintensity on T2-weighted and STIR images adjacent to the site of injury. This is most likely because of a combination of endoneurial fluid collection and vascular congestion, although the phenomenon is poorly understood. Mild muscular atrophy without gross signal change or denervation can also be seen in the muscles innervated by the affected nerves.[21,24]

Axonotmesis was characterized by Seddon as damage that results in axonal disruption, typically with good recovery, as the epineurium and supporting structures are preserved.[22] The Sunderland system further distinguishes 3 levels of axonotmesis, each with different clinical presentations that correlate with MRN findings.[23] Sunderland grade 2 injuries have axonal disruption with preserved endoneurium allowing the potential for good recovery. On MRN, this is observed as hyperintensity and enlargement of the nerve, as in Sunderland grade 1, along with effacement and disruption of the fascicular architecture.[24] Additionally, signs of muscle denervation and blurring of perivascular fat may be present. In Sunderland grade III injuries, the endoneurium is damaged, which leads to inappropriate routing of axons to targets, potentially as a result of fascicular scarring. Initially, MRN findings are similar to Sunderland grade 2, but when imaging is obtained subacutely or chronically, an area of hyperintense, fusiform enlargement, representing a neuroma-in-continuity, may be present. Sunderland grade 4 represents more severe nerve injury, including damage to the perineurium and poor prognosis for recovery without surgery. This consistently results in evidence of a neuroma-in-continuity on MRN, although not if imaging is obtained in the immediate postinjury period, as well as absence of fascicular appearance.[15]

Sunderland grade 5 corresponds to Seddon's neurotmesis, in which the entire nerve, including the epineurium, has been damaged.[22,23] To maximize diagnostic utility of MRN in suspected grade 5 injuries, imaging should be performed as soon as possible after injury, as the discontinuity fills with granulation tissue and fluid over time, leading to a swollen, thickened proximal ending of the nerve, which can diminish signal intensity and prevent diagnosis of a terminal neuroma.[15]

Recently, a practical classification of nerve injuries based primarily on interpretation of MRN imaging that is more similar to Seddon's original 3-tiered system has been proposed.[25] Neurapraxic-type stretch injury is identified by increased nerve signal intensity and mild to no enlargement compared with nearby nerves. In the next tier of injury, nerve enlargement and fascicular effacement are seen, with or without a neuroma-in-continuity. Finally, the most severe injuries show evidence of complete discontinuity, with either frank transection or terminal neuroma on imaging. Particularly when evaluating neuropathic pain, the identification of a terminal neuroma, such as can occur with a transected nerve following an amputation, can be important in guiding treatment (**Fig. 3**).

Changes visible on MRN in denervated muscle secondary to peripheral nerve injury may be important clues to the extent and chronicity of a peripheral nerve injury. In the subacute setting, denervated muscles can exhibit hyperintensity on T2-weighted imaging, particularly on STIR or similar sequences, often referred to as subacute denervation changes. More chronic denervation can result in atrophy with additional fatty infiltration of the muscle.[26]

Magnetic Resonance Neuropathy for Entrapment Neuropathies

Entrapment neuropathies are defined as chronic, pressure-induced compression injuries. The injury is thought to occur secondary to increased endoneurial fluid pressure, resulting in microvascular congestion, infarction, and fibrosis.[27] The criteria to diagnose a compression injury include close contact between a nerve and a compressive structure, the disappearance of the normal fat plane around an affected nerve, and a change in the nerve structure, including the fascicular architecture, nerve caliber, anatomic course, or signal intensity.[15] In general, compressed nerves demonstrate high signal intensity on T2-weighted or STIR images, with denervation changes of surrounding muscle if the compression is advanced. The caliber of the nerve can sometimes be observed to be small at the site of compression, but more commonly, what is visualized is enlargement of the nerve immediately proximal to the site of compression (**Fig. 4**). MRN imaging has been useful in cases of clinical ambiguity, where nerve function testing is indeterminate, or for postsurgical evaluation, as the hyperintense signal can normalize as soon as 8 weeks after neurolysis.[5,28]

Pitfalls of Magnetic Resonance Neuropathy

MRN has several pitfalls that clinicians and radiologists must bear in mind. MRN is limited by technical challenges inherent to MRI technology, such as the magic angle phenomenon, which can cause an increase in T2 signal that may falsely be interpreted as an injury.[29] Additionally, subclinical neuropathy may also present with increased T2 signal intensity within peripheral nerves, potentially misleading interpreters of MRN imaging to believe an injury exists, when, in fact, there is none.[14] In the case of MRN imaging for remote peripheral nerve injuries, it can be difficult to distinguish regenerating from chronically degenerating nerves, which may pose a challenge to the diagnostician.[30] Furthermore, the identification of a neuroma-in-continuity does not provide information about whether the degree of axonal regeneration across the site of injury will be sufficient to allow meaningful clinical recovery. Altogether, for its many advantages, the sensitivity of MRN at either 1.5 or 3.0 T is between 40% to 70%, suggesting that a normal or negative MRN study should not preclude further workup if clinical suspicion for a peripheral nerve injury is high.[31]

DIFFUSION TENSOR IMAGING
Introduction and Techniques

Diffusion tensor imaging (DTI) is a magnetic resonance-based imaging modality that exploits the preferential diffusion of water in directions that align with the shapes of highly asymmetrical

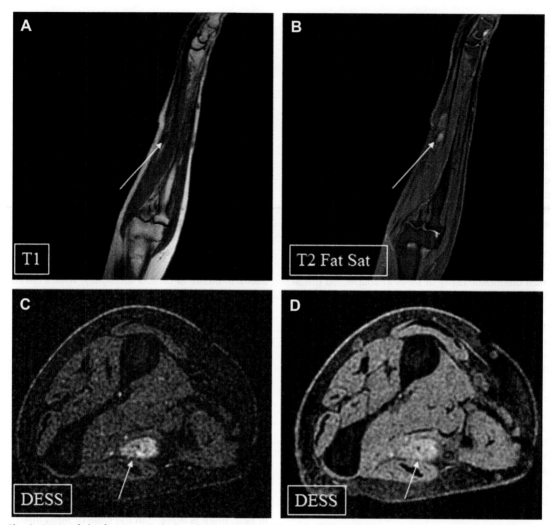

Fig. 3. MRN of the forearm, including (*A*) coronal T1, (*B*) coronal T2 with fat saturation, and (*C*) and (*D*) Axial DESS sequences, showing a terminal neuroma (*arrow*) at the transected end of the median nerve.

anatomic structures, such as peripheral nerves.[32] DTI allows for both qualitative and quantitative analysis of the integrity of peripheral nerves. Tractography relies on this property of water to trace the anatomic course of a peripheral nerve, while 4 parameters that are traditionally calculated and visualized in DTI sequences allow for quantitative microstructural analysis of peripheral nerves. Fractional anisotropy (FA) reflects the degree of alignment within fiber tracts; axial diffusivity (AD) is thought to correspond with axonal integrity and changes rapidly in axonal degeneration. Radial diffusivity (RD) reflects the potential of water to diffuse perpendicular to the axis of a nerve and may indicate myelin integrity, and the apparent diffusion coefficient (ADC) is a mathematical representation of the mean diffusivity of tissue.[33–35]

Applications for Peripheral Nerve Injury

DTI has been used to quantitatively measure peripheral nerve integrity immediately after injury and in a delayed fashion.[36–38] It allows for analysis of microstructural damage to peripheral nerves in pathologic conditions, such as demyelination, axonal degeneration, and Schwann cell necrosis and has been used to demonstrate normal and pathologically altered fiber trajectory in 1.5 and 3 T applications.[39–41] Changes in the diffusivity of water along the course of a damaged peripheral nerve are caused by blockage of axoplasmic flow, increased venous congestion, and distal Wallerian degeneration, all of which lead to widening of the space between axons and surrounding membranes, thought to be reflected by increases in ADC and corresponding decreases in FA.[42]

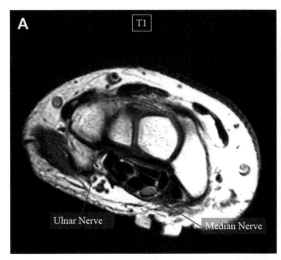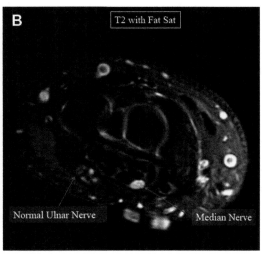

Fig. 4. MRN of the wrist, including (*A*) axial T1 and (*B*) axial T2 with fat saturation, showing enlargement and T2-hyperintensity of the median nerve within the carpal tunnel, consistent with a diagnosis of carpal tunnel syndrome.

Various pathologic entities have been imaged and described using DTI, including compressive neuropathies and nerve injuries. In carpal tunnel syndrome, the compressed median nerve exhibits decreased FA and increased ADC, which is at least partially mirrored by the decreased FA seen in the compressed ulnar nerve in cubital tunnel syndrome.[39,43–46] DTI also may be sensitive to transient, compression-induced neurapraxia. One group has shown decreased FA and decreased ADC of the median nerve along with increased FA and unchanged ADC of the radial nerve after brief tourniquet compression of the upper arm.[47]

Nerve fiber integrity may be assessed with DTI tractography after injury and during recovery. Tractography was used to track regenerating nerve fibers through a median nerve transection after surgical repair in 1 report. One month postoperatively, nerve fibers were seen at the site of transection, followed by regeneration distal to the point of transection after 2 months, with electrodiagnostic evidence of recovery.[48] Another group showed regenerating transected peroneal nerve fibers traveling through a sural nerve graft, forming a compact bundle of fibers through the graft 13 months after injury, again correlating with clinical and electrodiagnostic signs of recovery.[49]

Pitfalls in Diffusion Tensor Imaging

DTI is limited by many of the same factors that make MRN challenging:

Thin, superficial nerves that are difficult to track using current techniques

Poor contrast resolution or volume averaging relative to nearby blood vessels, muscles, or edematous tissue

High susceptibility to ghosting artifacts caused by adjacent fluid flow and organ motion

Technical considerations related to imaging structures not in or near the isocenter of the magnetic field in the MRI scanner[33,50]

Additionally, as quantitative analysis of nerve microstructure using DTI is relatively new, there is a dearth of consensus data regarding the normative ranges of diffusivity parameters, as well as significant inter-nerve differences, making assessment of pathology difficult.[51–56] More confusing still are findings by some groups that FA may not significantly decrease in peripheral nerve injury, and ADC may actually decrease.[44,57] The early and as-of-yet immature state of peripheral nerve DTI is reflected by a recent meta-analysis demonstrating sensitivity of 83% and specificity of 78% for identifying peripheral nerve injury.[58] More research and experience are needed to refine this technique before it can join ultrasound and MRN in the arsenal of routine clinical practice.

NEUROMUSCULAR ULTRASOUND
Introduction

Neuromuscular ultrasound (NMUS) has seen a rapidly growing body of literature and widening applications in nerve and muscle disorders. The technique can be used to supplement the history, physical examination, and EMG/NCS, and in some instances, it can be used as a standalone tool.

NMUS effectively evaluates nerve compression and trauma, identifies intraneural tumors and cysts, and screens for hereditary and inflammatory disorders. It is inexpensive and painless, and aids in real-time localization, diagnosis, and surgical decision making.[59]

The relative accuracy of ultrasound and MRI for focal neuropathies varies. Excluding carpal tunnel and cubital tunnel syndromes, ultrasound has been found to be as specific and perhaps more sensitive for detection of focal neuropathies, particularly for identification of multifocal lesions such as autoimmune nerve disorders.[60,61] Thus, for sonographically accessible regions of the body, NMUS is often proposed as the initial imaging modality.[61,62]

Technique

A linear transducer generating frequencies of 12 to 18 Hz is optimal, with higher frequencies providing the best images of cutaneous nerves. Piezoelectric elements within the transducer produce sound waves and capture reflected waves from echogenic body tissues. In nerve, the echogenic epineurium and perineurium highlight the outer boundaries of the nerve and fascicles. Individual axons are not visible. Ultrahigh frequency transducers up to 70 Hz have been explored for detailed images of individual fascicles, with potential utility for intraoperative evaluation.[63]

Elements of interest when assessing a peripheral nerve include nerve size (measured as cross-sectional area and sometimes diameter), echogenicity, and fascicular enlargement. Increased vascularity may be seen on Doppler. Anomalous structures are noted and may include cysts, tumors, intruding muscle, penetrating arteries, and foreign bodies.

Neuromuscular Ultrasound for Entrapment Neuropathies

In general, an entrapped nerve will demonstrate an enlarged cross-sectional area (CSA) proximal and distal to its compressive site. Loss of fascicular detail and increased vascularity may be present. Entrapment may be caused by passage through a fibro-osseous tunnel; enlargement or malpositioning of nearby structures (such as muscle or bone); postoperative changes such as scarring, foreign bodies, and hardware; and various other causes. The nerve of interest must always be imaged at noncompressive sites for comparison, and various ratios exist for determining carpal tunnel syndrome and ulnar neuropathy at the elbow. If the nerve is diffusely enlarged at noncompressive sites, an inflammatory or hereditary neuropathy should be considered.

Carpal tunnel syndrome

In carpal tunnel syndrome, NMUS has proven consistently accurate when compared with nerve conduction studies (NCS) and clinical examination (**Fig. 5**).[64] In some cases with typical symptoms and normal NCS, ultrasound may be more sensitive.[65] Although there are no formal guidelines for using NMUS in lieu of EMG/NCS, it may be considered in cases in which symptoms are classic and no other diagnoses requiring EMG/NCS (eg, radiculopathy, inflammatory neuropathy) are being considered. NMUS can also differentiate typical carpal tunnel syndrome from mimics, such as penetrating or thrombosed persistent median artery, cyst, or nerve tumor.

Ulnar neuropathy at the elbow

There are limitations to standard electrophysiologic testing for ulnar neuropathy. EMG/NCS may not always localize to the elbow or rule out cervical radiculopathy, and precise inching studies to pinpoint cubital tunnel versus retrocondylar groove pathology are time-consuming.[66] NMUS is an excellent adjunct. Nerve enlargement on NMUS confirms pathology at the elbow, correlates well with areas of motor nerve conduction slowing on NCS, and can distinguish cubital tunnel from retrocondylar pathology.[67,68] In patients with NMUS showing precise localization to the cubital tunnel, this finding is predictive of good clinical outcome after simple surgical decompression at this site.[69] Ultrasound can contribute to localization and potentially determine the choice of surgical intervention. Real-time imaging afforded by the use of ultrasound also allows the sonographer to assess for ulnar nerve subluxation with elbow range of motion and for snapping triceps syndrome, both of which potentially impact the surgical approach utilized.[70–72]

Peroneal neuropathy at the fibular head

In cases of purely compressive peroneal neuropathy without other anatomic factors such as ganglion cyst, NMUS is of varying utility. Some authors report normal nerve size in patients with marked conduction block on NCS testing, and nerve enlargement only when there is axonal involvement.[73] Others note an overall high incidence of nerve enlargement at the fibular head in idiopathic peroneal neuropathies.[74] Apart from this, NMUS is a reliable tool for identifying other anatomic contributors such as intraneural cysts, lipomas, or biceps femoris muscle anatomy that would change the treatment approach.[75] This is particularly true in patients without clear risk

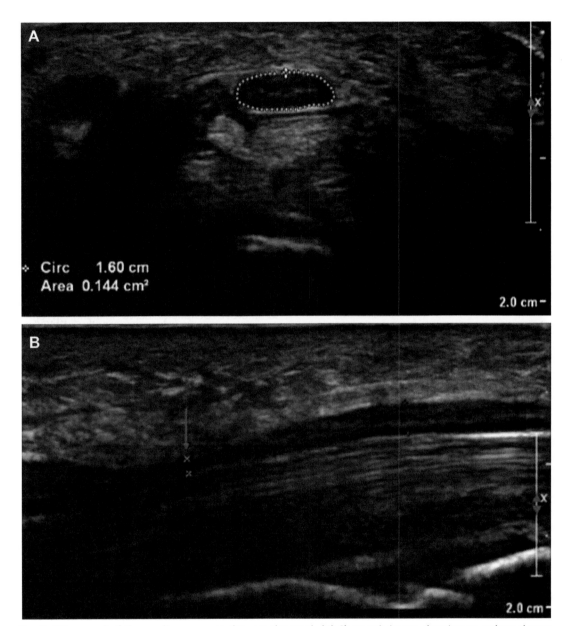

Fig. 5. Ultrasound of the median nerve at the carpal tunnel. (*A*) Short-axis image showing an enlarged cross-sectional area of the median nerve. (*B*) Long-axis image showing the notch sign (*red arrow*), suggesting compression of the median nerve at the carpal tunnel.

factors for entrapment. Given that intraneural ganglion cysts are likely under-recognized as a cause of common peroneal neuropathy, NMUS has value in differentiating idiopathic compression from the presence of an intraneural ganglion cyst.[76]

Other entrapment neuropathies

There is extensive literature on the use of NMUS to identify entrapments of nearly every major nerve. These include the median and anterior interosseous nerves at the forearm, radial nerve at the elbow, and superficial peroneal nerve.[77–79]

NMUS has also been described in entrapment of cutaneous nerves, including the medial brachial cutaneous nerve, superficial radial nerve, dorsal cutaneous branch of the ulnar nerve, palmar cutaneous branch of the median nerve, and lateral and posterior femoral cutaneous nerves.[80]

Neuromuscular Ultrasound for Traumatic Nerve Injuries

There are several goals when performing ultrasound after nerve injury:

Evaluate for nerve continuity, and, if possible, intraneural fascicular continuity.

If transection is present, identify transected ends and provide anatomic landmarks.

Identify the presence of a neuroma at the transected nerve end or neuroma-in-continuity of the intact nerve.

Identify foreign bodies and provide anatomic landmarks

Evaluate for nerve compression by fluid, scarring, hardware, or other mass.

NMUS has been used in a wide variety of cases of traumatic and iatrogenic nerve injury, always with the goals described previously. The paradigm shift to earlier nerve imaging after injury allows for earlier identification of these processes, particularly transection, and may alter the surgeon's choice of intervention and help guide incisions. After trauma, NMUS is particularly appealing, as it can be performed at the bedside by the clinician. Upper extremity and lower leg nerves can easily be imaged throughout their length, and experienced sonographers can evaluate even the brachial plexus for signs of injury.[81] NMUS is well-tolerated in instances of pain or when MRI is limited by hardware or patient movement.

Nerve continuity
Awareness of nerve transection may be delayed when suspicion is low or other injuries take precedence, and because the physical examination and EMG/NCS cannot diagnose transection. NMUS in the acute phase can identify transection and allow for early, direct nerve repair. Use of NMUS to locate the ends and measure the gap allows the surgeon to formulate an operative plan in advance (eg, graft length and type) and more accurately direct exploration.

Neuromas and intraneural discontinuity
With complete transection, the retracted ends can form neuromas, in which disorganized neural elements grow into a bulbous mass (**Fig. 6**). On ultrasound, these are hypoechoic, occasionally with internal hyperechoic features, and with little vascularity.[82] A neuroma-in-continuity may form after direct injury or traction injury when the epineurium remains in continuity but intraneural elements, including axons, endoneurium, and perineurium, do not. NMUS can evaluate for intact epineurium and perineurium with some accuracy, thus aiding in prognostication and surgical planning.[83]

Foreign bodies, compression, and other injury
The injured nerve will have an enlarged, hypoechoic appearance. Hyperechoic objects usually represent metallic hardware, particularly when they are more reflective than the bony surfaces. Staples, clips, screws, and plates can be identified along the path or adjacent to the nerve of interest. Wood, glass, and plastic are also hyperechoic, and any foreign body artifact may limit accurate measurement of nerve size and continuity.[84] Delayed deficits after injury or surgery may indicate seroma (anechoic) or hematoma (varying appearance depending on chronicity).[85] Over time, hyperechoic scarring of local tissue may be identified on NMUS as a source of nerve compression.

INVESTIGATIVE OPTIONS FOR NERVE IMAGING
7 T Magnetic Resonance Neurography

7 T magnetic resonance neurography (MRN) is becoming clinically available and has the potential to improve peripheral nerve imaging. In early studies, 7 T MRN has been shown to depict the fascicular structure better than comparable 3 T images.[86] Although the improved resolution may lead to better diagnosis, there will be a learning curve with interpreting 7 T images. More data, particularly on normal subjects, will be needed to establish norms. However, improved imaging at the fascicular level may allow for better identification of nerve injuries and may also help better characterize the severity of injury, allowing better predictive models and earlier surgery in appropriate cases. Furthermore, interpretation of MRN, whether 7 T or more standard 3 T or 1.5 T, may be improved with the utilization of artificial intelligence for interpretation and segmentation.[87]

Ultrasound Elastography

Ultrasound elastography is a promising technique for evaluating peripheral nerves. This technique utilizes ultrasound to quantify the stiffness of a given tissue. In many peripheral neuropathies, myelin, which is more compliant, is lost and replaced with connective tissue, which is stiffer. Thus, many peripheral neuropathies are associated with increased stiffness of the nerve, which can be measured using elastography.[88] As this technique continues to develop, its applications will continue to be defined.

Positron Emission Tomography

Positron emission tomography (PET) imaging utilizes radiotracers to assess activity at a cellular level or potentially expression of specific receptors. As novel radiotracers are developed, it may allow for assessment of injury to peripheral nerves. At their

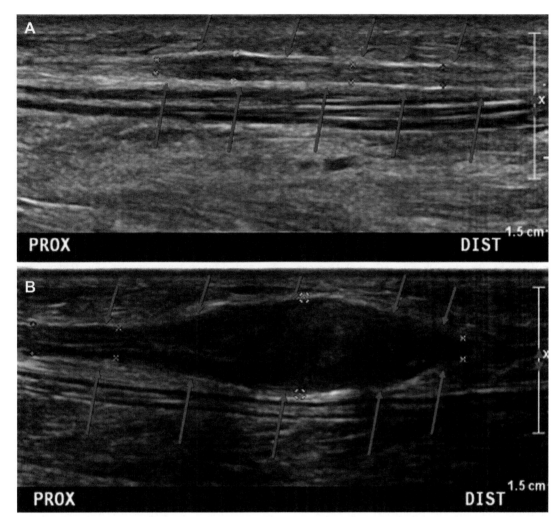

Fig. 6. Ultrasound of the sural nerve (outlined in *red arrows*) 9 years after sural nerve biopsy, showing (*A*) the cut distal end of the sural nerve and (*B*) a terminal neuroma on the cut proximal end of the nerve. The cut ends of the nerve were found to be approximately 6.5 cm apart.

institution, the authors are utilizing PET imaging to evaluate a novel radiotracer, [18F]-FTC-146, to assess the expression of sigma-1 receptors, thought to be upregulated in chronic pain (ClinicalTrials.gov; NCT03556137).[89–93] This may allow improved localization of neuropathic pain generators.

Surgical Applications of Imaging

As resolution improves, particularly with ultrasound, the real-time imaging that ultrasound affords will be taken advantage of in order to develop more minimally invasive surgical techniques for the treatment of nerve injuries and neuropathic pain. One example is the development of minimally invasive techniques that are ultrasound driven for neurectomy in cases of saphenous or lateral femoral cutaneous neuropathy.[94] Surely additional techniques will continue to be developed utilizing ultrasound and potentially other imaging techniques.

SUMMARY

Nerve imaging is an important part of the evaluation of damaged nerves. MRN and ultrasound are the most widely used techniques for nerve imaging. As techniques continue to improve, these improvements have the potential to transform the way we approach the evaluation of nerve injuries, entrapment neuropathies, neuropathic pain, and a variety of other nerve pathologies. In addition to improvements in MRN and ultrasound, an array of other promising imaging modalities are under investigation, making this an exciting time in the field of nerve imaging.

CONFLICTS OF INTEREST

None.

REFERENCES

1. Sandroni P, Benrud-Larson LM, McClelland RL, et al. Complex regional pain syndrome type I: incidence and prevalence in Olmsted county, a population-based study. Pain 2003;103(1–2):199–207.
2. Weiss KL, Beltran J, Shamam OM, et al. High-field MR surface-coil imaging of the hand and wrist. Part I. Normal anatomy. Radiology 1986;160(1):143–6.
3. Middleton WD, Kneeland JB, Kellman GM, et al. MR imaging of the carpal tunnel: normal anatomy and preliminary findings in the carpal tunnel syndrome. AJR Am J Roentgenol 1987;148(2):307–16.
4. Howe FA, Saunders DE, Filler AG, et al. Magnetic resonance neurography of the median nerve. Br J Radiol 1994;67(804):1169–72.
5. Cudlip SA, Howe FA, Clifton A, et al. Magnetic resonance neurography studies of the median nerve before and after carpal tunnel decompression. J Neurosurg 2002;96(6):1046–51.
6. Bilbey JH, Lamond RG, Mattrey RF. MR imaging of disorders of the brachial plexus. J Magn Reson Imaging 1994;4(1):13–8.
7. Blair DN, Rapoport S, Sostman HD, et al. Normal brachial plexus: MR imaging. Radiology 1987; 165(3):763–7.
8. Magill ST, Brus-Ramer M, Weinstein PR, et al. Neurogenic thoracic outlet syndrome: current diagnostic criteria and advances in MRI diagnostics. Neurosurg Focus 2015;39(3):E7.
9. Posniak HV, Olson MC, Dudiak CM, et al. MR imaging of the brachial plexus. AJR Am J Roentgenol 1993;161(2):373–9.
10. Rapoport S, Blair DN, McCarthy SM, et al. Brachial plexus: correlation of MR imaging with CT and pathologic findings. Radiology 1988;167(1):161–5.
11. Robbins NM, Shah V, Benedetti N, et al. Magnetic resonance neurography in the diagnosis of neuropathies of the lumbosacral plexus: a pictorial review. Clin Imaging 2016;40(6):1118–30.
12. Chhabra A, Williams EH, Wang KC, et al. MR neurography of neuromas related to nerve injury and entrapment with surgical correlation. AJNR Am J Neuroradiol 2010;31(8):1363–8.
13. Hayes CE, Tsuruda JS, Mathis CM, et al. Brachial plexus: MR imaging with a dedicated phased array of surface coils. Radiology 1997;203(1):286–9.
14. Husarik DB, Saupe N, Pfirrmann CW, et al. Elbow nerves: MR findings in 60 asymptomatic subjects—normal anatomy, variants, and pitfalls. Radiology 2009;252(1):148–56.
15. Binaghi D, Socolovsky M. Magnetic resonance neurography and peripheral nerve surgery. In: Socolovsky M, Rasulic LG, Midha R, et al, editors. Manual of peripheral nerve surgery: from the basics to complex procedures. Stuttgart: Thieme; 2018. p. 59–64.
16. Petchprapa CN, Rosenberg ZS, Sconfienza LM, et al. MR imaging of entrapment neuropathies of the lower extremity. Part 1. The pelvis and hip. Radiographics 2010;30(4):983–1000.
17. Freund W, Brinkmann A, Wagner F, et al. MR neurography with multiplanar reconstruction of 3D MRI datasets: an anatomical study and clinical applications. Neuroradiology 2007;49(4): 335–41.
18. Viallon M, Vargas MI, Jlassi H, et al. High-resolution and functional magnetic resonance imaging of the brachial plexus using an isotropic 3D T2 STIR (short term inversion recovery) SPACE sequence and diffusion tensor imaging. Eur Radiol 2008; 18(5):1018–23.
19. Gasparotti R, Ferraresi S, Pinelli L, et al. Three-dimensional MR myelography of traumatic injuries of the brachial plexus. AJNR Am J Neuroradiol 1997;18(9):1733–42.
20. Somashekar D, Yang LJ, Ibrahim M, et al. High-resolution MRI evaluation of neonatal brachial plexus palsy: a promising alternative to traditional CT myelography. AJNR Am J Neuroradiol 2014;35(6): 1209–13.
21. Chhabra A, Madhuranthakam AJ, Andreisek G. Magnetic resonance neurography: current perspectives and literature review. Eur Radiol 2018;28(2): 698–707.
22. Seddon HJ. A classification of nerve injuries. Br Med J 1942;2(4260):237–9.
23. Sunderland S. A classification of peripheral nerve injuries producing loss of function. Brain 1951;74(4): 491–516.
24. Chhabra A, Andreisek G, Soldatos T, et al. MR neurography: past, present, and future. AJR Am J Roentgenol 2011;197(3):583–91.
25. Chhabra A, Ahlawat S, Belzberg A, et al. Peripheral nerve injury grading simplified on MR neurography: as referenced to Seddon and Sunderland classifications. Indian J Radiol Imaging 2014;24(3): 217–24.
26. Deshmukh SD, Samet J, Fayad LM, et al. Magnetic resonance neurography of traumatic pediatric peripheral nerve injury: beyond birth-related brachial palsy. Pediatr Radiol 2019;49(7):954–64.
27. Garwood ER, Duarte A, Bencardino JT. MR imaging of entrapment neuropathies of the lower extremity. Radiol Clin North Am 2018;56(6): 997–1012.
28. Dailey AT, Tsuruda JS, Filler AG, et al. Magnetic resonance neurography of peripheral nerve degeneration and regeneration. Lancet 1997;350(9086): 1221–2.

29. Chappell KE, Robson MD, Stonebridge-Foster A, et al. Magic angle effects in MR neurography. AJNR Am J Neuroradiol 2004;25(3):431–40.

30. Grant GA, Britz GW, Goodkin R, et al. The utility of magnetic resonance imaging in evaluating peripheral nerve disorders. Muscle Nerve 2002;25(3):314–31.

31. Crim J, Ingalls K. Accuracy of MR neurography in the diagnosis of brachial plexopathy. Eur J Radiol 2017;95:24–7.

32. Martin Noguerol T, Barousse R, Socolovsky M, et al. Quantitative magnetic resonance (MR) neurography for evaluation of peripheral nerves and plexus injuries. Quant Imaging Med Surg 2017;7(4):398–421.

33. Jeon T, Fung MM, Koch KM, et al. Peripheral nerve diffusion tensor imaging: overview, pitfalls, and future directions. J Magn Reson Imaging 2018;47(5):1171–89.

34. Morisaki S, Kawai Y, Umeda M, et al. In vivo assessment of peripheral nerve regeneration by diffusion tensor imaging. J Magn Reson Imaging 2011;33(3):535–42.

35. Song SK, Sun SW, Ju WK, et al. Diffusion tensor imaging detects and differentiates axon and myelin degeneration in mouse optic nerve after retinal ischemia. Neuroimage 2003;20(3):1714–22.

36. Breckwoldt MO, Stock C, Xia A, et al. Diffusion tensor imaging adds diagnostic accuracy in magnetic resonance neurography. Invest Radiol 2015;50(8):498–504.

37. Heckel A, Weiler M, Xia A, et al. Peripheral nerve diffusion tensor imaging: assessment of axon and myelin sheath integrity. PLoS One 2015;10(6):e0130833.

38. Gallagher TA, Simon NG, Kliot M. Diffusion tensor imaging to visualize axons in the setting of nerve injury and recovery. Neurosurg Focus 2015;39(3):E10.

39. Baumer P, Pham M, Ruetters M, et al. Peripheral neuropathy: detection with diffusion-tensor imaging. Radiology 2014;273(1):185–93.

40. Khalil C, Hancart C, Le Thuc V, et al. Diffusion tensor imaging and tractography of the median nerve in carpal tunnel syndrome: preliminary results. Eur Radiol 2008;18(10):2283–91.

41. Tasdelen N, Gurses B, Kilickesmez O, et al. Diffusion tensor imaging in carpal tunnel syndrome. Diagn Interv Radiol 2012;18(1):60–6.

42. Takagi T, Nakamura M, Yamada M, et al. Visualization of peripheral nerve degeneration and regeneration: monitoring with diffusion tensor tractography. Neuroimage 2009;44(3):884–92.

43. Guggenberger R, Eppenberger P, Markovic D, et al. MR neurography of the median nerve at 3.0T: optimization of diffusion tensor imaging and fiber tractography. Eur J Radiol 2012;81(7):e775–82.

44. Lindberg PG, Feydy A, Le Viet D, et al. Diffusion tensor imaging of the median nerve in recurrent carpal tunnel syndrome - initial experience. Eur Radiol 2013;23(11):3115–23.

45. Stein D, Neufeld A, Pasternak O, et al. Diffusion tensor imaging of the median nerve in healthy and carpal tunnel syndrome subjects. J Magn Reson Imaging 2009;29(3):657–62.

46. Iba K, Wada T, Tamakawa M, et al. Diffusion-weighted magnetic resonance imaging of the ulnar nerve in cubital tunnel syndrome. Hand Surg 2010;15(1):11–5.

47. Jengojan S, Kovar F, Breitenseher J, et al. Acute radial nerve entrapment at the spiral groove: detection by DTI-based neurography. Eur Radiol 2015;25(6):1678–83.

48. Meek MF, Stenekes MW, Hoogduin HM, et al. In vivo three-dimensional reconstruction of human median nerves by diffusion tensor imaging. Exp Neurol 2006;198(2):479–82.

49. Simon NG, Narvid J, Cage T, et al. Visualizing axon regeneration after peripheral nerve injury with magnetic resonance tractography. Neurology 2014;83(15):1382–4.

50. Conturo TE, McKinstry RC, Aronovitz JA, et al. Diffusion MRI: precision, accuracy and flow effects. NMR Biomed 1995;8(7–8):307–32.

51. Hiltunen J, Suortti T, Arvela S, et al. Diffusion tensor imaging and tractography of distal peripheral nerves at 3 T. Clin Neurophysiol 2005;116(10):2315–23.

52. Jambawalikar S, Baum J, Button T, et al. Diffusion tensor imaging of peripheral nerves. Skeletal Radiol 2010;39(11):1073–9.

53. Simon NG, Lagopoulos J, Gallagher T, et al. Peripheral nerve diffusion tensor imaging is reliable and reproducible. J Magn Reson Imaging 2016;43(4):962–9.

54. Yao L, Gai N. Median nerve cross-sectional area and MRI diffusion characteristics: normative values at the carpal tunnel. Skeletal Radiol 2009;38(4):355–61.

55. Zhou Y, Kumaravel M, Patel VS, et al. Diffusion tensor imaging of forearm nerves in humans. J Magn Reson Imaging 2012;36(4):920–7.

56. Zhou Y, Narayana PA, Kumaravel M, et al. High resolution diffusion tensor imaging of human nerves in forearm. J Magn Reson Imaging 2014;39(6):1374–83.

57. Hiltunen J, Kirveskari E, Numminen J, et al. Pre- and post-operative diffusion tensor imaging of the median nerve in carpal tunnel syndrome. Eur Radiol 2012;22(6):1310–9.

58. Wang CK, Jou IM, Huang HW, et al. Carpal tunnel syndrome assessed with diffusion tensor imaging: comparison with electrophysiological studies of patients and healthy volunteers. Eur J Radiol 2012;81(11):3378–83.

59. Oni G, Chow W, Ramakrishnan V, et al. Plastic surgeon-led ultrasound. Plast Reconstr Surg 2018; 141(2):300e–9e.

60. Bignotti B, Assini A, Signori A, et al. Ultrasound versus MRI in common fibular neuropathy. Muscle Nerve 2017;55(6):849–57.

61. Zaidman CM, Seelig MJ, Baker JC, et al. Detection of peripheral nerve pathology: comparison of ultrasound and MRI. Neurology 2013;80(18):1634–40.

62. Padua L, Hobson-Webb LD. Ultrasound as the first choice for peripheral nerve imaging? Neurology 2013;80(18):1626–7.

63. Cartwright MS, Baute V, Caress JB, et al. Ultrahigh-frequency ultrasound of fascicles in the median nerve at the wrist. Muscle Nerve 2017;56(4): 819–22.

64. Cartwright MS, Hobson-Webb LD, Boon AJ, et al. Evidence-based guideline: neuromuscular ultrasound for the diagnosis of carpal tunnel syndrome. Muscle Nerve 2012;46(2):287–93.

65. Aseem F, Williams JW, Walker FO, et al. Neuromuscular ultrasound in patients with carpal tunnel syndrome and normal nerve conduction studies. Muscle Nerve 2017;55(6):913–5.

66. Practice parameter: electrodiagnostic studies in ulnar neuropathy at the elbow. American Association of Electrodiagnostic Medicine, American Academy of Neurology, and American Academy of Physical Medicine and Rehabilitation. Neurology 1999;52(4): 688–90.

67. Alrajeh M, Preston DC. Neuromuscular ultrasound in electrically non-localizable ulnar neuropathy. Muscle Nerve 2018;58(5):655–9.

68. Omejec G, Podnar S. Neurologic examination and instrument-based measurements in the evaluation of ulnar neuropathy at the elbow. Muscle Nerve 2018;57(6):951–7.

69. La Torre D, Raffa G, Pino MA, et al. A novel diagnostic and prognostic tool for simple decompression of ulnar nerve in cubital tunnel syndrome. World Neurosurg 2018;118:e964–73.

70. Chuang HJ, Hsiao MY, Wu CH, et al. Dynamic ultrasound imaging for ulnar nerve subluxation and snapping triceps syndrome. Am J Phys Med Rehabil 2016;95(7):e113–4.

71. Cornelson SM, Sclocco R, Kettner NW. Ulnar nerve instability in the cubital tunnel of asymptomatic volunteers. J Ultrasound 2019;22(3):337–44.

72. Kang JH, Joo BE, Kim KH, et al. Ultrasonographic and electrophysiological evaluation of ulnar nerve instability and snapping of the triceps medial head in healthy subjects. Am J Phys Med Rehabil 2017; 96(8):e141–6.

73. Tsukamoto H, Granata G, Coraci D, et al. Ultrasound and neurophysiological correlation in common fibular nerve conduction block at fibular head. Clin Neurophysiol 2014;125(7):1491–5.

74. Bignotti B, Cadoni A, Assini A, et al. Fascicular involvement in common fibular neuropathy: evaluation with ultrasound. Muscle Nerve 2016;53(4): 532–7.

75. Grant TH, Omar IM, Dumanian GA, et al. Sonographic evaluation of common peroneal neuropathy in patients with foot drop. J Ultrasound Med 2015; 34(4):705–11.

76. Wilson TJ, Hebert-Blouin MN, Murthy NS, et al. Recognition of peroneal intraneural ganglia in an historical cohort with "negative" MRIs. Acta Neurochir (Wien) 2017;159(5):925–30.

77. Choi SJ, Ahn JH, Ryu DS, et al. Ultrasonography for nerve compression syndromes of the upper extremity. Ultrasonography 2015;34(4):275–91.

78. Xiao TG, Cartwright MS. Ultrasound in the evaluation of radial neuropathies at the elbow. Front Neurol 2019;10:216.

79. Nwawka OK, Lee S, Miller TT. Sonographic evaluation of superficial peroneal nerve abnormalities. AJR Am J Roentgenol 2018;211(4):872–9.

80. Chang KV, Mezian K, Nanka O, et al. Ultrasound imaging for the cutaneous nerves of the extremities and relevant entrapment syndromes: from anatomy to clinical implications. J Clin Med 2018;7(11) [pii:E457].

81. Baute V, Strakowski JA, Reynolds JW, et al. Neuromuscular ultrasound of the brachial plexus: a standardized approach. Muscle Nerve 2018;58(5): 618–24.

82. Abreu E, Aubert S, Wavreille G, et al. Peripheral tumor and tumor-like neurogenic lesions. Eur J Radiol 2013;82(1):38–50.

83. Zhu J, Liu F, Li D, et al. Preliminary study of the types of traumatic peripheral nerve injuries by ultrasound. Eur Radiol 2011;21(5):1097–101.

84. Tantray MD, Rather A, Manaan Q, et al. Role of ultrasound in detection of radiolucent foreign bodies in extremities. Strategies Trauma Limb Reconstr 2018;13(2):81–5.

85. Ryu JK, Jin W, Kim GY. Sonographic appearances of small organizing hematomas and thrombi mimicking superficial soft tissue tumors. J Ultrasound Med 2011;30(10):1431–6.

86. Yoon D, Biswal S, Rutt B, et al. Feasibility of 7T MRI for imaging fascicular structures of peripheral nerves. Muscle Nerve 2018;57(3):494–8.

87. Balsiger F, Steindel C, Arn M, et al. Segmentation of peripheral nerves from magnetic resonance neurography: a fully-automatic, deep learning-based approach. Front Neurol 2018;9:777.

88. Wee TC, Simon NG. Ultrasound elastography for the evaluation of peripheral nerves: a systematic review. Muscle Nerve 2019;60(5):501–12.

89. Cipriano PW, Lee SW, Yoon D, et al. Successful treatment of chronic knee pain following localization by a sigma-1 receptor radioligand and PET/MRI: a case report. J Pain Res 2018;11:2353–7.

90. Hjornevik T, Cipriano PW, Shen B, et al. Biodistribution and radiation dosimetry of (18)F-FTC-146 in humans. J Nucl Med 2017;58(12): 2004–9.

91. James ML, Shen B, Nielsen CH, et al. Evaluation of sigma-1 receptor radioligand 18F-FTC-146 in rats and squirrel monkeys using PET. J Nucl Med 2014; 55(1):147–53.

92. Shen B, Behera D, James ML, et al. Visualizing nerve injury in a neuropathic pain model with [^{18}F]

FTC-146 PET/MRI. Theranostics 2017;7(11): 2794–805.

93. Shen B, Park JH, Hjornevik T, et al. Radiosynthesis and first-in-human PET/MRI evaluation with clinical-grade [(18)F]FTC-146. Mol Imaging Biol 2017; 19(5):779–86.

94. Henning PT, Wilson TJ, Willsey M, et al. Pilot study of intraoperative ultrasound-guided instrument placement in nerve transection surgery for peripheral nerve pain syndromes. Neurosurg Focus 2017;42(3):E6.

Ischemic Pain

Michael R. Romanelli, MD, Jacob A. Thayer, MD,
Michael W. Neumeister, MD, FRCSC*

KEYWORDS

• Ischemia • Ischemic pain • Ischemic surgical pain

KEY POINTS

- The sensation of ischemic pain is of neuropathic etiology, caused by the detection of acidosis in peripheral tissues.
- Ischemic pain signals ascend through spinothalamic and spinobrachial tracts to the cerebral cortex where they are interpreted.
- Upper extremity ischemic pain can present in the acute or chronic setting.
- Treatment revolves around restoring perfusion to the affected tissue, from surgical measures to conservative pharmacotherapy.

PATHOPHYSIOLOGY

Ischemic insults in the upper and lower extremities have many manifestations, the most significant being skin necrosis and pain. Ischemia results in a lack of oxygen and nutrients to tissues in cellular damage. Ischemic pain was once thought to be a result of direct nerve injury or stimulation, but is now thought to be a symptom of the breakdown of damaged tissue and subsequent local peripheral nerve receptor activation. When musculoskeletal tissue is deprived of oxygen, aerobic cellular metabolism is compromised resulting in the depletion of intracellular ATP. As a cons.equence, failure of the ATP-dependent sodium-potassium pump causes osmotic cellular swelling as sodium and water are retained within the cell. As the cell swells and becomes depolarized, the influx of calcium ions causes an overexcitation of the cell membrane, which results in the formation of reactive oxidative species. Reactive oxidative species cause damage to the cell, resulting in an overall extracellular acidosis. Although lactic acid also contributes to acidification of the extracellular space, it is not the primary source. During prolonged periods of ischemia, anaerobic pathways of metabolism predominate resulting in the additional build-up of lactic acid.[1]

The sensation of ischemic pain is of neuropathic etiology, caused by the detection of acidosis in peripheral tissues. This results in increased hydrogen ions, growth factors, and cytokines, which are detected by acid-sensing ion channels and sensory pathways. Acid-sensing ion channels are a voltage-insensitive, amiloride-sensitive sodium channel family of excitatory cation channels.[2] Once activated, these channels stimulate group III and IV muscle nerve afferent fibers, which are the muscular analogue of cutaneous $A\delta$ and C nerve fibers. This information passes to the spinal cord dorsal horn where signals are directed through the spinothalamic and spinobrachial tracts en route to the thalamus. They are then relayed to the cerebral cortex where they are interpreted as ischemic pain.[3]

PRESENTATION

Ischemic pain presents differently than other types of acute pain and is dependent on how quickly the perfusion is interrupted. Ischemic pain is classically associated with an insidious onset compared with acute pain associated with limb trauma. Lower extremity claudication is an example of the ischemic pain presenting with burning, muscle cramping, calf pain with exertion, or even calf pain at rest in

Department of Surgery, Institute for Plastic Surgery, Southern Illinois University School of Medicine, 747 North Rutledge Street, 3rd Floor, PO Box 19653, Springfield, IL 62794-9653, USA
* Corresponding author.
E-mail address: mneumeister@siumed.edu

Clin Plastic Surg 47 (2020) 261–265
https://doi.org/10.1016/j.cps.2019.11.002

plasticsurgery.theclinics.com

the later stages. Paresthesia and numbness, and motor weakness in the affected limb, have been observed. Other signs of ischemia include blanching or purple discoloration of digits, ulceration, and eventual tissue necrosis (gangrene).

ETIOLOGY

Upper extremity ischemic pain can present in the acute or chronic setting. Acute causes are diagnostically straightforward, and are often the result of traumatic penetrating injuries to arteries or vascular beds. Quantitative evidence of perfusion is available in the form of finger pressure readings in special circumstances where further evidence is desired. Digital brachial index values greater than 0.7 are widely held as evidence of adequate distal perfusion.[4]

Chronic ischemic pain is caused by two broad categories of occlusive arterial disease: atherosclerotic and nonatherosclerotic. Atherosclerotic etiologies comprise most ischemic disease and are associated with inflammatory and fibroproliferative changes within the vessel lumen incited by comorbidities including hypercholesterolemia, diabetes, smoking, and hypertension. The pathophysiology follows a sequence of increased plasma cholesterol levels leading to increased arterial wall permeability and then to the eventual accumulation of lipids within the subendothelial space.[5] Circulating monocytes follow into the arterial wall and eventually behave as foamy macrophages, expressing scavenger receptors leading to the mass import of cholesterol into the vessel wall. This leads to vascular changes including the development of intimal thickening, fatty streaks, fibroatheromas, and plaques, which serve to reduce overall flow through the vessel.[6]

Less common nonatheroma causes of ischemic pain in the upper extremity include vasospasm (Raynaud disease), vasoocclusive disorders, and vasculitis (**Table 1**). Vasospastic disease is a temporary restriction in distal perfusion compromise tissue perfusion. Raynaud disease is one such example, which like other vasospastic conditions is further divided into primary and secondary disorders. Primary vasospastic conditions can cause ischemic pain and associated dysesthesias but rarely cause ulcerations.[7] Secondary vasospastic conditions do cause ulcerations in the distal extremities and are coexistent with ischemic pain. These are caused by and related to a variety of other conditions (see **Table 1**). Maurice Reynaud's description of arterial insufficiency to the fingers in 1862 led to his name being the eponym of this condition. Raynaud described the process as a "local asphyxia of the extremities" as a result of

"increased irritability of the central parts of the cord presiding over vascular innervation." The asphyxia was vasospasm that resulted in anoxia to the distal digits. The anoxia manifest as paraesthesias, ischemic pain, discoloration, and eventually ulceration in many patients. Raynaud disease is often associated with an autoimmune connective tissue disorder.

Blunt trauma, as seen in ulnar hammer syndrome (hypothenar hammer syndrome), may also result in distal ischemia.[6,8] Repetitive blunt trauma commonly causes intimal damage, luminal thrombosis, intimal thickening, medial fibrosis, hypertrophy, and neovascularization. Occasionally (15% of total cases), intrinsic vasculopathies, such as fibromuscular dysplasia (ie smooth muscle disorganization), are found to contribute to hypothenar hammer syndrome.[9] Direct blunt trauma is not the only cause of traumatic thrombosis in vessels of the upper extremity. Arterial cannulation may also develop false or true aneurysms with subsequent traumatic embolus formation.

Vasculitis may cause ischemic pain but may also present with vague, nonspecific systemic symptoms including fevers, arthralgias, and weight loss. Pathologies are categorized based on the size of the lumen targeted, and cause inflammatory changes in the walls of the vessels they affect. Buerger disease affects small-to-medium-sized vessels, inciting intimal changes and tissue necrosis from tobacco products.[10,11] Collagen vascular diseases including rheumatoid arthritis, systemic lupus erythematosus, and scleroderma are mediated by collagen deposition within the vascular intima and surrounding soft tissues causing contracture and pain. Less common causes of vasculitis that should be considered include polyarteritis nodosa, medication and hypersensitivity vasculitis, and blood dyscrasias.[12]

TREATMENT

Treating pain related to ischemia is thought of as directed toward the fundamental goal of improving perfusion. Perfusion is improved through surgical and nonsurgical approaches. Acute arterial compromise with ischemia should be restored with direct surgical repair, vessel reconstruction, vessel bypass, or clot lysis.[10] In some instances of limb amputation, temporary arterial shunting may be required to control hemorrhage and perfuse distal tissue. This is helpful if critical limb ischemia time is being approached before replantation is complete.[11] For embolic vascular injury, surgical treatments include endovascular thrombectomy, embolectomy, or catheter-directed thrombolysis.[13]

Table 1
Raynaud phenomenon associated conditions

Category	Connective Tissue Disorders	Vasooclusive Disorders	Vasospastic Disorders	Pharmacologic	Occupational Exposures	Other
Examples	Scleroderma	Atherosclerosis	Pheochromocytoma	Beta-blockers	Vibration	Lyme disease
	Lupus	Thoracic outlet syndrome	Carcinoid syndrome	Cyclosporine	Mercury	Multiple sclerosis
	Rheumatoid arthritis	Buerger disease	Thyroid disease	Bromocriptine	Vinyl chloride	Pulmonary
	Ehlers-Danlos syndrome	Takayasu arteritis		Nicotine	Traumatic injury	hypertension
	Polymyositis	Thromboangiitis obliterans		Ergotamine		Frostbite
	Blood disorders	Angiocentric lymphoma		Cisplatin		Anorexia
	CREST syndrome			Vinblastine		
	Sjögren syndrome			Dextroamphetamine		
	Dermatomyositis			Methylphenidate		
				Bleomycin		
				Clonidine		
				Cocaine		
				Gemcitabine		
				Arsenic		
				Interferon alpha		
				Doxorubicin		
				Cyclophosphamide		

Conservative management for the purposes of increasing perfusion and reducing ischemic pain is largely focused on medical management and lifestyle modification. Medical comorbidity management of such diseases as diabetes and hypertension is paramount for the preservation of distal perfusion. Other conservative measures include elimination of risk factors. Smoking cessation and exercise are promoted to relax blood vessels and to limit the metabolic demand of obesity.

Numerous medications have been used to improve blood flow with vessels and capillary beds in attempts to diminish the ischemia (**Table 2**). Several studies have identified botulinum toxin-A as a favorable treatment of Raynaud disease in increasing perfusion and in decreasing pain.[14,15] The exact mechanism is yet to be elucidated but there seems to be some effect on the chronically irritated nerves that undergo biochemical and pathophysiologic alterations within the nerve and dorsal root ganglion where botulinum toxin-A may block ectopic pathways of pain.[16] Indeed, botulinum toxin-A has been used for many chronic pain syndromes, besides ischemic pain, from neuropathic, or arthritic, to inflammatory pain.[17]

As an adjunct therapy, gabapentin has proven to reduce levels of pain scores significantly in patients with critical limb ischemia.[18] For patients with depression and psychiatric comorbidities, the use of tricyclic antidepressants has been demonstrated for years in the treatment of neuropathic pain.[19] Although less efficacious, selective serotonin reuptake inhibitors and serotonin norepinephrine reuptake inhibitors also can improve neuropathic pain associated with comorbidities including diabetes mellitus. "Tricyclic antidepressants will relieve one in every 2 to 3 patients with peripheral neuropathic pain, serotonin norepinephrine reuptake inhibitors one in every 4 to 5, and selective serotonin reuptake inhibitors one in every 7 patients."[20] Despite the benefit of central effects on improved analgesia, the limitation in these studies is that there are no head-to-head comparisons between antidepressants and other analgesics. Less common modalities described by other authors include systemic anticoagulation and prostacyclin,[21] and corticosteroids, calcium channel blockers, cytotoxic medication, and colchicine for ischemia in the upper extremity.[22]

For those patients who do not respond to the previously mentioned pharmacologic treatments, sympathectomies (whether chemical or surgical) may provide benefit in the patient population with nonrevascularizable critical limb ischemia.[23] In addition to directly blocking a component of nociception, sympathectomies limit sympathetic tones influence on the vasculature of an ischemic limb to improve tissue oxygenation. Downstream effects have been shown to decrease tissue damage from ischemia and thus pain.

SUMMARY

Ischemic pain is the result of poor perfusion, lack of oxygen delivery, and subsequent metabolite damage to cells and tissues. The anoxic insult fosters lactic acidosis and pain receptor activation leading to pain. The management of patients with ischemic pain is often multimodal but ultimately directed at increasing tissue perfusion with oxygenated blood.

DISCLOSURE

The authors have nothing to disclose.

Table 2
Pharmacologic agents for the treatment of ischemic pain

Agent	Route
Narcotics	IV, PO
Local anesthetics	IV, intradermal
Ketamine	IV
Gabapentin	PO
Buprenorphine	Transdermal
Tricyclic antidepressants	PO
Selective serotonin reuptake inhibitors	PO
Selective norepinephrine reuptake inhibitors	IV, PO
Anticoagulants (heparin, coumadin)	IV
Prostaglandin (prostacyclin)	PO
Corticosteroids	PO
Calcium channel blockers	IV
Immunosuppressants (cytotoxic agents)	IV
Colchicine	PO

Abbreviations: IV, intravenous route; PO, oral route.

REFERENCES

1. Issberner U, Reeh PW, Steen KH. Pain due to tissue acidosis: a mechanism for inflammatory and ischemic myalgia? Neurosci Lett 1996;208(3):191–4.
2. Waldmann R, Champigny G, Bassilana F, et al. A proton-gated cation channel involved in acid-sensing. Nature 1997;386(6621):173–7.

3. Queme LF, Ross JL, Jankowski MP. Peripheral mechanisms of ischemic myalgia. Front Cell Neurosci 2017;11:419.

4. Higgins JP, McClinton MA. Vascular insufficiency of the upper extremity. J Hand Surg 2010;35(9): 1545–53 [quiz: 53].

5. Sakakura K, Nakano M, Otsuka F, et al. Pathophysiology of atherosclerosis plaque progression. Heart Lung Circ 2013;22(6):399–411.

6. Bergheanu SC, Bodde MC, Jukema JW. Pathophysiology and treatment of atherosclerosis: current view and future perspective on lipoprotein modification treatment. Neth Heart J 2017;25(4):231–42.

7. Netscher D. Raynaud's Syndrome. In: Berger RA, Weiss APC, editors. Hand surgery. Philadelphia: Lippincott Williams & Wilkins; 2004. p. 1643–62.

8. Shutze RA, Leichty J, Shutze WP. Palmar artery aneurysm. Proc (Bayl Univ Med Cent) 2017;30(1):50–1.

9. Larsen BT, Edwards WD, Jensen MH, et al. Surgical pathology of hypothenar hammer syndrome with new pathogenetic insights: a 25-year institutional experience with clinical and pathologic review of 67 cases. Am J Surg Pathol 2013;37(11):1700–8.

10. McClinton MA. Ischemic conditions of the hand. Plastic surgery. Philadelphia: WB Saunders; 2006.

11. Pederson WC. Acute ischemia of the upper extremity. Orthop Clin North Am 2016;47(3):589–97.

12. Rukwied R, Chizh BA, Lorenz U, et al. Potentiation of nociceptive responses to low pH injections in humans by prostaglandin E2. J Pain 2007;8(5):443–51.

13. Gifford SM, Aidinian G, Clouse WD, et al. Effect of temporary shunting on extremity vascular injury: an outcome analysis from the Global War on Terror vascular injury initiative. J Vasc Surg 2009;50(3): 549–55 [discussion: 55–6].

14. Van Beek AL, Lim PK, Gear AJ, et al. Management of vasospastic disorders with botulinum toxin A. Plast Reconstr Surg 2007;119(1): 217–26.

15. Neumeister MW. Botulinum toxin type A in the treatment of Raynaud's phenomenon. J Hand Surg 2010; 35(12):2085–92.

16. Neumeister MW, Chambers CB, Herron MS, et al. Botox therapy for ischemic digits. Plast Reconstr Surg 2009;124(1):191–201.

17. Singh JA. Botulinum toxin therapy for osteoarticular pain: an evidence-based review. Ther Adv Musculoskelet Dis 2010;2(2):105–18.

18. Morris-Stiff G, Lewis MH. Gabapentin (Neurontin) improves pain scores of patients with critical limb ischaemia: an observational study. Int J Surg 2010; 8(3):212–5.

19. Moore RA, Derry S, Aldington D, et al. Amitriptyline for neuropathic pain in adults. Cochrane Database Syst Rev 2015;(7):CD008242.

20. Sindrup SH, Finnerup NB, Jensen TS. Antidepressants in the treatment of neuropathic pain. Basic Clin Pharmacol Toxicol 2005;96(6):399–409.

21. Baguneid M, Dodd D, Fulford P, et al. Management of acute nontraumatic upper limb ischemia. Angiology 1999;50(9):715–20.

22. Sultan S, Evoy D, Eldin AS, et al. Atraumatic acute upper limb ischemia: a series of 64 patients in a Middle East tertiary vascular center and literature review. Vasc Surg 2001;35(3):181–97.

23. Sanni A, Hamid A, Dunning J. Is sympathectomy of benefit in critical leg ischaemia not amenable to revascularisation? Interact Cardiovasc Thorac Surg 2005;4(5):478–83.

Nerve Entrapments

Lauren Jacobson, MD[a], Jana Dengler, MD[b], Amy M. Moore, MD[c],*

KEYWORDS

- Nerve compression • Nerve entrapment • Carpal tunnel syndrome • Cubital tunnel syndrome
- Radial tunnel syndrome

KEY POINTS

- Nerve entrapment syndromes are a common cause of pain and disability.
- There are more than 2 dozen described nerve entrapment syndromes in the body.
- The mainstay of nonsurgical management includes activity modification, nerve gliding, and splinting.
- Surgical decompression involves releasing tight structures overlying the entrapped nerve.

INTRODUCTION

Nerve entrapment syndromes are common, and can lead to sensory disturbance, loss of motor function and pain. More than 2 dozen nerve entrapment syndromes have been described (**Table 1**). Although they can occur acutely as a result of trauma with subsequent swelling, most compression neuropathies are chronic in nature. Chronic, focal compression of a nerve can occur as a result of ordinary, everyday activities, such as sleeping position or repetitive movements at work.[1] Our understanding of these processes has evolved significantly over the past 40 years. Pain, although a common feature of nerve entrapment, has received less attention.

Here, we discuss the pathophysiology of nerve entrapment and its relationship to pain. We review the most common upper and lower extremity nerve entrapment syndromes and highlight their assessment and management. We also discuss several clinical scenarios where nerve entrapment is underdiagnosed. With a strong foundation and understanding of the biology of compression neuropathy, indications for surgical decompression will continue to expand to provide relief for patients suffering from pain.

MICROANATOMY

Peripheral nerves are composed of motor sensory, and autonomic fibers. Type A fibers are large myelinated nerve fibers and include afferent and efferent motor and sensory fibers. They exhibit the highest conduction velocity. Type B fibers are smaller myelinated fibers, and are made up of preganglionic autonomic nerve fibers. Type C fibers are the thinnest and unmyelinated, and include visceral and somatic pain fibers, as well as postganglionic autonomic nerve fibers. The fibers (known as axons), are grouped into fascicles, which are bundled with blood vessels and connective tissue to form the nerve (**Fig. 1**). There are 3 layers of connective tissue matrix. The innermost layer, the endoneurium, surrounds axons and Schwann cells and is resistant to injury by stretch.[2] The middle layer, the perineurium, surrounds fascicles and maintains the physiologic

[a] Division of Plastic and Reconstructive Surgery, Department of Surgery, Barnes-Jewish Hospital, Washington University School of Medicine, 660 South Euclid Avenue, Campus Box 8238, St Louis, MO 63110, USA; [b] Division of Plastic and Reconstructive Surgery, Department of Surgery, Sunnybrook Health Sciences Centre, M1-500, 2075 Bayview Avenue, Toronto, Ontario M4N 3M5, Canada; [c] Department of Plastic and Reconstructive Surgery, The Ohio State University Wexner Medical Center, 915 Olentangy River Road, Suite 2100, Columbus OH 43212, USA
* Corresponding author.
E-mail address: amy.m.moore@osumc.edu

Clin Plastic Surg 47 (2020) 267–278
https://doi.org/10.1016/j.cps.2019.12.006
0094-1298/20/© 2020 Elsevier Inc. All rights reserved.

Table 1
Summary of nerve entrapment syndromes

Involved Nerve	Site of Entrapment	Signs and Symptoms	Surgical Decompression
Upper extremity			
Median nerve	Carpal tunnel	Pain and paraesthesias in the *radial 3 and one-half digits* (sparing of PCM) and night-time wakening *APB weakness*, muscle atrophy	Release of transverse carpal ligament
Median nerve	Forearm	*Volar forearm pain* exacerbated by pronation and reproduced with supination and pressure over leading edge of pronator Paresthesias and sensory loss in median nerve distribution *including PCM* Weakness of muscles supplied by AIN (*FPL, FDP [1, 2], PQ*)	Release of lacertus fibrosis, deep head of pronator, flexor digitorum superficialis arch with or without ligament of Struthers with or without supracondylar process
Ulnar nerve	Cubital tunnel	Pain and paraesthesias in *ring and small fingers* *Aching medial elbow* into forearm *Clumsiness* and weak grip strength Atrophy *first dorsal interossei, abductor digiti minimi*	Release of cubital tunnel, heads of FCU, with or without arcade of Struthers with or without anconeus with or without transposition
Ulnar nerve	Guyon's canal	Pain and paraesthesias in *ring and small fingers* Clumsiness, clawing of ring and small fingers Atrophy *first dorsal interossei, abductor digiti minimi*	Release of antebrachial fascia, Guyon's canal, leading edge of hypothenar muscles
Radial nerve	Spiral groove	Radial nerve palsy (*weakness/loss of wrist/ elbow and finger/ thumb extension*), numbness dorsoradial aspect of hand	Neurolysis of radial nerve as travels around humerus in spiral groove
Radial nerve	Radial tunnel	Palsy of muscles supplied by *posterior interosseous nerve* (finger, thumb extensors) *Arm fatigue* and *pain dorsal forearm*, worsens with elbow extension and forearm rotation	Release of ECRB, Arcade of Frohse, with or without radial recurrent vessels (leash of Henry)

(*continued on next page*)

Table 1
(continued)

Involved Nerve	Site of Entrapment	Signs and Symptoms	Surgical Decompression
Superficial sensory branch of the radial nerve	Forearm: between brachioradialis, ECRL	Paraesthesias *dorsoradial aspect of the hand*, exquisite pain with ulnar flexion of the wrist or activities such as gripping and pinching	Release (with or without resection) of brachioradialis tendon, neurolysis of superficial sensory branch of the radial nerve
Axillary nerve	Quadrangular space	Pain *posterior shoulder*, weakness *shoulder abduction*, numbness *lateral arm*, point tenderness over quadrangular space	Release of lateral head of triceps tendon with or without teres minor fascia, neurolysis of axillary nerve
Suprascapular nerve	Suprascapular notch	*Deep, diffuse pain posterior and lateral shoulder* that may *refer* down the arm, to the neck, or to upper anterior chest wall. *Muscle weakness and atrophy of supraspinatus and infraspinatus* (external rotation)	Release of transverse scapular ligament, which forms the roof of the suprascapular notch
Brachial plexus	Thoracic outlet	*Proximal pain (shoulder/scapula)* with distal numbness with or without paresthesias (usually C8/T1 distribution). Symptoms brought on with *activity/overhead movement*	Anterior and middle scalenectomy with or without rib resection
Lateral antebrachial cutaneous nerve	Arm: biceps tendon	Pain, paresthesias lateral forearm	Neurolysis of the lateral antebrachial cutaneous nerve
Lower extremity			
Femoral nerve	Iliacus fascia, inguinal ligament	Weakness/atrophy *hip flexion, knee extension*, paraesthesias anteromedial thigh, medial leg, gait disturbance	Neurolysis femoral nerve, with or without (partial) release of inguinal ligament
Lateral cutaneous nerve of the thigh	Inguinal ligament (meralgia paresthetica)	*Pain, paresthesias anterolateral thigh*, exacerbated by standing, walking; relief with nerve block	Neurolysis of lateral femoral cutaneous nerve along its course
Obturator nerve	Medial thigh	Pain and paresthesias *medial thigh*, weakness of *thigh adduction, internal rotation*, gait disturbance; relief with nerve block	Release of adductor brevis fascia

(continued on next page)

Table 1
(continued)

Involved Nerve	Site of Entrapment	Signs and Symptoms	Surgical Decompression
Common peroneal nerve	Fibular neck	Pain and paraesthesias in *lateral leg and foot*, weakness dorsiflexion, *foot drop*	Release of 3 intermuscular septal planes of the lateral and anterior compartments
Superficial peroneal nerve	Distal third of leg	Pain and paraesthesias in *lateral leg and foot*	Release of deep fascia overlying superficial peroneal nerve
Deep peroneal nerve	Dorsum of foot	Weakness, pain, and paresthesias of the foot and ankle, specifically, in the *first web space*	Release of extensor retinaculum over anterior ankle, with or without release of extensor hallucis brevis
Posterior tibial nerve	Soleus arch	Calf pain, exacerbated by exercise	Release of tendinous leading edge of soleus
Posterior tibial nerve	Tarsal tunnel	Pain and paresthesias over *medial ankle and heel*, *sole of the foot*, and *toes*; and weakness and atrophy of *toe flexion* muscles	Release of the flexor retinaculum, as well as the superficial and deep fascia of the abductor muscle belly
Saphenous nerve	Adductor canal Gonyalgia paresthetica, minor causalgia	*Deep aching pain* medial thigh and knee, paresthesias *medial leg and foot*; relief with nerve block	Release of adductor canal
Plantar nerves	Morton's neuroma: between metatarsal heads	*Pain in the webspace with walking*; pain shoots into toes and is relieved at rest and with elevation; lateral web spaces more commonly involved	Release of deep transverse metatarsal ligament and overlying fascia
Head and neck			
Supraorbital and supratrochlear nerves	Supraorbital/frontal	Chronic headaches/migraines in *frontal region*; relief with injection of botulinum toxin or nerve block	Release of supraorbital notch/foramen, excision corrugator muscle with or without excision of supraorbital/trochlear vasculature
Zygomaticotemporal and auriculotemporal nerve	Temporal	Chronic headaches/migraines in *temporal region*; relief with injection of botulinum toxin or nerve block	Release deep fascial bands with or without release of temporalis muscle with or without ligation superficial temporal artery
Greater, lesser and third occipital nerves	Occipital	Chronic headaches/migraines in *occipital region*; relief with injection of botulinum toxin or nerve block	Release of semispinalis capitis muscle, with or without trapezial tunnel plus sternocleidomastoid fascia/muscle

(continued on next page)

Table 1
(continued)

Involved Nerve	Site of Entrapment	Signs and Symptoms	Surgical Decompression
Sphenopalatine ganglion	Nasal	Chronic headaches/ migraines in frontal region; relief with injection of botulinum toxin or nerve block	–

milieu and the blood–nerve barrier.[3] The external layer, the epineurium, provides structural support and protects against compression[3]; it is most abundant where a nerve crosses a joint.[4] The blood supply is 2-fold: intrinsic vessels run within the endoneurial space, and anastomose with the extrinsic plexus of the epineurial space.

PATHOPHYSIOLOGY OF NERVE ENTRAPMENT

Nerve entrapment occurs at sites of fibroosseous or fibromuscular tunnels.[5] Owing to the limited volume within these tunnels, any insult that leads to an increase in the size of the nerve or a decrease in the volume of the tunnel will cause compression of the nerve and affect the intrinsic and extrinsic blood flow.[4] Pressure increases of as little as 20 mm Hg can lead to venous stasis and subsequent extraneural edema; at 80 mm Hg, all intraneural blood flow ceases.[6] Stretching of nerves can also lead to venous stasis. When a nerve is stretched by 8% of its resting length, venous outflow is blocked.[7] Over time, venous outflow obstruction leads to fibrosis and scarring, which further worsens endoneurial edema.[6,7] The

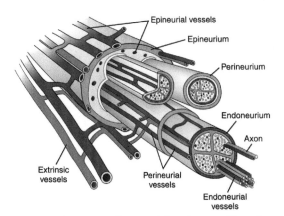

Fig. 1. Architecture of the peripheral nerve. (*From* Power HA, Moore AM. Basic science of nerve compression. In: Skirven T et al. (Eds), Rehabilitation of the Hand and Upper Extremity, 7th edition. Philadelphia: Elsevier, 2020; with permission.)

intact perineurium prevent this increased pressure from being relieved, causing a miniature compartment syndrome within the nerve.[8] The resultant hypoxia leads to further inflammation, fibrosis, demyelination, and eventually, axonal degeneration.[9,10]

These intraneural physiologic changes are accompanied by predictable clinical symptoms. Patients with mild or intermittent nerve entrapment experience intermittent paraesthesias, aching and weakness in the distribution of the affected nerve. These symptoms are usually relieved by a change in position or the shaking out one's hand or arm. However, as neural hypoxia becomes severe or chronic in nature, symptoms progress to constant paraesthesias, atrophy, and pain.[10]

PAIN IN NERVE ENTRAPMENT

There are 4 proposed mechanisms for neuropathic pain, which may explain the pain phenomena of nerve entrapment: denervation, ectopic activity, peripheral sensitization, and central sensitization.[11] With partial nerve damage, pain can occur as a result of injured and uninjured afferents supplying the affected region.[12] Damaged afferent pathways are responsible for sensory loss owing to denervation, but can also contribute to ongoing pain from ectopic activity in the dorsal root ganglia that results from the loss of trophic support.[11] Undamaged afferent nociceptors, in contrast, can be peripherally sensitized by the inflammatory process (macrophage infiltration, T-cell activation, increased expression of proinflammatory cytokines) that ensues after nerve damage, and cause hyperalgesia from enhanced trophic support in the dorsal root ganglia.[12,13] Both input from damaged and undamaged nociceptors can produce central sensitization, which can also cause hyperalgesia. Ongoing pain may be the only manifestation of nerve entrapment (owing to ectopic activity), but in many cases altered perception to evoked pain (hyperalgesia owing to denervation, peripheral sensitization, and central sensitization) may be present.[12]

Nerve entrapment causes a disturbance of fast axonal transport along the nerve in the area of compression, and leads to ectopic expression of the transduced proteins, which is thought to result in the Tinel sign, where patients experience paraesthesias or dysesthesias when the area over the irritated nerve is tapped.[12] An increase in substance P immunoreactivity has been noted in the dorsal root ganglia after nerve injury,[14] as well as at sites of nerve entrapment,[15] and has been proposed as the cause of the reflexive collapse response noted in the scratch collapse test.[16]

ACUTE VERSUS CHRONIC NERVE ENTRAPMENT

There are 2 key differences in acute traumatic compression neuropathy and chronic compression neuropathy. First, axonal degeneration is noted early in acute nerve entrapment, although it is a late finding in chronic nerve entrapment. Histologically, axonal degeneration in chronic nerve entrapment is not visualized until muscle atrophy is clinically evident. Instead, chronic nerve entrapment first results in demyelination and slowing of nerve conduction, followed by subsequent thinner remyelination.[17] Second, Schwann cell proliferation in chronic compression is independent of macrophages and instead is induced by mechanical forces.[18] In contrast, acute entrapment shows greater infiltration of macrophages into the nerve.[19]

THE DOUBLE CRUSH

Upton and McComas[20] first introduced the theory of the double crush phenomenon in 1973. They proposed that compression of a nerve at a proximal point will compromise axoplasmic flow, thus making the same nerve increasingly susceptible to injury at another, more distal point. For example, a patient with cervical radiculopathy or thoracic outlet syndrome may develop carpal tunnel syndrome (CTS) more easily. In 2004, Lundborg[21] described the reverse double crush syndrome, in which a site of distal nerve entrapment predisposes the nerve to more proximal compression injury. He hypothesized that compression of a nerve at a distal site would decrease flow of neurotrophic substances back to the neuron body, with subsequent alteration of axoplasmic flow. Both theories suggest that entrapment of a nerve can affect axoplasmic transport and render other areas of the nerve more susceptible to entrapment.

MEDIAN NERVE ENTRAPMENT
Carpal Tunnel Syndrome

The median nerve (C6–T1) can become compressed at multiple points along its course from the distal humerus to the wrist (**Fig. 2**). The most common site of entrapment is at the carpal tunnel, where the nerve travels under the transverse carpal ligament. With a prevalence ranging from 3.72% to 6.80% in the United States, CTS is the

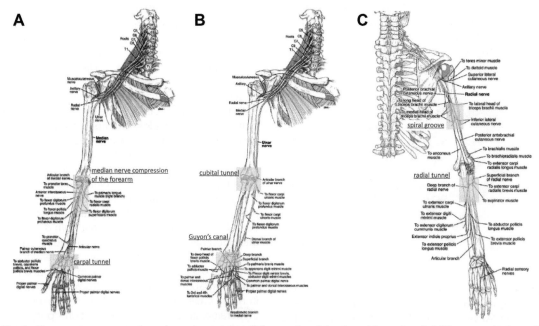

Fig. 2. Nerve entrapment points along the course of the median (*A*), ulnar (*B*), and radial (*C*) nerves. (*Adapted from* Mackinnon SE. Nerve Surgery. New York, NY: Thieme Medical Publishers, Inc.; 2015; with permission.)

most common nerve entrapment syndrome in the body.[22] Classic symptoms of CTS include intermittent pain and parenthesis in the radial three and a half digits and night-time wakening. Symptoms are often exacerbated by gripping and certain hand positions; symptoms are relieved by shaking out the hand. On examination, patients exhibit decreased sensation in the median nerve distribution with sparing of the palmar cutaneous nerve distribution over the thenar eminence. Provocative tests include the Tinel test,[23] the Phalen test,[23] the median nerve compression test,[24] and recently the scratch collapse test.[25] Over time, paraesthesias progress to become constant. In late CTS, weakness and thenar muscle atrophy are noted. Diagnosis can usually be made by history and physical examination alone. If examination is equivocal, electrodiagnostic studies (EDX) can be helpful in establishing the diagnosis. A negative EDX, however, does not preclude the diagnosis of CTS. EDX only evaluates large myelinated fibers, and will thus be normal in mild or early CTS, when only small or unmyelinated nerve fibers are affected.[26]

Nonsurgical management includes adaptive behaviors, night-time wrist splinting, corticosteroid injections, and nerve gliding exercises. When these interventions fail, or in the setting of advanced CTS, surgical decompression of the carpal tunnel (carpal tunnel release [CTR]) is recommended. Controversy regarding open versus endoscopic CTR continues. A meta-analysis demonstrated that although irreversible nerve injury is rare with either technique, there is a higher incidence of reversible nerve injury in endoscopic CTR.[27] We recommend the surgeon chose the technique she or he is most comfortable with and offers the best visualization of the median nerve to minimize risk of injury.

Pronator Syndrome

When pain, numbness, and tingling extend proximally into the forearm, arm, or shoulder, more proximal nerve compression should be considered. In pronator syndrome, the median nerve is compressed by the deep head of pronator teres, the fibrinous edge of the flexor digitorum superficialis, the bicipital aponeurosis (laceratus fibrosus), and/or the ligament of Struthers. Patients present with predominant symptoms of volar forearm pain. When present, paraesthesias include the distribution of the palmar cutaneous branch. Pronator syndrome and CTS may present concurrently in up to 6% of patients,[28] suggesting a double crush syndrome. EDX is not helpful in establishing a diagnosis of pronator syndrome.

Nonsurgical management is similar to that for CTS. Surgical decompression can involve release of only the laceratus fibrosis[29] or all potential sites of compression.[26] Decompression has shown to significantly improve quick Disabilities of the Arm, Shoulder, and Hand scores.[30] For patients who have incomplete resolution of symptoms with CTR, release of the median nerve in the forearm has proven successful at alleviating symptoms.[31]

ULNAR NERVE ENTRAPMENT
Cubital Tunnel Syndrome

The ulnar nerve (C8–T1) also has multiple potential sites of compression along its course from the distal humerus to the wrist (see **Fig. 2**). It is most commonly entrapped at the elbow within the cubital tunnel, with prevalence in the United States of 1.8% to 5.9%.[32] Cubital tunnel syndrome can be a result of repetitive elbow flexion, anomalous musculature, or direct compression. Elbow flexion can decrease the volume of the cubital tunnel by as much as 55%.[33] Patients commonly present with pain and numbness in the ring and small fingers, and endorse an aching sensation at the medial elbow into the forearm. Sensory deficit in the dorsal ulnar cutaneous nerve distribution can help confirm proximal nerve entrapment (as opposed to entrapment at Guyon's canal, described elsewhere in this article). In more advanced stages, patients exhibit clumsiness and weak grip strength. Weakness and atrophy is most easily appreciated in the first dorsal interossei and the abductor digiti minimi muscles. Patients with chronic compression may have difficulty with index cross-over, and a positive Froment and/or a Wartenberg sign. Although cubital tunnel syndrome is a clinical diagnosis, EDX is helpful in establishing the location and severity of compression. Slowing of the conduction velocity across the elbow of less than 50 m/s confirms the diagnosis of cubital tunnel syndrome,[26] and compound muscle action potential amplitude helps to determine the severity.[34]

Nonsurgical management is most successful in patients with dynamic ischemia, where symptoms are relieved with a change in position.[35] Activity modifications and preventing elbow flexion during sleep have demonstrated improvement in mild to moderate cubital tunnel syndrome.[36] Other modalities include stretching and nerve gliding exercises. Surgical decompression should be offered to patients who fail nonsurgical management or who present with severe compression. Decompression procedures vary (in situ decompression, subcutaneous transposition, submuscular transposition), with success rates of 65% to 75%.[37]

Guyon's Canal Compression

Compression of the ulnar nerve within Guyon's canal occurs less frequently than at the cubital tunnel, and can be caused by trauma resulting in hypothenar hammer syndrome,[38] distal radius/carpal dislocations,[39] or fractures of the hook of the hamate.[40] Other causes include activities such as cycling, which places the nerve under continuous stretch and compression,[41] ganglion cysts,[42] vascular malformations,[43] and anomalous musculature. This diagnosis should be included in instances of proximal nerve injury (double crush), severe proximal compression, and/or persistent symptoms despite proximal ulnar nerve decompression. EDX cannot pick up abnormalities at Guyon's canal, but a Tinel sign on clinical examination can help to confirm the diagnosis.

Nonsurgical management includes splinting the wrist in a neutral position and may provide benefit after an acute, closed insult.[26,35] Surgical decompression of Guyon's canal involves release of the antebrachial fascia overlying the ulnar nerve at the wrist, and release of the tendinous leading edge of the hypothenar muscles which can compress the motor branch.[44] Notably, patients with symptoms of ulnar nerve entrapment at the wrist can experience symptom relief with CTR, likely owing to the relief of pressure within Guyon's canal following release of the transverse carpal ligament and proximal antebrachial fascia.[45]

RADIAL NERVE ENTRAPMENT
Radial Tunnel Syndrome

The radial nerve (C5–T1) can become compressed at the spiral groove, the radial tunnel, and in the distal forearm (see **Fig. 2**). Compression of the radial nerve in the proximal forearm causes a posterior interosseous nerve palsy. Patients present with arm fatigue and pain on the dorsal forearm that worsens at night and with activities of forceful elbow extension and forearm rotation.[46] Radial tunnel syndrome symptoms can mimic lateral epicondylitis, which presents with tenderness on direct palpation of the lateral epicondyle.[46] EDX is rarely useful in the diagnosis of radial tunnel syndrome and clinical suspicion with a directed physical examination is needed.[26] Patients exhibit reproducible tenderness with compression over the radial tunnel and pain with elbow extension, forearm pronation, or wrist flexion. Patients may also exhibit decreased sensation of the dorsum of the hand.

Nonsurgical management relies heavily on nerve gliding exercises and treatment of other concomitant issues, such as lateral epicondylitis. Wrist immobilization and anti-inflammatories have also been suggested, although the success of these modalities remains to be determined.[47] Surgical decompression can be performed through various approaches, including the transmuscular brachioradialis-splitting approach, the posterior (Henry or Thompson) approach, and the anterior (modified Henry) approach. Release of the arcade of Frohse (leading edge of the supinator) and ligation of the radial recurrent vessels, is essential.[46] Decompression has been shown to be highly effective in achieving pain relief, with several studies supporting excellent outcomes in up to 95% of patients.[46,48,49]

Superficial Radial Nerve Entrapment

Wartenberg first described compression of the radial sensory nerve (superficial branch of the radial nerve) in the forearm in 1932.[50] The nerve travels under brachioradialis, and exits in the majority of people between the tendons of ECRL and brachioradialis in the distal forearm, making it vulnerable to compression and trauma. In 3% to 10% of people, it pierces through the brachioradialis.[26] Traction on the superficial radial nerve can occur with movement from radial extension to ulnar flexion, and with pronation/supination. Patients present with paraesthesias over the dorsoradial aspect of the hand, and exquisite, life-altering pain with ulnar flexion of the wrist or activities such as gripping and pinching.

Activity modification is a mainstay of nonsurgical management. Injection of a corticosteroid has been found to be effective.[51] During surgical decompression (release of the brachioradialis tendon), caution is required to avoid damaging branches of the superficial branch of the radial nerve.[44] Decompression has been shown to be successful in the majority of patients.[51]

LOWER EXTREMITY NERVE ENTRAPMENT
Peroneal Neuropathy

Peroneal neuropathy is the most common nerve entrapment in the lower extremity, owing to the anatomic course of the peroneal nerve around the bony fibular head. The common peroneal nerve (L4–S1) divides into superficial and deep branches distal to the fibular head, which can also become compressed. Entrapment of the common peroneal nerve can be caused by pressure from prolonged immobilization (ie, cast immobilization or inadequate padding during surgery), habitual leg crossing, direct trauma, or surrounding masses such as ganglion cysts.[52] In its most severe and clinically recognized form, compression causes foot drop. In less severe entrapment, peroneal neuropathy presents with pain and paraesthesias in the lateral leg and dorsum of the foot.[53] The superficial branch can become entrapped, where it exits the deep fascia to run in the subcutaneous plane at the junction of the middle and distal thirds of the leg. Compression here causes pain and paraesthesias only. EDX studies can be helpful to localize compression of the peroneal nerve, eliminating confounding by more proximal lesions that can mimic peroneal neuropathy, such as sciatic nerve injury, radiculopathy, or generalized disorders like amyotrophic lateral sclerosis.[52,54] EDX can also provide information on the severity of axonal injury[52] and prognosis.[55,56]

Nonsurgical management includes activity modifications, patient education, and the use of an ankle–foot orthosis for foot drop. Surgical intervention is usually reserved for refractory cases. Decompression of the common peroneal nerve involves release of 3 intermuscular septal planes of the lateral and anterior compartments, and has shown good recovery in both sensory and motor function.[57] Nerve and tendon transfers are available to restore ankle dorsiflexion, if decompression is unsuccessful.[54]

Tarsal Tunnel

Compression of the posterior tibial nerve at the tarsal tunnel is rare. The tarsal tunnel is a fibroosseous tunnel created by the flexor retinaculum at the medial side of the ankle. Compression of the nerve can occur with repetitive movements (eversion and plantarflexion), soft tissue inflammation or edema, and bony or vascular lesions.[52] Symptoms of compression include pain and paresthesias over the medial ankle and heel, sole of the foot, and toes; and weakness and atrophy of toe flexion muscles. Mimickers include calcaneal spurs, bursitis, tendonitis of the flexor tendons, plantar fasciitis, polyneuropathy, and radiculopathy.[58] Provocative maneuvers to localize the site of compression include the dorsiflexion–eversion test,[59] the Trepman test (plantar flexion–inversion test),[60] and the Tinel test. Diagnosis can be confirmed by EDX, which show delayed latencies or low amplitude compound muscle action potentials of the medial and lateral plantar nerves across the ankle and denervation of tibial-innervated intrinsic muscles.[61] However, a high incidence of abnormal nerve conduction studies can be seen in normal individuals.[62]

Nonsurgical management is the mainstay for tarsal tunnel syndrome. This includes custom orthoses, stretching, taping, massage, and anti-inflammatories.[52] If nonsurgical management fails, surgical intervention may be indicated. An open technique with release of the flexor retinaculum, as well as the superficial and deep fascia of the abductor muscle belly is the preferred technique. The success rate of decompression is reported from 75% to 91%.[63]

CLINICAL SCENARIOS

There are several clinical scenarios in which nerve entrapment may be contributing to pain, and release of compression can significantly improve symptoms. We discuss 3 of these conditions here, because they have traditionally received little attention: complex regional pain syndrome (CRPS), burns, and hemodialysis.

Complex Regional Pain Syndrome

CRPS is a chronic pain syndrome that can result from nerve damage (type II, previously called causalgia), or in the absence of nerve damage (type I, previously called reflex sympathetic dystrophy). Patients present with a constellation of symptoms, including severe throbbing or burning pain, increased temperature of the affected extremity, excessive swelling, stiffness, and alteration of skin blood flow. Multiple studies have demonstrated that compression of one or more nerves coexists in CRPS, the median nerve being most common, followed by the ulnar nerve at the elbow and the posterior interosseous nerve.[64,65] Surgical decompression has traditionally not been widely recommended, and findings show that this delay in surgical intervention may result in worse outcomes after eventual decompression.[66] Placzek and colleagues[66] performed nerve decompression on patients diagnosed with CRPS after upper extremity surgery. After surgical decompression, patients noted significant pain relief, with pain scores decreasing from 7.5 to 3.5 in the immediate postoperative period. Functional improvement was noted with Disabilities of the Arm, Shoulder, and Hand scores decreasing from 71 before surgery to 30 at the time of follow-up.[66] All patients noted immediate relief of somatic symptoms.[66] Multiple studies now propose the need for a paradigm shift in the management of patients with CRPS.[66–68]

Burns

A frequent, but often undiagnosed or overlooked, neuromuscular sequela of burn injury is peripheral neuropathy.[69,70] Compression of the ulnar nerve at the elbow is most common. Onset of symptoms, such as pain, paraesthesias, and weakness can occur in the first week of injury, but can also present up to 6 months later.[71] Peripheral neuropathies in burns can be classified as mono-neuropathy, mononeuropathy multiplex, and poly-neuropathy. Mononeuropathy is the involvement of a single nerve distribution and relates to local factors, such as edema from escharotomy, fasciotomy, or direct injury of electrical burns.[70,72] Mononeuropathy multiplex is the involvement of 2 or more nerves in unrelated areas of the body. It occurs in 56% to 69% of burn patients.[73] Polyneuropathy is characterized by symmetric distal sensory loss and weakness. Treatment depends on the timing of symptom onset. Acute management involves the treatment of the burns with concomitant nerve decompression.[69] Delayed presentation is a result of edema, progressive scarring, heterotopic ossification, and exacerbation of chronic compression.[71] Some studies suggest that physical therapy may be sufficient to allow functional recovery in delayed neuropathy.[74,75] However, surgical decompression has shown a high potential for functional improvement with a low risk of complications,[69] and should be considered in patients with unrelenting symptoms.

Hemodialysis

Neurologic conditions are common in patients undergoing hemodialysis, usually related to uremia or diabetes.[76] However, nerve injury, CRPS, ischemic neuropathy, and nerve entrapment need to also be considered in patients presenting with pain and paraesthesias. Direct injury to nerves, particularly sensory nerves, can occur during creation of an adjacent arteriovenous fistula.[76] Although believed to be underreported, the effects of these injuries are usually mild and transient, but progression to CRPS can occur.[77] Ischemic neuropathy occurs in the setting of chronic neural microvascular disease, which is further aggravated by steal syndrome.[76] It typically affects all 3 motor nerves of the forearm (median, radial, and ulnar) and presents with severe postoperative pain and progressive sensory and motor deficits.[78] Treatment is division of the arteriovenous fistula and decompression of the affected nerves. CTS is the most common nerve entrapment syndrome in patients on hemodialysis, with an incidence up to 10 times greater than in the general population,[76] and has been reported in 50% of patients after 10 years of hemodialysis.[79] EDX studies can help to confirm the diagnosis.

SUMMARY

Nerve entrapments syndromes are abundant and can lead to debilitating pain. Clinical suspicion and a thorough physical examination remain the key diagnostic tools in identifying opportunities to treat patient with nerve entrapment. Although a clinical diagnosis, EDX studies can be useful in assisting the clinician to assess severity and location. Nonsurgical interventions should be used first, but surgical decompression has a strong history of success and should be considered in patients with persistent pain and identifiable sources of entrapment.

DISCLOSURE

The authors have nothing to disclose.

REFERENCES

1. Roth bettlach CL, Hasak JM, Krauss EM, et al. Preferences in sleep position correlate with nighttime paresthesias in healthy people without carpal tunnel syndrome. Hand (N Y) 2019;14(2):163–71.
2. Sunderland S. The connective tissues of peripheral nerves. Brain 1965;88(4):841–54.
3. Shanthaveerappa TR, Bourne GH. Perineural epithelium: a new concept of its role in the integrity of the peripheral nervous system. Science 1966;154(3755):1464–7.
4. Power HA, Moore AM. Basic science of nerve compression. In: Skirven T, Osterman A, Fedorczyk J, et al, editors. Rehabilitation of the Hand and Upper Extremity. 7th edition. Philadelphia: Elsevier; 2020. in press.
5. Dong Q, Jacobson JA, Jamadar DA, et al. Entrapment neuropathies in the upper and lower limbs: anatomy and MRI features. Radiol Res Pract 2012;2012:230679.
6. Rydevik B, Lundborg G, Bagge U. Effects of graded compression on intraneural blood blow. An in vivo study on rabbit tibial nerve. J Hand Surg Am 1981;6:3–12.
7. Lundborg G, Rydevik B. Effects of stretching the tibial nerve of the rabbit. A preliminary study of the intraneural circulation and the barrier function of the perineurium. J Bone Joint Surg Br 1973;55(2):390–401.
8. Lundborg G, Myers R, Powell H. Nerve compression injury and increased endoneurial fluid pressure: a "miniature compartment syndrome. J Neurol Neurosurg Psychiatr 1983;46:1119–24.
9. O'brien JP, Mackinnon SE, Maclean AR, et al. A model of chronic nerve compression in the rat. Ann Plast Surg 1987;19(5):430–5.
10. Mackinnon SE. Pathophysiology of nerve compression. Hand Clin 2002;18(2):231–41.
11. Vollert J, Magerl W, Baron R, et al. Pathophysiological mechanisms of neuropathic pain: comparison of sensory phenotypes in patients and human surrogate pain models. Pain 2018;159(6):1090–102.

12. Campbell JN, Meyer RA. Mechanisms of neuropathic pain. Neuron 2006;52:77–92.

13. Costigan M, Scholz J, Woolf CJ. Neuropathic pain: a maladaptive response of the nervous system to damage. Annu Rev Neurosci 2009;32:1–32.

14. Noguchi K, Dubner R, De Leon M, et al. Axotomy induces preprotachykinin gene expression in a subpopulation of dorsal root ganglion neurons. J Neurosci Res 1994;37(5):596–603.

15. Ozturk N, Erin N, Tuzuner S. Changes in tissue substance P levels in patients with carpal tunnel syndrome. Neurosurgery 2010;67:1655–60 [discussion: 1660–1].

16. Kahn LC, Yee A, Mackinnon SE. Important details in performing and interpreting the scratch collapse test. Plast Reconstr Surg 2018;141(2):399–407.

17. Ludwin SK, Maitland M. Long-term remyelination fails to reconstitute normal thickness of central myelin sheaths. J Neurol Sci 1984;64(2):193–8.

18. Tapadia M, Mozaffar T, Gupta R. Compressive neuropathies of the upper extremity: update on pathophysiology, classification, and electrodiagnostic findings. J Hand Surg Am 2010;35(4):668–77.

19. Bendszus M, Stoll G. Caught in the act: in vivo mapping of macrophage infiltration in nerve injury by magnetic resonance imaging. J Neurosci 2003; 23(34):10892–6.

20. Upton AR, McComas AJ. The double crush in nerve entrapment syndromes. Lancet 1973;2:359–62.

21. Lundborg G. Nerve injury and repair: regeneration, reconstruction, and cortical remodeling. 2nd edition. New York: Elsevier; 2004.

22. Papanicolaou GD, Mccabe SJ, Firrell J. The prevalence and characteristics of nerve compression symptoms in the general population. J Hand Surg Am 2001;26(3):460–6.

23. Popinchalk SP, Schaffer AA. Physical examination of upper extremity compressive neuropathies. Orthop Clin North Am 2012;43(4):417–30.

24. Williams TM, Mackinnon SE, Novak CB, et al. Verification of the pressure provocative test in carpal tunnel syndrome. Ann Plast Surg 1992;29:8–11.

25. Cheng CJ, Mackinnon-Patterson B, Beck JL, et al. Scratch collapse test for evaluation of carpal and cubital tunnel syndrome. J Hand Surg Am 2008;33: 1518–24.

26. Mackinnon SE, Novak CB. Compression neuropathies. In: Wolfe SW, Hotchkiss RN, Pederson WC, et al, editors. Green's operative hand surgery. Seventh Edition. Philadelphia: Elsevier Inc; 2016. p. 921–58.

27. Thoma A, Veltri K, Haines T, et al. A meta-analysis of randomized controlled trials comparing endoscopic and open carpal tunnel decompression. Plast Reconstr Surg 2004;114(5):1137–46.

28. Hsiao CW, Shih JT, Hung ST. Concurrent carpal tunnel syndrome and pronator syndrome: a retrospective study of 21 cases. Orthop Traumatol Surg Res 2017;103(1):101–3.

29. Lalonde D. Lacertus syndrome: a commonly missed and misdiagnosed median nerve entrapment syndrome. BMC Proc 2015;9(Suppl 3):A74.

30. Hagert E. Clinical diagnosis and wide-awake surgical treatment of proximal median nerve entrapment at the elbow: a prospective study. Hand (N Y) 2013;8(1):41–6.

31. Olehnik WK, Manske PR, Szerzinski J. Median nerve compression in the proximal forearm. J Hand Surg Am 1994;19(1):121–6.

32. An TW, Evanoff BA, Boyer MI, et al. The prevalence of cubital tunnel syndrome: a cross-sectional study in a U.S. Metropolitan cohort. J Bone Joint Surg Am 2017;99(5):408–16.

33. Apfelberg DB, Larson SJ. Dynamic anatomy of the ulnar nerve at the elbow. Plast Reconstr Surg 1973;51(1):76–81.

34. Power HA, Sharma K, El-Haj M, et al. Compound muscle action potential amplitude predicts the severity of cubital tunnel syndrome. J Bone Joint Surg Am 2019;101(8):730–8.

35. Dy CJ, Mackinnon SE. Ulnar neuropathy: evaluation and management. Curr Rev Musculoskelet Med 2016;9(2):178–84.

36. Shah CM, Calfee RP, Gelberman RH, et al. Outcomes of rigid night splinting and activity modification in the treatment of cubital tunnel syndrome. J Hand Surg Am 2013;38:1125–30.

37. Caliandro P, La Torre G, Padua R, et al. Treatment for ulnar neuropathy at the elbow. Cochrane Database Syst Rev 2016;(11):CD006839.

38. Conn J, Bergan JJ, Bell JL. Hypothenar hammer syndrome: posttraumatic digital ischemia. Surgery 1970;68(6):1122–8.

39. Vance RM, Gelberman RH. Acute ulnar neuropathy with fractures at the wrist. J Bone Joint Surg Am 1978;60:962–5.

40. Foucher G, Schuind F, Merle M, et al. Fractures of the hook of the hamate. J Hand Surg Br 1985;10:205–10.

41. Brubacher JW, Leversedge FJ. Ulnar neuropathy in cyclists. Hand Clin 2017;33(1):199–205.

42. Kwak KW, Kim MS, Chang CH, et al. Ulnar nerve compression in Guyon's canal by ganglion cyst. J Korean Neurosurg Soc 2011;49:139–41.

43. Kim SS, Kim JH, Kang HI, et al. Ulnar nerve compression at Guyon's canal by an arteriovenous malformation. J Korean Neurosurg Soc 2009;45:57–9.

44. Mackinnon SE. Nerve surgery. New York: Thieme Medical Pub; 2015.

45. Ablove RH, Moy OJ, Peimer CA, et al. Pressure changes in Guyon's canal after carpal tunnel release. J Hand Surg Br 1996;21:664–5.

46. Moradi A, Ebrahimzadeh MH, Jupiter JB. Radial tunnel syndrome, diagnostic and treatment dilemma. Arch Bone Jt Surg 2015;3(3):156–62.

47. Cleary CK. Management of radial tunnel syndrome: a therapist's clinical perspective. J Hand Ther 2006;19(2):186–91.

48. Bolster MA, Bakker XR. Radial tunnel syndrome: emphasis on the superficial branch of the radial nerve. J Hand Surg Eur 2009;34(3):343–7.

49. Sotereanos DG, Varitimidis SE, Giannakopoulos PN, et al. Results of surgical treatment for radial tunnel syndrome. J Hand Surg Am 1999;24(3):566–70.

50. Wartenber R. Cheiralgia paresthetica. Neuritis des ramus superficialis nervi radialis. Z Neurol 1932; 141:145–55.

51. Mackinnon SE, Dellon AL. Experimental study of chronic nerve compression. Clinical implications. Hand Clin 1986;2(4):639–50.

52. Bowley MP, Doughty CT. Entrapment neuropathies of the lower extremity. Med Clin North Am 2019; 103(2):371–82.

53. Corriveau M, Lescher JD, Hanna AS. Peroneal nerve decompression. Neurosurg Focus 2018; 44(VideoSuppl1):V6.

54. Marciniak C. Fibular (peroneal) neuropathy: electrodiagnostic features and clinical correlates. Phys Med Rehabil Clin N Am 2013;24(1):121–37.

55. Derr JJ, Micklesen PJ, Robinson LR. Predicting recovery after fibular nerve injury: which electrodiagnostic features are most useful? Am J Phys Med Rehabil 2009;88:547–53.

56. Smith T, Trojaborg W. Clinical and electrophysiological recovery from peroneal palsy. Acta Neurol Scand 1986;74:328–35.

57. Fabre T, Piton C, Andre D, et al. Peroneal nerve entrapment. J Bone Joint Surg Am 1998;80(1): 47–53.

58. McSweeney SC, Cichero M. Tarsal tunnel syndrome- A narrative literature review. Foot (Edinb) 2015; 25(4):244–50.

59. Kinoshita M, Okuda R, Morikawa J, et al. The dorsiflexion-eversion test for diagnosis of tarsal tunnel syndrome. J Bone Joint Surg Am 2001;83-A(12): 1835–9.

60. Trepman E, Kadel NJ, Chisholm K, et al. Effect of foot and ankle position on tarsal tunnel compartment pressure. Foot Ankle Int 1999;20(11):721–6.

61. Mondelli M, Giannini F, Reale F. Clinical and electrophysiological findings and follow-up in tarsal tunnel syndrome. Electroencephalogr Clin Neurophysiol 1998;109(5):418–25.

62. Patel AT, Gaines K, Malamut R, et al. Usefulness of electrodiagnostic techniques in the evaluation of suspected tarsal tunnel syndrome: an evidence-based review. Muscle Nerve 2005;32(2):236–40.

63. Sammarco GJ, Chang L. Outcome of surgical treatment of tarsal tunnel syndrome. Foot Ankle Int 2003; 24(2):125–31.

64. Grundberg AB, Reagan DS. Compression syndromes in reflex sympathetic dystrophy. J Hand Surg 1991;16A:731–6.

65. Monsivais JJ, Baker J, Monsivais D. The association of peripheral nerve compression and reflex sympathetic dystrophy. J Hand Surg 1993;18B:337–8.

66. Placzek JD, Boyer MI, Gelberman RH, et al. Nerve decompression for complex regional pain syndrome type II following upper extremity surgery. J Hand Surg Am 2005;30(1):69–74.

67. Dellon L, Andonian E, Rosson GD. Lower extremity complex regional pain syndrome: long-term outcome after surgical treatment of peripheral pain generators. J Foot Ankle Surg 2010;49(1):33–6.

68. Koh SM, Moate F, Grinsell D. Co-existing carpal tunnel syndrome in complex regional pain syndrome after hand trauma. J Hand Surg Eur 2010;35(3):228–31.

69. Tu Y, Lineaweaver WC, Zheng X, et al. Burn-related peripheral neuropathy: a systematic review. Burns 2017;43(4):693–9.

70. Strong AL, Agarwal S, Cederna PS, et al. Peripheral neuropathy and nerve compression syndromes in burns. Clin Plast Surg 2017;44(4):793–803.

71. Ferguson JS, Franco J, Pollack J, et al. Compression neuropathy: a late finding in the postburn population: a four-year institutional review. J Burn Care Res 2010;31(3):458–61.

72. Smith MA, Muehlberger T, Dellon AL. Peripheral nerve compression associated with low-voltage electrical injury without associated significant cutaneous burn. Plast Reconstr Surg 2002;109(1):137–44.

73. Khedr EM, Khedr T, el-Oteify MA, et al. Peripheral neuropathy in burn patients. Burns 1997;23(7–8): 579–83.

74. Gabriel V, Kowalske KJ, Holavanahalli RK. Assessment of recovery from burn related neuropathy by electrodiagnostic testing. J Burn Care Res 2009; 30:668–74.

75. Dagum AB, Peters WJ, Neligan PC, et al. Severe multiple mononeuropathy in patients with major thermal burns. J Burn Care Rehabil 1993;14(4):440–5.

76. Gibbons CP. Neurological complications of vascular access. J Vasc Access 2015;16(Suppl 9):S73–7.

77. Weise WJ, Bernard DB. Reflex sympathetic dystrophy syndrome of the hand after placement of an arteriovenous graft for hemodialysis. Am J Kidney Dis 1991;18(3):406–8.

78. Miles AM. Vascular steal syndrome and ischaemic monomelic neuropathy: two variants of upper limb ischaemia after haemodialysis vascular access surgery. Nephrol Dial Transplant 1999;14(2):297–300.

79. Harris SA, Brown EA. Patients surviving more than 10 years on haemodialysis. The natural history of the complications of treatment. Nephrol Dial Transplant 1998;13(5):1226–33.

Neuroma

Michael W. Neumeister, MD, FRCSC[a],*, James N. Winters, MD[b]

KEYWORDS

• Neuroma • Pain • Neuroma treatment • Neuroma formation

KEY POINTS

- Neuroma formation occurs because of some degree of nerve injury followed by improper intrinsic nerve repair.
- The cause of neuroma pain is incompletely understood, but appears to be multifactorial in nature, including local and system changes.
- The pathophysiology and genesis of neuroma formation are reviewed.

INTRODUCTION AND HISTORY OF NEUROMA

The peripheral nervous system is delicate and susceptible to injury. Nerve injury occurs from multiple mechanisms: pressure, stretch, chronic irritation, ischemia, crush, sharp transection, iatrogenic, and poor repair of prior injuries.[1] Peripheral nerve injuries resulting in abnormal axonal regeneration and organization lead to neuroma formation. One of the earliest reports on neuromas came from Abroise Pare, in 1634, describing treatment of this entity with massage.[2] In 1811, Odier provided the first gross description of a neuroma as a sensitive bulbous stump of a severed nerve.[3] The first pathologic studies of neuromas followed closely, by Wood in 1828.[4] Neuroma formation represents a challenging scenario for both the patient and the surgeon. Painful symptoms can be both physically and psychologically debilitating, leading to lifestyle modifications and decreased productivity. A multitude of research has been devoted to eliciting the mechanism of neuroma formation, preventative techniques, and treatments.

NERVE ANATOMY

To comprehend nerve injury and neuroma formation, a general knowledge of peripheral nerve anatomy is required. A basic review of the peripheral nerve and its cross-sectional anatomy is highlighted in this article. A more detailed description of the anatomy and physiology of the peripheral nerve, including microscopic and macroscopic structures, can be found in an article by Topp and Boyd.[5]

Nerves are composed of neural, vascular, and connective tissues. Peripheral nerves arise from the central nervous system and may contain both motor and sensory nerve fibers. The cell body of the nerve resides in the brainstem, spinal cord, or dorsal/ventral root ganglia. Individual nerve fibers, known as axons, extend from the cell body to the periphery of the body. The axons may be unmyelinated or surrounded by Schwann cells and a myelin sheath. In cross-section, the axon represents the basic subunit of the nerve. The axon is surrounded by endoneurium, a type of connective tissue. Axons with the same end organ target are grouped together into fascicles, or bundles of axons. Fascicles are surrounded by connective tissue called perineurium. Groups of fascicles make up a peripheral nerve and are surrounded by an internal and external covering of epineurium. Vascular supply to the nerve courses within the nerve's connective tissue and in a longitudinal fashion outside of the epineurium.

NERVE INJURY CLASSIFICATION

Nerve injury can occur because of systemic and local pathologic conditions. Typically, local

a Department of Surgery, Institute for Plastic Surgery, Southern Illinois University School of Medicine, 747 North Rutledge, Suite 357, Baylis Building, Springfield, IL 62702, USA; b Institute for Plastic Surgery, Southern Illinois University School of Medicine, 747 North Rutledge, Suite 357, Baylis Building, Springfield, IL 62702, USA
* Corresponding author.
E-mail address: mneumeister@siumed.edu

Clin Plastic Surg 47 (2020) 279–283
https://doi.org/10.1016/j.cps.2019.12.008
0094-1298/20/Published by Elsevier Inc.

pathologic conditions, such as compression, stretch, blunt and sharp trauma, or iatrogenic injuries, are of greater interest to the surgeon. Injury to a nerve may vary in severity and involve one or more anatomic components: myelin, axon, or connective tissue. The 2 most commonly used nerve injury grading systems are the Seddon and Sunderland classifications.[6]

In 1943, Seddon[7] classified nerve injuries into 3 groups: neurapraxia, axonotmesis, and neurotmesis. Neurapraxia involves local myelin damage; however, the axon is preserved, and no distal degeneration occurs. Axonotmesis results as a loss of continuity of axons with varying degrees of connective tissue damage. Neurotmesis involves complete transection of the nerve with damage to axons, endoneurium, perineurium, and epineurium. Wallerian degeneration of the distal nerve occurs with both axonotmesis and neurotmesis.

In 1951, Sunderland[8] further expanded this classification system to involve 5 degrees of neural injury. Sunderland's first- and fifth-degree nerve injuries are equivalent to neurapraxia and neurotmesis, respectively. Second-, third-, and fourth-degree nerve injuries are variations of Seddon's axonotmesis based off an inside-out injury pattern. Second-degree injury involves axonal injury with preservation of endoneurium, perineurium, and epineurium. Full recovery is expected from second-degree injury. Third-degree injury includes disruption of the axon and endoneurium, with partial recovery expected. In fourth-degree injury, the axon, endoneurium, and perineurium all incur damage, but the epineurium remains intact. Fourth- and fifth-degree injuries require surgical repair because little to no recovery can be expected.

Mackinnon and Dellon[9] later added a sixth degree of nerve injury to Sunderland's classification. Sixth-degree injury represents a mixed picture nerve injury. Along a given segment of nerve, 1 section might sustain a first-degree injury, but another portion of the nerve sustained a fourth-degree injury. The exact pattern of nerve injury is often difficult to determine, relying on both clinical examination and electromyography findings.

NERVE DEGENERATION AND REGENERATION

Axonal transection triggers a sequence of events within the nerve proximally and distally to the injury site. Proximally, the cell body undergoes chromatolysis, a reorganization of rough endoplasmic reticulum and shift in metabolic production from neurotransmitters to structural materials for axon growth and repair.[6,10] The proximal axon undergoes traumatic degeneration to the next node of Ranvier. Distally the transected nerve undergoes Wallerian degeneration. Macrophages and Schwann cells phagocytize the myelin debris at the distal axon.[11]

Schwann cells align in columns to form bands of Bugner with nerve growth factor receptors present on the surface acting as a scaffold or tunnel for the regenerating axon.[12–14] The distal nerve and surrounding cells produce a gradient of neurotrophic factors and neurite-promoting factors to guide axon regeneration in a process known as neurotropism.[15] The regenerating axon detects permissive or inhibitory signals from the microenvironment via sprouts and growth cones, which guide direction of growth based off motor versus sensory, topographic, tissue, and end-organ signaling specificity.[16] The neurotrophic growth factors important for nerve survival are transported retrogradely to the cell body. Neurite-promoting factors, laminin and fibronectin, promote growth extension of the axons toward the distal target.[17–19] Additional growth factors and contact factors promote cell migration and nerve generation. The process of nerve generation proceeds at roughly 1 mm/d or 1 inch/mo.[20–22]

PATHOPHYSIOLOGY AND CLASSIFICATION OF NEUROMA FORMATION

Nerve injuries can result from pressure, stretch, chronic irritation, ischemia, crush injury, sharp transection, iatrogenic, and poor repair of prior injuries.[1] All neuroma formation occurs because of some degree of nerve injury followed by improper intrinsic nerve repair.[23]

Neuromas can be divided into 2 main categories: terminal neuromas and neuroma-in-continuity (NIC). Terminal neuromas result from complete transection of a nerve or amputation of a distal extremity. This injury pattern is classified as neurotmesis or fifth-degree Sunderland. In this case, the distal axon is too far away for neurotrophic and neurite-promoting factors to be sensed by the proximal axon. The proximal axon cannot progress toward its distal target, resulting in unorganized fascicular overgrowth at its end.[24] NIC results from damage to the perineurium in a Sunderland fourth-degree or Mackinnon mixed injury. Damage to the perineurium allows fascicular escape and disorganized nerve repair of axons in the surrounding epineurial tissue, along with deposition of scar tissue by fibroblasts.[25] An NIC following nerve graft repair is also possible secondary to defect length, scarring, or mismatched fascicles, permitting only some fascicles to regenerate appropriately.[26] Disorganized patterns of axons with accompanying proliferating fibroblasts, Schwann cells, and blood vessels are characteristic findings of neuroma on microscopic analysis.[27]

The exact incidence of neuroma formation after injury is unknown. However, postoperative, painful neuroma rates range from 1% to 30%.[28–31] The amount of axoplasmic flow, ratio of fascicles to epineurial tissue, and nutritional status of the peripheral nerve appear to affect neuroma formation.[32–34] Diagnosis of neuroma is clinically characterized by pain associated with scar, altered sensation within the given nerve distribution, and a Tinel sign. Ultrasound sonography can help determine the exact location of neuroma and reproduce symptoms.[3]

Neuropathic pain associated with neuroma can be classified into 4 types according to Sood and Elliot[35]: spontaneous pain, pain with pressure over neuroma, pain on movement of adjacent joints, and hypersensitivity with light skin touch. The cause of neuroma pain is incompletely understood as well, but appears to be multifactorial in nature, including local and system changes. Repetitive mechanical irritation owing to tethering scar tissue or compression in an area of thin overlying tissue can result in persistent pain. Increased scarring and myofibroblast proliferation have been associated with neuropathic pain. Myofibroblasts have been postulated to cause pain by direct contraction around surrounding nerve tissue and release of alpha smooth muscle actin.[36–38] Abnormal accumulation of sodium and potassium channels within the neuroma has been found to account for hyperexcitability and spontaneous discharge from injured nerves.[39–42] Local tissue damage surrounding neuromas can result in an inflammatory response thought to chemically sensitize nociceptive A-delta and C fibers resulting in transmission of painful stimuli.[43–46] Melzack and Wall[47] proposed another mechanism for neuroma pain termed gate control theory representing a complex interplay between the substantia gelatinosa, dorsal column of the spinal cord, and T cells in the dorsal horn. Reorganization and release of inflammatory cytokines, such as tumor necrosis factor-alpha and interleukin-1, within the central nervous system have also been proposed as mechanisms for neuroma pain.[48–51]

The pain pathway surrounding symptomatic neuromas remains complex and poorly understood. Multiple pharmacologic therapies have been used to try to break this chronic and unpredictable pain cycle. Topical therapy and neuromodulation are often attempted before any surgical intervention. More than 150 surgical interventions have been used to attempt neuroma prevention, treatment, and pain control. Burying the proximal severed nerve end in muscle or bone was the traditional mainstay of neuroma prevention. Neurolysis, nerve wrapping, neuroma resection, and reconstruction. Emerging techniques involving targeted muscle reinnervation and regenerative peripheral nerve interfaces have shown promising results in neuroma prevention and management and are discussed in subsequent articles.[52–54] A comprehensive understanding of nerve anatomy, injury, and repair techniques should be used when dealing with neuroma formation and its physical manifestations.

In summary, neuroma formation occurs after nerves are subject to significant damage. The injury may be from a sharp object, blunt trauma, or a traction injury. Complete nerve injuries result in end neuromas, where, as partial injuries, result in NICs . Sprouting axons engulfed in a disarray of fibrosis form a disorganized mass of small, unmyelinated minifascicles. The painful neuromas are associated with enhanced alpha smooth muscle actin.[37] The greater the intensity of the alpha smooth muscle actin, the more painful the neuroma. Also, the size of the neuroma is influenced by the nutritional status of the nerve, the axoplasmic flow, and the extent of Schwann cell and myofibroblast proliferation.[33]

DISCLOSURE

Nothing to disclose.

REFERENCES

1. Watson J, Gonzalez M, Romero A, et al. Neuromas of the hand and upper extremity. J Hand Surg 2010;35(3):499–510.
2. Vernadakis AJ, Koch H, MacKinnon SE. Management of neuromas. Clin Plast Surg 2003;30:247–68.
3. Provost N, Bonaldi VM, Sarazin L, et al. Amputation stump neuroma: ultrasound features. J Clin Ultrasound 1997;25:85–9.
4. Burchiel KJ, Ochoa J. Surgical management of posttraumatic neuropathic pain. Neurosurg Clin N Am 1991;2:117–26.
5. Topp KS, Boyd BS. Peripheral nerve: from the microscopic functional unit of the axon to the biomechanically loaded macroscopic structure. J Hand Ther 2012;25:142–52.
6. Lee SK, Wolfe SW. Peripheral nerve injury and repair. J Am Acad Orthop Surg 2000;8:243–52.
7. Seddon HJ. Surgical disorders of the peripheral nerves. Baltimore (MD): Williams & Wilkins; 1972. p. 68–88.

8. Sunderland S. Nerve injuries and their repair: a critical appraisal. New York: Churchill Livingstone; 1991.

9. Mackinnon SE, Dellon AL. Surgery of the peripheral nerve. New York: Thieme Medical Publishers; 1988. p. 115–29.

10. Grafstein B. The nerve cell body response to axotomy. Exp Neurol 1975;48:32–51.

11. Stoll G, Muller HW. Nerve injury, axonal degeneration and neural regeneration: basic insights. Brain Pathol 1999;9(2):313–25.

12. Johnson EM Jr, Taniuchi M, DiStefano PS. Expression and possible function of nerve growth factor receptors on Schwann cells. Trends Neurosci 1988;11:299–304.

13. Taniuchi M, Clark HB, Johnson EM Jr. Induction of nerve growth factor receptor in Schwann cells after axotomy. Proc Natl Acad Sci U S A 1986;83:4094–8.

14. Taniuchi M, Clark HB, Schweitzer JB, et al. Expression of nerve growth factor receptors by Schwann cells of axotomized peripheral nerves: ultrastructural location, suppression by axonal contact, and binding properties. J Neurosci 1988;8:664–81.

15. Cajal RS. Degeneration and regeneration of the nervous system, vol. 1. London: Oxford University Press; 1928.

16. Lundborg G. A 25-year perspective of peripheral nerve surgery: evolving neuroscientific concepts of clinical significance. J Hand Surg 2000;25A:391–414.

17. Davis GE, Engvall E, Varon S, et al. Human amnion membrane as a substratum for cultured peripheral and central nervous system neurons. Brain Res 1987;430:1–10.

18. Manthorpe M, Engvall E, Ruoslahti E, et al. Laminin promotes neuritic regeneration from cultured peripheral and central neurons. J Cell Biol 1983;97:1882–90.

19. Davis GE, Manthorpe M, Williams LR, et al. Characterization of a laminin-containing neurite-promoting factor and a neuronotrophic factor from peripheral nerve and related sources. Ann N Y Acad Sci 1986;486:194–205.

20. Yan Y, Johnson PJ, Glaus SW, et al. A novel model for evaluating nerve regeneration in the composite tissue transplant: the murine heterotopic limb transplant. Hand (N Y) 2011;6:304–12.

21. Morisaki S, Kawai Y, Umeda M, et al. In vivo assessment of peripheral nerve regeneration by diffusion tensor imaging. J Magn Reson Imaging 2011;33:535–42.

22. Lehmann HC, Zhang J, Mori S, et al. Diffusion tensor imaging to assess axonal regeneration in peripheral nerves. Exp Neurol 2010;223:238–44.

23. Brogan DM, Kakar S. Management of neuromas of the upper extremity. Hand Clin 2013;29:409–20.

24. Maggi SP, Lowe JB 3rd, Mackinnon SE. Pathophysiology of nerve injury. Clin Plast Surg 2003;30(2):109–26.

25. Yüksel F, Kişlaoğlu E, Durak N, et al. Prevention of painful neuromas by epineural ligatures, flaps and grafts. Br J Plast Surg 1997;50:182–5.

26. Meek MF, Coert JH, Robinson PH. Poor results after nerve grafting in the upper extremity: quo vadis? Microsurgery 2005;25(5):396–402.

27. Badalamente MA, Hurst LC, Ellstein J, et al. The pathobiology of human neuromas: an electron microscopic and biochemical study. J Hand Surg 1985;10(1):49–53.

28. Fisher GT, Boswick JA Jr. Neuroma formation following digital amputations. J Trauma 1983;23(2):136–42.

29. Lacoux PA, Crombie IK, Macrae WA. Pain in traumatic upper limb amputees in Sierra Leone. Pain 2002;99(1–2):309–12.

30. Geraghty TJ, Jones LE. Painful neuromata following upper limb amputation. Prosthet Orthot Int 1996;20(3):176–81.

31. Van der Avoort DJ, Hovius SE, Selles RW, et al. The incidence of symptomatic neuroma in amputation and neurorrhaphy patients. J Plast Reconstr Aesthet Surg 2013;66(10):1330–4.

32. Mackinnon SE, Dellon AL, Hudson AR, et al. Alteration of neuroma formation by manipulation of its microenvironment. Plast Reconstr Surg 1985;76(3):345–53.

33. Nath RK, Mackinnon SE. Management of neuromas in the hand. Hand Clin 1996;12(4):745–56.

34. Dellon AL, Mackinnon SE. Susceptibility of the superficial sensory branch of the radial nerve to form painful neuromas. J Hand Surg 1984;9(1):42–5.

35. Sood MK, Elliot D. Treatment of painful neuromas of the hand and wrist by relocation into the pronator quadratus muscle. J Hand Surg Br 1998;23(2):214–9.

36. Mavrogenis AF, Pavlakis K, Stamatoukou A, et al. Current treatment concepts for neuromas-in-continuity. Injury 2008;39(Suppl 3):S43–8.

37. Yan H, Gao W, Pan Z, et al. The expression of α-SMA in the painful traumatic neuroma: potential role in the pathobiology of neuropathic pain. J Neurotrauma 2012;29(18):2791–7.

38. Weng W, Zhao B, Lin D, et al. Significance of alpha smooth muscle actin expression in traumatic painful neuromas: a pilot study in rats. Sci Rep 2016;6:23828.

39. Burchiel KJ, Ochoa JL. Pathophysiology of injured axons. Neurosurg Clin N Am 1991;2:105–16.

40. England JD, Happel LT, Kline DG, et al. Sodium channel accumulation in humans with painful neuromas. Neurology 1996;47:272–6.

41. England JD, Happel LT, Liu ZP, et al. Abnormal distributions of potassium channels in human neuromas. Neurosci Lett 1998;255:37–40.

42. Devor M, Govrin-Lippmann R, Angelides K. Na+ channel immunolocalization in peripheral mammalian axons and changes following nerve injury and neuroma formation. J Neurosci 1993;13: 1976–92.

43. Orza F, Boswell MV, Rosenberg SK. Neuropathic pain: review of mechanisms and pharmacologic management. NeuroRehabilitation 2000;14:15–23.

44. Nicholson B. Gabapentin use in neuropathic pain syndromes. Acta Neurol Scand 2000;101:359–71.

45. Zimmerman M. Review–pathobiology of neuropathic pain. Eur J Pharmacol 2001;429:23–37.

46. Dahl JB, Mathiesen O, Moiniche S. 'Protective premedication': an option with gabapentin and related drugs? A review of gabapentin and pregabalin in the treatment of post-operative pain. Acta Anaesthesiol Scand 2004;48:1130–6.

47. Melzack R, Wall PD. Pain mechanisms: a new theory. Science 1965;150:971–9.

48. Pruimboom L, van Dam AC. Chronic pain: a non-use disease. Med Hypotheses 2007;68:506–11.

49. Sorkin LS, Doom CM. Epineurial application of TNF elicits an acute mechanical hyperalgesia in the awake rat. J Peripher Nerv Syst 2000;5:96–100.

50. Sommer C, Schmidt C, George A. Hyperalgesia in experimental neuropathy is dependent on the TNF receptor 1. Exp Neurol 1998;151:138–42.

51. Ignatowski TA, Covey WC, Knight PR, et al. Brain-derived TNF alpha mediates neuropathic pain. Brain Res 1999;841:70–7.

52. Valerio IL, Dumanian GA, Jordan SW, et al. Preemptive treatment of phantom and residual limb pain with targeted muscle reinnervation at the time of major limb amputation. J Am Coll Surg 2019;228(3): 217–26.

53. Dumanian GA, Potter BK, Mioton LM, et al. Targeted muscle reinnervation treats neuroma and phantom pain in major limb amputees: a randomized clinical trial. Ann Surg 2019;270(2):238–46.

54. Woo SL, Kung TA, Brown DL, et al. Regenerative peripheral nerve interfaces for the treatment of postamputation neuroma pain: a pilot study. Plast Reconstr Surg Glob Open 2016;4(12):e1038.

Targeted Muscle Reinnervation for Treatment of Neuropathic Pain

Ava G. Chappell, MD, Sumanas W. Jordan, MD, PhD,
Gregory A. Dumanian, MD*

KEYWORDS

- Neuropathic pain • Neuroma • Targeted muscle re innervation • Chronic postoperative pain
- Phantom limb pain

KEY POINTS

- Targeted muscle reinnervation (TMR) is a reproducible technique for effective treatment and prevention of neuropathic pain.
- The fundamental concept of TMR is to give severed nerve endings a place to go and something to do, which facilitates healing of these severed peripheral nerves.
- Methods to encourage normal healing of severed peripheral nerves instead of burying the nerve ending in surrounding tissue, will lead to improved outcomes of neuroma treatment.
- Neuropathic pain is a surgically treatable condition.

INTRODUCTION

Chronic pain after surgery leads to significant disability worldwide. Although there are numerous established causes of chronic postsurgical pain, neuropathic pain due to peripheral nerve injury is a known contributor. In some proportion of peripheral nerve injuries, symptomatic neuromas—disorganized axons encased in scar—form and may be exquisitely painful to light touch, pressure, vibration, and extreme temperatures or even at rest. Many management strategies have been proposed, yet symptomatic neuromas remain a challenge.[1] Pharmacologic therapy with antidepressants, anticonvulsants, opioids, and topical anesthetics have variable efficacy and places patients at risk for opioid dependence.[2–5] Behavioral strategies include desensitization protocols, cognitive behavioral therapy, and group psychotherapy.[6] Interventional methods for neuropathic pain include minimally invasive treatments of the injured nerve with radiofrequency ablation, perineural injection with alcohol or corticosteroids, regional blocks, spinal cord stimulation, transcutaneous electrical nerve stimulation, and direct operative handling of the injured nerves.[7–11]

Whenever possible, nerve injuries should be repaired. When this is not feasible, such as in the case of an absent distal nerve stump or in the case of a failed reconstruction, direct operative handling of the injured nerve is preferred. For decades, the standard surgical approach for symptomatic neuroma has been neuroma excision and relocation to a more favorable position, commonly buried into bone or muscle, with the hope that the recurrent neuroma would be hidden and asymptomatic.[12,13] In contrast, more recent strategies are based on the concept of providing severed axons an end organ—somewhere to go and something to do. One such technique is targeted muscle reinnervation (TMR), a nerve transfer procedure that treats pain via direct nerve to nerve healing.

First performed by the senior author G.A. Dumanian in 2002, TMR is defined as the coaptation of

Division of Plastic Surgery, Department of Surgery, Northwestern Feinberg School of Medicine, 675 North Street Clair, Suite 19-250, Chicago, IL 60611, USA
* Corresponding author.
E-mail address: gdumania@nm.org
Twitter: @gregdumanian (G.A.D.)

Clin Plastic Surg 47 (2020) 285–293
https://doi.org/10.1016/j.cps.2020.01.002

Table 1
Classifications of peripheral nerve injury

Seddon (1947)[38]	Sunderland (1951)[39]	Mackinnon (1988)[40]	Summary
Neuropraxia	1		Local conduction block with possible segmental demyelination. No injury to axons, so no regeneration. Remyelination and complete recovery by 12 wk postinjury.
Axonotmesis	2		Axonal injury occurs. Intact endoneurium, perineurium, and epineurium. Distal segment undergoes wallerian degeneration. Proximal nerve fibers regenerate at 1mm/day. Full recovery possible unless distance of injury from motor end plate far and prolonged denervation of the receptor prevents motor recovery.
	3		Axonal injury occurs. Wallerian degeneration combined with fibrosis of endoneurium. Perineurium and epineurium intact. Incomplete recovery likely, due to scar within endoneurium hinders regenerating fibers interaction with correct end organs.
	4		Nerve-in-continuity but injury causes complete scar block. Only epineurium intact. Recovery only possible if scar is surgically removed and nerve repaired or grafted.
Neurotmesis	5		Nerve completely divided and must be surgically repaired before regeneration can occur.
		6	Mixed nerve injury. Combination of any of the types of injuries 1–5, and different levels of injury occur at different regions of the nerve.

cut peripheral nerves to a newly divided nearby motor nerve branch.[14] The fascicles of the proximal nerve grow into motor end plates, and likely into proprioceptors and other sensory end organs, to reinnervate the target muscle.[15,16] TMR has evolved from a technique to improve intuitive prosthesis control in amputees to a technique to treat and prevent neuropathic pain from peripheral neuroma. A recent randomized clinical trial in the treatment of chronic postamputation pain demonstrated that healing a nerve ending with TMR had better patient-reported outcomes for residual limb pain and phantom limb pain at 18 months of follow-up, compared with neuroma excision and muscle burying.[17] Furthermore, a cohort study of patients who underwent TMR at the time of amputation compared with unselected amputees from the general population demonstrated significantly fewer TMR patients with moderate to severe residual limb and phantom limb pain by multiple measures.[9] Additional clinical data have shown that pain outcomes from nonamputees with neuroma pain who were treated with TMR are better than those who were treated with standard neuroma excision and hiding.[18–20] There is growing acceptance for TMR as an effective surgical strategy for management of neuropathic pain. TMR may be performed by any surgeon with knowledge of peripheral nerve anatomy and nerve dissection experience.

PATHOPHYSIOLOGY

Traumatic neuromas are regions of nerve swelling/inflammation that can occur in any part of the body after nerve injury. Nerve injury can be direct—transection during dissection, or indirect—stretched or crushed during retraction. The physiologic response to axonal injury is axon sprouting and regeneration from the proximal segment and wallerian degeneration of the distal segment. Seddon's classification distinguishes types of nerve injury in terms of neuropraxia, axonotmesis, and

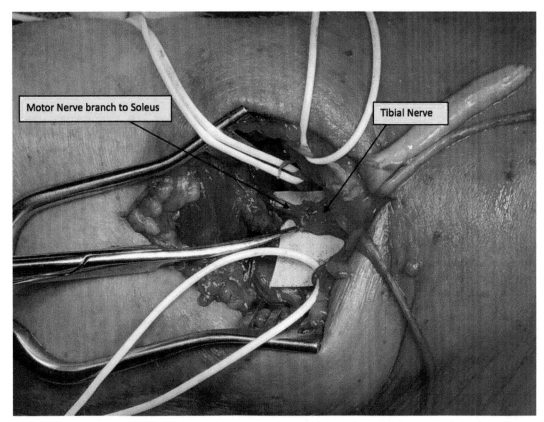

Fig. 1. TMR nerve transfers for BKA. Under loupe magnification (2.5×), the tibial nerve was divided and coapted to the motor nerve to the soleus with 6-0 Prolene interrupted sutures (*yellow background*). The common peroneal nerve was transposed medial to lateral gastrocnemius tendon and coapted to the lateral gastrocnemius motor nerve and the motor nerve to the lateral gastrocnemius (*vessel loops at the top*). The 2 components of the sural nerve were coapted to 2 separate motor nerves to the medial gastrocnemius muscle. The total tourniquet time was 45 minutes.

neurotmesis.[21] Sunderland further grades nerve injury based on expected recovery. With intact or repaired perineurium and epineurium, sprouting axons find a distal target and eventually prune excess axons. For Sunderland grade 4 or greater, however, sprouting axons fail to connect to a distal segment or target organ and become encased in scar, thus forming neuromas, specifically neuroma-in-continuity in axonotmesis or end neuroma in neurotmesis (**Table 1**).[21]

Within the neuroma bulb, the authors' data have shown that the axons are sensory, with no motor staining found.[22] The model is that the sensory nerves continue to seek a distal nerve attempting to heal and reinnervate, whereas without Schwann cells and other trophic factors, the motor axons recede back toward the spine.[22] This is consistent with clinical peripheral nerve surgery that motor outcomes tend to be less successful than sensory recoveries for mixed nerve repairs. Furthermore, it has been the authors' experience that cut pure motor nerves do not form neuromas, a key to TMR.

Histologically, TMR restores axon count, size, and myelination in a rabbit amputation model.[23] In the authors' clinical experience, reestablishment of muscle function can be detected clinically in more than 95% of nerve transfers.[23] Electromyography after transhumeral TMR has demonstrated physiologic synaptic inputs to reinnervated muscles.[24] What is unclear is the fascicles that fail to find a distal target after nerve transfer due to obvious mismatch in size and fascicle numbers between donor and recipient nerves. This size mismatch undoubtedly led to the slow adoption of TMR as a surgical technique. It is hypothesized that the large denervated block of muscle near the nerve coaptation site is a source of additional end organs to soak up escaping axons.

PRESENTATION AND DIAGNOSIS

A typical patient presenting with a symptomatic neuroma may describe the pain as electric, shooting, or burning. The pain may be associated with light touch or pressure or changes in weather and temperature or be without any provocation at all. Neuropathic pain may affect sleep quality, such as the common complaint of night waking in carpal tunnel syndrome; mood; ambulation; and, for the amputee, prosthetic use. Patients may present with high opioid tolerances. For the amputee, postamputation pain may include residual limb (or stump) pain, phantom limb pain, back pain, and hip pain.[25,26] To clarify distinctions between pain syndromes, residual limb pain is defined as pain local to the residual limb, often due to a neuroma[27]; phantom limb pain is defined as unpleasant or painful sensations perceived in the missing limb, thought to be a complex interplay between the neuroma and several levels of the central nervous system[28–30]; and chronic pain is defined as pain lasting greater than 6 months and causing physical debilitation and decreased quality of life.[31] A simple history for pain includes an assessment of intensity on an 11-point numerical rating scale (0 is no pain and 10 is the worst pain imaginable) and an assessment of frequency.

For the patient who presents with intolerable symptomatic neuroma, the clinician must address the nerve injury. Symptomatic neuromas by definition are associated with injury to a mixed or sensory nerve. The clinical diagnosis is made as a combination of the chief complaint as chronic pain postamputation/surgery/injury and a focused physical examination. The clinician asks patients to point to a location on their extremity where the pain is the greatest, and the patients can quickly identify this painful spot. There likely is a Tinel sign when this spot is tapped by the clinician, or patients may experience severe acute pain when this region is palpated. The nerve leading to this neuroma often is excitable to palpation along its length. Imaging typically is not necessary or recommended for the work-up of intolerable neuropathic pain.

Injections with local anesthesia may be performed to confirm that treatment of the injured nerve will lead to a change in symptoms. An inability to improve symptoms temporarily with an anesthetic injection should give both surgeon

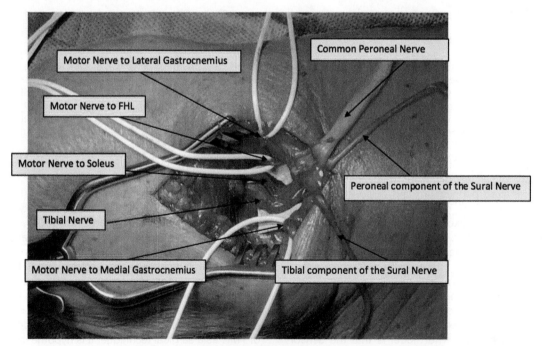

Fig. 2. Case example, a 68-year-old woman one year post op left below knee amputation presented with persistent left leg pain in the common peroneal nerve distribution. Despite medical treatment with hydrocodone and gabapentin, her residual limb pain and phantom limb pain were severe, and she was unable to tolerate wearing a prosthesis. After discussion of risks and benefits, she wished to pursue with TMR surgery for her chronic postamputation pain and phantom limb pain. Prior to nerve transfers from a midline posterior incision, donor nerves are prepared (*right, from top of figure to bottom*): the common peroneal nerve, the peroneal component of the sural nerve, and the tibial component of sural nerve. The tibial nerve in the center of the field has not undergone neurotomy. Recipient motor branches are shown with vessel loops (*from top to bottom*): motor nerve to the lateral gastrocnemius, motor nerve to the flexor hallucis longus (FHL), and 2 motor branches to the medial gastrocnemius. The motor nerve to the soleus is in the center of the field.

and patient pause before beginning surgery. A few patients have centralization of their pain, with a complete lack of pain reduction after neuroma treatment. Fortunately, these completely centralized pain patients are infrequent but may be more common as the time from amputation or injury increases over decades. Diagnostic nerve blocks are even more important as the surgeon attempts to localize neuromas of the head and neck, trunk, or in nonamputees. Injections can be done for thin patients in the office, but heavier patients may require interventional radiology for an ultrasound-guided procedure.

SURGICAL TECHNIQUE
Targeted Muscle Reinnervation for the Amputee (ie, Treatment of End Neuroma)

The procedural method of TMR has been well described in the literature for the various levels of upper and lower extremity amputation.[22,32–34] The fundamental technical steps of TMR are (1) nerve identification and preparation to healthy fascicles, (2) recipient motor nerve identification, and (3) tension-free coaptation. Common nerve transfers are listed in **Tables 2–8** for convenience.

In the preoperative area, the location of painful Tinel signs are marked. In amputees or patients who have undergone previous peripheral nerve manipulation, the locations of the neuromas may not be intuitive from anatomy alone. Although neuroma excision is not necessary because the nerves are treated proximally, the trajectory of the nerve toward the Tinel sign can be helpful during nerve identification. Smooth Gerald forceps work well for handling larger nerves and microsurgical forceps are used for small motor branches. Once the donor nerves are identified, nearby motor nerve branches are identified via anatomy and/or a handheld nerve stimulator (Checkpoint

Table 2
Donor nerves and potential motor nerve targets for delayed below-knee amputation (prone, 1-incision approach, posterior midline only)

Nerve	Primary Muscle Target
Common peroneal, possible sparing of motor nerve to anterior tibial	Lateral gastrocnemius
Tibial	Soleus
Medial sural	Soleus, or medial gastrocnemius
Lateral sural	Flexor hallucis longus

Table 3
Donor nerves and potential motor nerve targets for acute below-knee amputation (supine)

Nerve	Primary Muscle Target
Deep peroneal	Tibialis anterior
Superficial peroneal	Peroneus longus
Tibial	Soleus, or flexor digitorum longus
Medial sural[a]	Medial gastrocnemius
Lateral sural[a]	Lateral gastrocnemius

[a] Indicated when significant soft tissue dissection is not required.

Surgical, Cleveland, Ohio). These nerve stimulators are recommended becuase they do not exhaust motor nerves, can locate intramuscular motor points, and enable stimulation of motor nerves at more than 45 minutes tourniquet time. These motor points serve as potential recipients of TMR nerve transfer. Sometimes, finding motor points involves intramuscular dissection. The motor nerve branches are divided 1 mm to 2 mm from the muscle entry point. The mixed nerve proximal segment is coapted to the surgically divided distal segment of the motor nerve branch using standard technique, under loupe magnification with 2 to 3 6-0 or 7-0 polypropylene epineural sutures. The coaptation should be under no tension with minimal redundancy. Size mismatch is common. If encountered, pure sensory nerves are treated in the similar manner.

In the acute setting, the major peripheral nerves have been exposed and divided by the resecting team. It is important to communicate to the resecting team not to perform a traction neurectomy if that is their standard practice. Access to known motor nerves may require a position change, or intramuscular dissection may be performed to identify nearby motor points, which is a term

Table 4
Donor nerves and potential motor nerve targets for above-knee amputations

Nerve	Primary Muscle Target
Saphenous	Vastus medialis
Peroneal component of sciatic	Biceps femoris
Tibial component of sciatic	Semitendinosus/ semimembranosus
Posterior femoral cutaneous	Biceps femoris (distal motor branch)

Table 5
Donor nerves and possible motor nerve targets for shoulder disarticulation nerve transfer

Nerve	Primary Muscle Target
Radial	Thoracodorsal
Musculocutaneous	Superior pectoral to clavicular head
Median	Middle pectoral
Ulnar	Lateral pectoral

Table 7
Donor nerves and possible motor nerve targets for transradial nerve transfer

Donor Nerve	Primary Muscle Target
Median	Flexor digitorum superficialis Flexor digitorum profundus Brachioradialis
Ulnar	Flexor carpi ulnaris
Radial nerve: superficial branch	Pronator quadratus Flexor digitorum profundus

used to describe tiny excitable nerve fascicles found within a muscle. The decision to stay within the wound to perform TMR or to perform a position change and to use a new incision is left to the discretion of the TMR surgeon, with pros and cons to both strategies (**Fig. 1** and **2**).

Targeted Muscle Reinnervation for the Nonamputee (ie, Treatment of End Neuroma and Unreconstructable Neuroma-in-Continuity)

TMR for the nonamputee is indicated for patients with neuroma formation and failed prior reconstruction or nerve gaps greater than 3 cm to 5 cm. Again, the neuroma is located by palpation with the assistance of the patient preoperatively. The injured nerves are exposed proximally, and nearby motor targets are identified, as described previously. For the lower leg, for example, the authors recommend TMR to the extensor digitorum longus for nerves in the lateral compartment and the lateral gastrocnemius in the superficial posterior compartment.[34] Because the deep posterior compartment is inaccessible in the nonamputee patient, this is not used as a motor target for TMR.

Further illustrating the utility and principles of TMR to treat symptomatic neuroma, the authors have performed TMR to treat chronic abdominal wall pain due to ilioinguinal nerve injury after inguinal hernia repair. Chronic abdominal wall neuroma pain is an underrecognized condition. Whereas the standard procedure is ilioinguinal neurectomy, an alternative approach is to treat the injured nerve by giving the nerve somewhere to go and something to do. Recently, the use of processed nerve allograft has been described to serve as interposition graft after neuroma excision when the neuroma can be located.[17] When the nerve cannot be reconstructed, the ilioinguinal nerve is dissected proximally toward the spine and coapted to a motor nerve to the internal oblique and transversus abdominis, that is, TMR. This procedure has shown excellent pain outcomes in the authors' hands (see **Fig. 3** for clinical photograph of abdominal wall TMR).

POSTOPERATIVE CARE

For patients presenting for chronic pain or prosthetic control, patients typically are observed overnight for pain control and discharged to home. Postoperative blocks may be performed at the discretion of the regional anesthesia team. If a patient's pain is well controlled on oral pain medication and the patient wishes to be discharged on the same day of surgery, there is no contraindication. Postoperative swelling is minimized with

Table 6
Donor nerves and possible motor nerve targets for transhumeral nerve transfer

Nerve	Primary Muscle Target
Median	Medial head of biceps
Ulnar	Brachialis
Radial	Lateral head of triceps
Medial antebrachial cutaneous/lateral antebrachial cutaneous	Any local muscles

Table 8
Donor nerves and possible motor nerve targets for the nonamputee with an unreconstructable neuroma

Donor Sensory Nerve	Primary Muscle Target
Deep peroneal	Extensor digitorum longus
Superficial peroneal	Peroneus longus
Lateral sural	Lateral gastrocnemius
Medial sural	Lateral or medial gastrocnemius

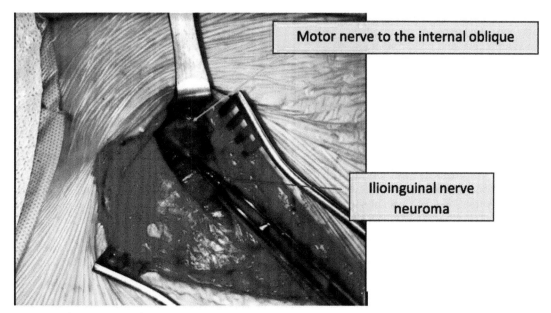

Fig. 3. TMR for treatment of recurrent ilioinguinal neuroma. The neuroma is excised and the freshened ending of the ilioinguinal nerve coapted to a freshly divided motor nerve to the internal oblique.

compressive dressings. A splint or other additional form of immobilization is not needed. Patients can restart wearing their original prosthesis when their surgical incisions are healed and postoperative edema has resolved, at approximately 4 weeks to 6 weeks after surgery.[35] It is important that patients are informed prior to surgery that after surgery they may experience numbness in the residual limb, dysesthesia, and even transfer sensation in the skin over reinnervated muscles. Additionally, for patients with phantom limb pain, some may have an exacerbation of symptoms lasting up to 4 weeks to 6 weeks after surgery until new nerve connections have formed.[32] Internal data support the improvement in established phantom limb pain approximately 6 months after TMR.

For patients presenting for TMR at the time of amputation, postoperative care and discharge planning are dictated by needs related to the amputation itself. No special instructions are necessary because of the TMR portion of the case. Once evidence of muscle reinnervation has occurred, the patient may practice contracting the reinnervated muscles.

DISCUSSION

Postamputation pain syndromes may include residual limb pain, phantom limb pain, back pain, and hip pain and are a significant concern for the amputee population, with prevalence ranging between 50% and 90% of amputees.[25,26] Symptomatic neuromas are a major driver of residual limb pain and phantom limb pain.[36] Moreover, symptomatic neuromas may occur with any injury to mixed and sensory peripheral nerves. Fundamentally, the injured sensory axons are sprouting in an attempt to find an end organ. Modern techniques, including nerve repair, nerve autografts and allografts, regenerative peripheral nerve interfaces, and TMR, all aim to satisfy the need for an end organ.[8,10,18] TMR resolves sprouting and associated painful symptoms by direct nerve-to-nerve healing.

Recent studies have shown that TMR can address the chronic postamputation pain problem. TMR results in clinically meaningful improvement in residual limb and phantom limb pain by an average of 3.7 and 3.6 of 10 points, respectively, at last follow-up.[17] TMR has shown improvement in postamputation neuroma pain even months to years after the initial amputation, although learned behaviors from chronic pain are difficult to reverse.[17,37] As a prophylactic measure, TMR performed at the time of initial amputation leads to significantly lower residual limb and phantom limb pain scores (1 of 10 for both) compared with the general amputee population (4 of 10 and 5 of 10, respectively).[9] TMR more than doubled the proportion of amputees reporting zero pain and nearly halved the proportion of amputees reporting severe pain (7–10 of 10).[9] Thus, the indication for TMR extends beyond prosthesis control for upper extremity amputees and includes the treatment and prevention of symptomatic neuroma pain in amputees and nonamputees.

SUMMARY

Postoperative neuropathic pain causes chronic disability to many people globally. As access to surgical care increases, clinicians must be aware of the potential postoperative pain complications. Chronic neuroma pain frequently is misdiagnosed, overlooked, or masked with opioids. Surgical techniques and principles from TMR can apply to successfully treat neuroma pain at sites of amputation as well as other postsurgical sites.

CODING

International Classification of Diseases, Tenth Revision	D36.10 Neuroma
Current Procedural Terminology	64905 Nerve pedicle transfer, first stage 64910 Neuroma excision

DISCLOSURE

Dr G.A. Dumanian has consulted for the Checkpoint Surgical Company and has received support for his teaching course for Targeted Muscle Reinnervation. Dr S.W. Jordan and Dr A.G. Chappell have nothing to disclose.

REFERENCES

1. Vernadakis AJ, Koch H, Mackinnon SE. Management of neuromas. Clin Plast Surg 2003;30(2): 247–68, vii.
2. Huse E, Larbig W, Flor H, et al. The effect of opioids on phantom limb pain and cortical reorganization. Pain 2001;90(1–2):47–55.
3. Baron R. Neuropathic pain: a clinical perspective. Handb Exp Pharmacol 2009;(194):3–30.
4. Moore A. Gabapentin and post tonsillectomy pain-the next best thing? Arch Trauma Res 2013;1(4): 188–90.
5. Wiffen PJ, Derry S, Moore RA, et al. Carbamazepine for chronic neuropathic pain and fibromyalgia in adults. Cochrane Database Syst Rev 2014;(4): CD005451.
6. Eccleston C, Hearn L, Williams AC. Psychological therapies for the management of chronic neuropathic pain in adults. Cochrane Database Syst Rev 2015;(10):CD011259.
7. Bittar RG, Otero S, Carter H, et al. Deep brain stimulation for phantom limb pain. J Clin Neurosci 2005; 12(4):399–404.
8. Kubiak CA, Kemp SWP, Cederna PS. Regenerative peripheral nerve interface for management of post-amputation neuroma. JAMA Surg 2018;153(7): 681–2.
9. Valerio IL, Dumanian GA, Jordan SW, et al. Preemptive treatment of phantom and residual limb pain with targeted muscle reinnervation at the time of major limb amputation. J Am Coll Surg 2019;228(3): 217–26.
10. Woo SL, Kung TA, Brown DL, et al. Regenerative peripheral nerve interfaces for the treatment of postamputation neuroma pain: a pilot study. Plast Reconstr Surg Glob Open 2016;4(12):e1038.
11. Kung TA, Langhals NB, Martin DC, et al. Regenerative peripheral nerve interface viability and signal transduction with an implanted electrode. Plast Reconstr Surg 2014;133(6):1380–94.
12. Mackinnon SE, Dellon AL, Hudson AR, et al. Alteration of neuroma formation by manipulation of its microenvironment. Plast Reconstr Surg 1985;76(3): 345–53.
13. Boldrey E. Amputation neuroma in nerves implanted in bone. Ann Surg 1943;118(6):1052–7.
14. hijiawi JKT, Lipschutz. An improved brain-machine interface accomplished using multiple nerve transfers. Plast Reconstr Surg 2006;118:1573–8.
15. Kuiken TA, Dumanian GA, Lipschutz RD, et al. The use of targeted muscle reinnervation for improved myoelectric prosthesis control in a bilateral shoulder disarticulation amputee. Prosthet Orthot Int 2004; 28(3):245–53.
16. Kuiken TA, Miller LA, Lipschutz RD, et al. Targeted reinnervation for enhanced prosthetic arm function in a woman with a proximal amputation: a case study. Lancet 2007;369(9559):371–80.
17. Bi A, Park E, Dumanian GA. Treatment of painful nerves in the abdominal wall using processed nerve allografts. Plast Reconstr Surg Glob Open 2018; 6(3):e1670.
18. Eberlin KR, Ducic I. Surgical algorithm for neuroma management: a changing treatment paradigm. Plast Reconstr Surg Glob Open 2018;6(10). https://doi.org/10.1097/GOX.0000000000001952.
19. Wolvetang NHA, Lans J, Verhiel S, et al. Surgery for symptomatic neuroma: anatomic distribution and predictors of secondary surgery. Plast Reconstr Surg 2019;143(6):1762–71.
20. Guse DM, Moran SL. Outcomes of the surgical treatment of peripheral neuromas of the hand and forearm: a 25-year comparative outcome study. Ann Plast Surg 2013;71(6):654–8.
21. Kaya Y, Sarikcioglu L. Sir Herbert Seddon (1903-1977) and his classification scheme for peripheral nerve injury. Childs Nerv Syst 2015;31(2):177–80.

22. Agnew SP, Ko J, De La Garza M, et al. Limb transplantation and targeted reinnervation: a practical comparison. J Reconstr Microsurg 2012;28(1):63–8.

23. Kim PS, Ko JH, O'Shaughnessy KK, et al. The effects of targeted muscle reinnervation on neuromas in a rabbit rectus abdominis flap model. J Hand Surg Am 2012;37(8):1609–16.

24. Farina D, Castronovo AM, Vujaklija I, et al. Common synaptic input to motor neurons and neural drive to targeted reinnervated muscles. J Neurosci 2017; 37(46):11285–92.

25. Ephraim PL, Wegener ST, MacKenzie EJ, et al. Phantom pain, residual limb pain, and back pain in amputees: results of a national survey. Arch Phys Med Rehabil 2005;86(10):1910–9.

26. Sadosky A, McDermott AM, Brandenburg NA, et al. A review of the epidemiology of painful diabetic peripheral neuropathy, postherpetic neuralgia, and less commonly studied neuropathic pain conditions. Pain Pract 2008;8(1):45–56.

27. Buchheit T, Van de Ven T, Hsia HL, et al. Pain phenotypes and associated clinical risk factors following traumatic amputation: results from Veterans Integrated Pain Evaluation Research (VIPER). Pain Med 2016;17(1):149–61.

28. Flor H, Elbert T, Knecht S, et al. Phantom-limb pain as a perceptual correlate of cortical reorganization following arm amputation. Nature 1995;375(6531): 482–4.

29. Flor H, Nikolajsen L, Staehelin Jensen T. Phantom limb pain: a case of maladaptive CNS plasticity? Nat Rev Neurosci 2006;7(11):873–81.

30. Jensen TS, Krebs B, Nielsen J, et al. Phantom limb, phantom pain and stump pain in amputees during the first 6 months following limb amputation. Pain 1983;17(3):243–56.

31. Rudy TE, Lieber SJ, Boston JR, et al. Psychosocial predictors of physical performance in disabled individuals with chronic pain. Clin J Pain 2003;19(1): 18–30.

32. Gart MS, Souza JM, Dumanian GA. Targeted muscle reinnervation in the upper extremity amputee: a technical roadmap. J Hand Surg Am 2015;40(9): 1877–88.

33. Morgan EN, Kyle Potter B, Souza JM, et al. Targeted muscle reinnervation for transradial amputation: description of operative technique. Tech Hand Up Extrem Surg 2016;20(4):166–71.

34. Fracol ME, Janes LE, Ko JH, et al. Targeted muscle reinnervation in the lower leg: an anatomical study. Plast Reconstr Surg 2018;142(4):541e–50e.

35. Kuiken TA, Li G, Lock BA, et al. Targeted muscle reinnervation for real-time myoelectric control of multifunction artificial arms. JAMA 2009;301(6):619–28.

36. Vaso A, Adahan HM, Gjika A, et al. Peripheral nervous system origin of phantom limb pain. Pain 2014;155(7):1384–91.

37. Souza JM, Cheesborough JE, Ko JH, et al. Targeted muscle reinnervation: a novel approach to postamputation neuroma pain. Clin Orthop Relat Res 2014;472(10):2984–90.

38. Seddon HJ. The use of autogenous grafts for the repair of large gaps in peripheral nerves. The British Journal of Surgery 1947;35(138):151–67.

39. Sunderland S. Nerve Injuries and Their Repair: A Critical Appraisal. New York: Churchill Livingstone; 1991.

40. Mackinnon S, Dellon AL. Diagnosis of nerve injury. Surgery of the peripheral nerve. New York: Thieme; 1988. p. 74–8.

Migraine Treatment

Danielle Olla, MD[a], Justin Sawyer, MD[a], Nicole Sommer, MD[a,*],
John B. Moore IV, MD[b,c]

KEYWORDS

- Migraine • Migraine headaches • Botulinum toxin type A • Migraine surgery
- Migraine trigger zones

KEY POINTS

- Migraine headaches affect 35 million American and are ranked the third-highest cause of disability worldwide, resulting in serious economic burdens, with loss of work days and productivity.
- There are 4 types of migraine headaches, with well-described trigger sites associated with each type of migraine headache.
- Migraines headaches often are refractory to medical therapy and may respond well to botulinum toxin type A administered to specific trigger sites.
- Literature found an average success rate of 90% with either elimination or greater than 50% improvement of migraine headaches after migraine surgery.

MIGRAINE HEADACHE TREATMENT
Introduction

Migraine headaches cause significant suffering and disability at the national and global levels. Headaches and migraines are leading causes of outpatient and emergency department visits and remain an important public health problem.[1] In the Global Burden of Disease Study 2010, migraine headache was ranked the third most prevalent disorder in the world. In 2015, it was ranked the third-highest cause of disability worldwide in both men and women under the age of 50 years.[2] Approximately 35 million Americans suffer from migraine headaches, approximately 1 out of every 7. This includes 19% of all women and 9% of all men.[1] This results in extreme economic consequences. There are 112 million collective workdays lost, an estimated $1 billion in medical costs, and $16 billion productivity loss in the United States annually.[3–5] The theory behind migraine pathophysiology has evolved over the past several decades, and literature is rapidly accumulating supporting that migraine headaches are the consequence of compression or traction and subsequent irritation to peripheral nerves in the head and neck. Advances in the underlying pathophysiology have led to newer and promising treatment modalities, such as botulinum toxin type A (BTX-A) injections and migraine surgery, both of which provide relief to the peripheral nerves associated with the migraine.

Diagnostic Criteria for Migraine Headaches

In 2018, the Headache Classification Committee of the International Headache Society released the *International Classification of Headache Disorders*, 3rd edition, with diagnostic criteria for migraine headaches. This helps delineate migraine headaches from other headaches, such as cluster or tension headaches.

To be diagnosed with migraine headaches there must be at least 5 attacks meeting the following criteria[6]:

- Headache attacks lasting 4 hours to 72 hours (when untreated or unsuccessfully treated)
- Headaches having 2 of the following 4 characteristics:

[a] Institute for Plastic Surgery, Southern Illinois University, 747 North Rutledge Street #3, Springfield, IL 62702, USA; [b] Midwest Migraine Surgery Center & KS Hand Center, 20375 West 151st Street, Suite #370, Olathe, KS 66061, USA; [c] KU Med Center, 3901 Rainbow Boulevard, Kansas City, KS 66160, USA
* Corresponding author.
E-mail address: nsommer@siumed.edu

Clin Plastic Surg 47 (2020) 295–303
https://doi.org/10.1016/j.cps.2020.01.003
0094-1298/20/© 2020 Elsevier Inc. All rights reserved.

- Unilateral location
- pulsating quality
- moderate/severe pain intensity
- aggravation by or causing avoidance of routine physical activity (eg, walking or climbing stairs)
- During headache at least 1 of the following:
  - Nausea and/or vomiting
  - Photophobia and phonophobia
- Not better accounted for by another diagnosis or disorder

Nonsurgical Treatment

Nonsurgical treatment of migraine headaches consists of 2 categories, nonpharmacologic and pharmacologic. Nonpharmacologic treatment of migraine headaches consists of behavior modifications, such as avoidance of triggers.[7,8] Other nonpharmacologic treatments like application of pressure, cold or heat, and acupuncture can mitigate or abort the migraine headaches.[9,10]

Current forms of pharmacologic treatments of migraine headaches include prophylactic and abortive medications.[10]

- Prophylactic: lessen the frequency and severity of the migraine attacks
  - Antihypertensives
    - β-blockers
    - Calcium channel blockers
    - Angiotensin-converting enzyme inhibitors
  - Antidepressants
  - Anticonvulsants
  - Antihistamines
- Abortive: prevent a migraine attack or to stop it once it starts
  - Triptans
  - Nonsteroidal anti-inflammatory drugs
  - Acetaminophen
  - Combination (acetaminophen, caffeine, and aspirin)
  - Narcotics

Pathophysiology

Over the past 20 years there have been advances in the understanding of migraine headaches and their cause. There has been a shift from a vascular theory to neuronal theory involving the central nervous system, peripheral nervous system, or both as the cause of migraine headaches.[11] These newer theories have brought forth the concept of peripheral trigger points involving branches of the trigeminal nerve and greater occipital nerve and their muscular investments and surrounding structures.

Pain from migraine headaches is thought to be the result of increased activity of nociceptors that innervate the meninges and their blood vessels. The peripheral branches of the trigeminal and occipital nerve encounter muscles at defined trigger points. Subsequent muscle contraction causes compression or traction of the nerve branches leading to nerve irritation. Although compression of the nerves is the most widely believed cause of nerve irritation, it has been noted that the involved nerves do not show the classic appearance of a compressed nerve, as would be seen in the median nerve of carpal tunnel syndrome, such as the hourglass deformity or color change from myelin loss. Because of this, another theory for nerve irritation suggests traction on the nerve branches rather than a pure nerve compression.

In the trigger point theory, the activation is mechanical stimulation of branches of the trigeminal nerve, which causes the nerve fibers to release vasoactive chemicals, such as substance P and calcitonin gene–related peptide (CGRP). The theory is that these vasoactive substances are released in the cell bodies of the trigeminal nerve and travel proximally, causing local meningitis and dilation of trigeminal nerve-innervated vessels and dura mater and project to the trigeminal nucleus caudalis.[12–14] Studies of peptide release have shown, however, that substance P is not elevated but CGRP is elevated in patients during migraine attacks. This observation has given rise to development and testing of medical therapies that target CGRP, the most abundant neuropeptide in the trigeminal nerve.[15] The theory is that the more specific action on the trigeminal pain system will more effectively treat migraine pain with little to no adverse effects, as is common with many of the current day pharmacologic treatments. CGRP antagonists, known as gepants, are used for acute relief of migraines. Monoclonal antibodies against CGRP or targeting the CGRP receptor prevent migraine attacks. There have been promising results in phase 3 trials.[16,17]

Types of Migraine Headaches

Frontal migraine headaches

Frontal migraine headaches are characterized by frontal pain, typically occur in the late afternoon, and are associated with stress. Patients with these headaches tend to have hypertrophy of the furrowing muscles, including the corrugator supercilii. Eyebrow ptosis and eyelid ptosis are other possible clinical manifestations of frontal migraines.[18,19]

Frontal migraines originate secondary to irritation of supraorbital and supratrochlear nerves. Frontal trigger is the most common trigger site. The supra-orbital nerves have 3 muscular trigger sites: the corrugator supercilii, depressor supercilii, and procerus muscles. There are 4 branching types of the supraorbital nerve relative to the corrugator muscle. The supraorbital nerve also may be irritated by the supraorbital artery and at the entrance into the brow through the supraorbital forearm or a narrow supraorbital notch. The supratrochlear nerve has 3 branching patterns relative to the corrugator muscles. Additional points of irritation include corrugator supercilii and the frontal notch.[19,20]

Temporal migraine headache

Temporal migraine headaches are located in the temple area, lateral and superior to the lateral canthus. They frequently occur in the morning, are related to stress, and are associated with clenching of teeth. Patients often wake up in the morning with pain after grinding teeth while asleep and may have worn dental facets on examination. Migraine headaches in this location also are associated with trigger point tenderness as well as temporomandibular joint pain.[10,18]

Temporal migraine headaches are caused by compression or traction of the zygomaticotemporal branch of the trigeminal nerve (ZTBTN). Trigger sites include the exit point of the nerve through the zygomatic bone, 17 mm lateral to and 7 mm superior to the lateral canthus. In addition, the ZTBTN may be compressed by temporalis muscle, deep temporal fascia and superficial temporal artery. The temporal trigger is the second most common trigger area.[21] Temporal region migraines occasionally are caused by the irritation of the auriculotemporal nerve (ATN) as it runs superior to the ear.

Occipital migraine headaches

The pain of occipital migraines is located in the upper neck and occipital region. These headaches are associated with stress, upper neck and occipital pain, muscle tightness, and trigger point tenderness and may be related to heavy exercise. Patients may have a history of whiplash.[10,18]

Compression of the greater occipital nerve by the semispinalis capitis is thought to be responsible for migraine headaches at this location. The occipital nerve is compressed as it pierces the semispinalis capitis muscles. Mosser and colleagues[22] performed an anatomic study of the nerve's relation to the muscle, demonstrating that the nerve can reliably be found 3 cm inferior to the occipital protuberance and 1.5 cm lateral to the midline. The nerve also may be compressed by trapezius, obliquus capitis muscles, and nuchal fascia.[23,24]

Rhinogenic migraine headaches

Rhinogenic migraine headaches are characterized by retrobulbar pain behind the eye. They often occur in the early morning and are related to weather, allergies, and hormones. The headaches often are cyclic in nature. A trial of nasal sprays can be used.[10]

Intranasal triggers lead to impingement and irritation of the terminal trigeminal branches and can be diagnosed by evidence of nasal septum deviation, turbinate hypertrophy, and/or mucosal inflammation on an intranasal examination. Further diagnostic support of these migraine headaches may be provided by computed tomography (CT) of the face with evidence of contact points, including septal spurs or septal deviation.[18]

Nonsurgical Treatment of Migraine Pain

Nonsurgical treatment of migraines consists of chemodenervation with BTX-A.

BTX-A has a defined intracellular mechanism of action, impairing the soluble N-ethylmaleimide-sensitive factor attachment protein receptor (SNARE)-mediated synaptic vesicle fusion to nerve terminals.[25] BTX-A prevents the release of acetylcholine at the neuromuscular junction, thus inhibiting initiation of the action potential and firing of the affected muscle. It is thought that the inhibition of muscle contraction that follows then reduces compression and irritation of the nerve associated with the trigger point.

The entire mode of action of BTX-A in migraine headaches, however, is not fully understood. Studies have shown that in addition to the extracranial effects, BTX-A may effect modulation of neurotransmitter release and changes in surface expression of receptors and cytokines as well as enhancement of opioidergic transmission.[26] There is reduced sensory transduction of suprathreshold mechanical stimuli associated with processing mechanical pain but not sensory transduction of threshold tactile mechanosensitivity.[25] The peripherally delivered BTX-A is taken up by sensory afferents and may undergo transcytosis to cleave SNAREs in second-order neurons in the ganglion and trigeminal nucleus caudalis or in adjacent afferent terminals and prevent evoked afferent release and downstream activation.[27]

BTX-A was first demonstrated to reduce the severity and frequency of migraines headaches by Binder and colleagues,[28] in 2000, in their landmark study that demonstrated complete resolution of migraines in 55% of migraine patients and partial reduction in 38%. This study came after years of successful treatment with BTX-A in other ailments associated with muscular dystonia. The study was followed by a double-blind randomized trial of 123 patients with moderate to severe migraines and provided further evidence for the ability of BTX-A to alleviate migraines.[29] A great deal of work has been done to study the role for BTX-A in migraine headaches, however, likely none more impactful than the 2010 Phase III Research Evaluating Migraine Prophylaxis Therapy 1 trial that provided the convincing and rigorous evidence for the efficacy of BTX-A as a prophylactic treatment of migraine headaches, which was largely responsible for the subsequent Food and Drug Administration (FDA) approval of the therapy in 2010.[30,31]

Low doses of BTX-A (**Table 1**) are injected directly into the muscle site that has been identified as a trigger point. Trigger points are identified during the initial work-up through history, physical examination, and often a headache diary, in which the patient keeps track of headaches for at least 1 month, carefully recording the characteristics of the migraines. The trigger points then are systematically injected from most to least likely source, and the results are logged by the patient. An added benefit of this approach is that it can provide a reliable source of the trigger point for future surgical intervention if indicated.

Complications of Botulinum Toxin Type A for Migraine Headache

- Atrophy of muscles
- Ptosis of eyelids if injected around glabellar region
- Antibody development, which can render BTX-A ineffective[32,33]
  - Occurs in approximately 7% of patients
  - Keeping 3-month cumulative dose under 400 U can help avoid this complication.

Presurgical Work-up and Treatment of Migraine Headaches

Step 1: initial screening

Patients considered for BTX-A must have been seen by a neurologist and have a diagnosis of migraine headaches, a history of chronic migraines treated by a physician for at least 3 months, history of failure to respond to conservative abortive and prophylactic medical treatments, and no contraindications for BTX-A. Insurance preauthorization is required before injection, or private pay options can be discussed. Onabotulinum A (Botox) is FDA approved for the treatment of migraine headaches. Patients keep a pre–BTX-A diary that is returned 1 week prior to appointment and is scored.

Table 1
Migraine types by location and the nerves associated with their trigger points, their injection sites with dosing for BTX-A therapy and complications associated with each site.

Migraine Zone	Nerve	Trigger Points	Injection Site	Botulinum Toxin Type A Dose	Complications
Frontal	Supraorbital Supratrochlear	Glabellar group Corrugator supercilii Depressor supercilii Fascial band and bony tunnel in supraorbital rim Supraorbital artery Frontal notch	Corrugator muscles	12.5 U/side	Eyelid ptosis (10%)[34] glabellar muscle atrophy
Temporal	ZTBTN	Temporalis muscle Deep temporal fascia Forearm in zygomatic bone Superficial temporal artery	The ZTBTN emergence from deep temporal fascia Inject BTX-A 2 cm posterolateral to emergence point just through the deep temporal fascia[18]	18.75 U/side	Temple hollowing (23%)[34]
Occipital	Greater occipital	Semispinalis capitis Obliquus capitis Trapezius	3 cm inferior/1.5 cm lateral to occipital protuberance[20]	25 U/side	Neck weakness (27%)[34]

Common insurance criteria for BTX-A for treatment of migraine headaches:

- History of chronic migraine (not approved for episodic use)
- Greater than 15 migraines per month
- Greater than 4 hours' average duration
- Nausea and/or vomiting OR sensitivity to both light and sound
- Aggravation of and/or avoidance of routine activity
- Greater than 18 years of age
- Failed 3-month trial of at least 3 medications from 2 prophylactic therapy classes (antihypertensives, antidepressants, and anticonvulsants)
- Must not be using opioids greater than 10 days per month
- Must not be using CGRP antagonists

Step 2: office visit

A thorough examination is performed. The migraine diary and neurology and primary care physician records are reviewed to determine the most likely migraine trigger point. Pre–BTX-A photos are taken and informed consent is obtained. Temporal injections can result in noticeable temporal hollowing that does not always resolve when BTX-A injections are stopped, so patients should be made aware of this side effect.

BTX-A is injected in a systematic manner into the most common and severe trigger sites based on the patient's migraine diary and physical examination. The frontal areas are injected bilaterally due to asymmetry that would develop if only 1 side were treated. If occipital or temporal areas are unilateral, only that side is injected. Patient is scheduled for return follow-up in 12 weeks and must keep a post–BTX-A diary that is returned 1 week before follow-up visit. This diary helps track the success of BTX-A in decreasing the frequency, intensity, and duration of the symptoms at the injected trigger sites. It also tracks occurrence of new trigger points that may arise after the successful treatment of areas of initial concern.

Table 1 contains migraine types by location and the nerves associated with their trigger points, their injection sites, and dosing for BTX-A therapy as well as complications associated with BTX-A injections at each site.

Step 3: the post–botulinum toxin type A visit

The pre–BTX-A and post–BTX-A migraine headache diaries are compared to assess BTX-A effect on migraine headaches. Positive response wasdefined as a 50% or greater decrease in frequency, intensity, or duration of migraine headaches. For continued insurance coverage of chemodenervation treatment, documentation of a decrease by 7 migraines per month, decrease in duration greater than 100 hours per month, or 50% decrease in patient-reported severity may be required.

Because BTX-A temporarily inhibits muscle contraction, usually for approximately 3 months, it can be used as a trial to see if a patient's migraine headaches go away or become less intense after injection. A BTX-A treatment is successful in preventing migraines or lessening their severity, and then surgery to remove the trigger is likely to achieve the same result or better on a more permanent basis. Some patients may wish to continue with the temporary relief of BTX-A rather than undergo surgery whereas some desire the more permanent relief with surgery. Others may develop breakthrough migraines at 9 weeks, and because they are unable to undergo insurance covered injection until 12 weeks, they must experience 3 weeks of debilitating migraines 4 times a year. These patients often decide to have a more permanent treatment with surgical release of the triggers. Nerve blocks with local anesthesia with/or without steroid also can be performed to help diagnose trigger sites amenable to surgical decompression or neurectomy. The patient must be experiencing a migraine at the time of local injection for this to be effective.

The sphenopalatine ganglion modulates input from the nose and midface. Blocking this collection of nerve cell bodies may eliminate or prevent migraine headaches and has become an adjunctive treatment. This treatment involves injection of the sphenopalatine ganglion through a tactile, transnasal, endoscopic, or image-guided approach (**Figs 1-3**).

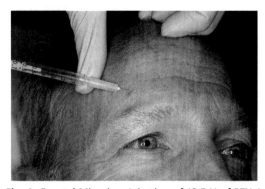

Fig. 1. Frontal Migraine: Injection of 12.5 U of BTX-A in retrograde fashion from the medial to lateral aspect of the corrugators.

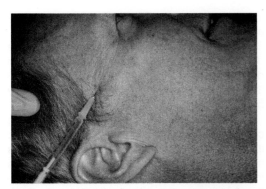

Fig. 2. Temporal Migraine: Injection of 18.75 U of BTX-A in fanning fashion just deep to temporal fascia into the temporalis muscle.

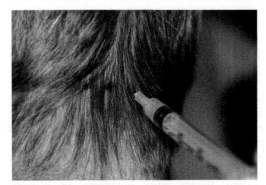

Fig. 3. Occipital Migraine: Injection of 25 U of BTX-A 3cm inferior to occipital protuberance and 1.5cm lateral from midline burying needle deep into the semispinalis muscle.

Migraine Surgery

Migraine surgery was documented by Dandy in 1931[34] when he removed the inferior cervical and first thoracic sympathetic ganglion for treatment of migraine headaches. An association between migraine relief and surgery was noted by Dr Bahman Guyuron at Case Western Reserve University. Patients reported disappearance of migraines after forehead rejuvenation surgery, which included resection of the corrugator supercilii muscles. He found that 31 of 39 patients reported preoperative migraine disappearance or improvement at 47-month follow-up.[35] Since that time, migraine surgery has been established as a successful treatment modality for migraine headaches.

Migraine surgery is best suited for patients unresponsive to medical or pharmacologic therapies but with positive response to BTX-A or local anesthetic injections of trigger sites. The trigger sites include

- Frontal (supraorbital, supratrochlear, and zygomaticofacial nerves)

- Temporal (zygomaticotemporal and auriculotemporal nerves)
- Occipital (greater occipital, lesser occipital, and third occipital nerves)
- Rhinogenic

Migraine surgery is performed under general anesthesia, typically done as an outpatient procedure, and on average takes 1.5 hours to 2 hours bilaterally per migraine trigger area. For best surgical outcomes, it is recommended that migraine patients are weaned off narcotics before surgery.

Frontal migraine procedure

Frontal migraine headaches are treated with release of the trigger sites of the supraorbital and supratrochlear nerves. The main objective is a partial versus complete resection of the glabellar muscle group, including the corrugator supercilii, depressor supercilii, and procerus muscles and release of other trigger points, including the supraorbital and supratrochlear artery and vein, myofascial sleeve, and supraorbital foramen.[10,18,19] Muscle resection and supraorbital foraminotomy are performed endoscopically or open, through a transpalpebral or conventional direct brow lift approach.

An endoscopic approach is preferred for the patients who have optimal or short forehead length. Five or 6 incisions are placed within the hair-bearing skin. The endoscope is introduced and the dissection is carried down in the subperiosteal plane to the superior and lateral orbital rims. The periosteum is incised to expose the supraorbital nerves, supratrochlear nerves, and corrugator muscle groups. The periosteum is then released, leaving the central portion intact over the midglabellar area to prevent elevation of the medial brow. The supratrochlear and supraorbital nerve branches are preserved while the corrugator and depressor muscles are removed via piecemeal. The supraorbital rim can be evaluated through an upper eyelid counter-incision, for sites of bony compression, which are released with an osteotome. Harvested fat from the temple is placed at the corrugator site to prevent contour deformity.[10,18]

The transpalpebral approach starts with a transpalpebral incision followed by dissection to the plane between the orbicularis oculi muscle and the septum. This dissection plane is carried superiorly toward the superior orbital rim where the depressor supercilii muscle is encountered first and is removed. The corrugator supercilii muscle, which is lighter in color, is then identified above the supraorbital rim. The corrugator supercilii muscle is removed in a medial to lateral fashion while the nerves are preserved. The supraorbital notch is evaluated for sites of compression. Harvested fat from the upper eyelid is placed at the corrugator site to prevent contour deformity.[10,18,20,36]

Temporal migraine procedure

Temporal migraine headaches triggers are treated with neurectomy of the ATN or zygomaticotemporal nerve (ZTN). Less commonly, these nerves are decompressed and left in situ.

ZTN neurectomy or avulsion is performed endoscopically through the same endoscopic incisions used for the frontal surgery or through a temporal hairline incision. The main objective is to remove the nerve to eliminate irritation. Postoperatively, patients usually have a temporary small area of numbness in the parietal scalp.[10,18]

The estimated position of the ZTN is marked on the skin by identifying the zygoma and lateral orbital rim and bisecting at 45° angle. It is approximately 15 mm to 20 mm lateral and 5 mm to 10 mm superior to the lateral canthus, often near the sentinel vein. A 3-cm incision is made parallel to the hairline either at the hairline or 1 cm posterior to the hairline for improved camouflage. Skin dissection is performed carefully to avoid injury to the hair follicles. The dissection is continued through the superficial temporal fascia down to the deep temporal fascia. A plane immediately superficial to the deep temporal fascia is exposed, leaving no fat on the fascia. The endoscope is introduced and a periosteal elevator is used to dissect the plane medially until the ZTBTN is identified lateral and superior to the lateral canthus; 30% of the time there are multiple ZTN branches. The sentinel vein may need to be transected to allow visualization of the ZTN. The ZTBTN is oriented more vertically than the zygomaticofacial branch of the facial nerve. At least 2 cm of nerve is avulsed with a long hemostat to prevent recoaptation.[10,18,36]

Temporal migraines can be triggered separately by the ATN, which can be diagnosed by relief of symptoms with local anesthetic injection superior to the ear in line with the nerve. ATN is decompressed or a segment removed through the same posterior hairline incision. The superficial temporal artery may need to be resected or ligated if it intersects with the ATN.

Occipital migraine procedure

Occipital migraine headache triggers are treated with release of the greater occipital nerve primarily but occasionally the lesser occipital and third occipital nerves. Greater occipital nerve release with fat flap transposition is performed through a 4-cm to 5-cm posterior midline incision. The main objective is to decompress the greater occipital nerve at 6 points along the path of the nerve, including obliquus capitis, semispinalis, trapezial tunnel, occipital artery, and nuchal fascia.[10,18]

The posterior midline incision is within the hairline at the caudal most portion of the occipital area. Trapezius fascia is incised approximately 0.5 cm to 1 cm lateral to midline. Dissection is carried through the oblique fibers of the trapezius down to the semispinalis capitis fascia and underlying vertically oriented muscle fibers. Blunt dissection is performed subfascial and superficial to the muscle until the trunk of occipital nerve is identified approximately 1.5 cm from the midline and 3 cm to 3.5 cm caudal to occipital protuberance.[22,36] The nerve is isolated and the segment of semispinalis muscle medial to the nerve is dissected away from the nerve, separated from the midline raphe and excised. The path of the nerve is then followed laterally and cephalically, assuring release of all overlying fascia up to the subcutaneous plane to ensure release of all potential compression points along the course of nerve.[23] If the occipital artery is passing over or entangled with the nerve, it is ligated and transected. A 2-cm × 2-cm subcutaneous flap, based caudally, is elevated and passed under the nerve and drain placed. If the occipital artery is passing over or entangling the nerve it should be ligated and transected.

Rhinogenic migraine procedure

Septoplasty and turbinectomy are performed to relieve intranasal contact points impinging on the terminal branches of the trigeminal nerve. Surgery is based on the structures identified on examination or CT scan.[18] Standard mucoperichondrial flaps are raised to allow for partial septal resection, leaving an L-shaped 1.5-cm anterior and 1-cm caudal strut. If present, deviated portions of the perpendicular and vomer plates are removed. The inferior, middle, and/or superior turbinates are reduced and outfractured or resected as needed, depending on the touch points elicited on CT scan as well as intraoperatively.

Results of Migraine Surgery

There is expanding literature demonstrating the reliable success for patients who undergo migraine surgery. Guyuron and colleagues[37] found that of BTX-A responders who have surgery, 90% have a reduction of at least 50% in frequency, severity, or duration of migraine headaches and 35% actually have complete elimination of migraine headaches. They later published a placebo-controlled surgical trial of 75 patients for the treatment of migraine headaches in 2009: 57.1% of patients had complete elimination in migraine headaches after actual migraine surgery versus 3.8% who had a sham surgery (P<.001) and 83.7% significant improvement in migraine headaches after actual migraine surgery versus 57.7% of those who underwent sham surgery (P<.05).[36]

In 2014, a systematic review of current evidence in the surgical treatment of migraine headaches was published. It reviewed the 17 clinical articles regarding migraine headache surgery. This included 3 case series, 8 retrospective cohort studies, 3 prospective cohort studies, and 2 randomized controlled trials. All but 1 study had greater than 1-year follow-up. The investigators found an average success rate of 90% with either elimination or 50% or greater improvement of migraine headaches. These results were reproduced by different institutions and multiple surgeons.[38]

There also has been proved socioeconomic benefit. Faber and colleagues[39] published a study in 2012 showing a median total cost reduction of $3949/y. This included decrease in medication costs, number of workdays missed, and number of primary care visits. The expense of medical treatment of migraine headaches exceeded the cost of surgery a little after 2 years. The average surgical cost was $8378.[39]

SUMMARY

Migraine headaches are prevalent among Americans and cause significant morbidity and economic consequences. Understanding of the pathophysiologic basis of migraines has evolved over the past several decades. There is now a large body of evidence suggesting that migraines can be triggered by irritation of peripheral nerves of the head and neck at well-defined trigger points. This understanding has led to newer treatment options, such as BTX-A injections at the identified trigger points as well as surgical release of the sites of compression associated with the nerves. A systematic review of the migraine surgery literature found an average success rate of 90% with either elimination or greater than 50% improvement of migraine headaches after migraine surgery.

DISCLOSURE

The authors have nothing to disclose.

REFERENCES

1. Burch RC, Loder S, Loder E, et al. The prevalence and burden of migraine and severe headache in the united states: updated statistics from government health surveillance studies. Headache 2015; 55(1):21–34.
2. Leonardi M, Raggi A. Burden of migraine: international perspectives. Neurol Sci 2013;34(Suppl 1):S117–8.
3. Hu XH, Markson LE, Lipton RB, et al. Burden of migraine in the United States: disability and economic costs. Arch Intern Med 1999;159(8):813–8.
4. Stewart WF, Lipton RB, Celentano DD, et al. Prevalence of migraine headache in the United States. relation to age, income, race, and other sociodemographic factors. JAMA 1992;267(1):64–9.
5. Goldberg LD. The cost of migraine and its treatment. Am J Manag Care 2005;11(2 Suppl):S62–7.
6. Headache classification committee of the international headache society (IHS) the international classification of headache disorders, 3rd edition. Cephalalgia 2018;38(1):1–211.
7. Charles A. The pathophysiology of migraine: implications for clinical management. Lancet 2017. https://doi.org/10.1016/S1474-4422(17)30435-0.
8. Dodick D. Migraine. Lancet 2018;391:1315–30.
9. Da Silva AN. Acupuncture for migraine prevention. Headache 2015;55(3):470–3.
10. Totonchi A, Guyuron B. Surgical treatment of migraine headaches. In: Losee J, editor. Plastic surgery: volume 3: craniofacial, head and neck surgery and pediatric plastic surgery. 4th edition. Canada: Elsevier Inc; 2018. p. 82–91.
11. Puledda F, Messina R, Goadsby PJ. An update on migraine: current understanding and future directions. J Neurol 2017;264(9):2031–9.
12. Olesen J, Burstein R, Ashina M, et al. Origin of pain in migraine: evidence for peripheral sensitisation. Lancet Neurol 2009;8(7):679–90.
13. Lv X, Wu Z, Li Y. Innervation of the cerebral dura mater. Neuroradiol J 2014;27(3):293–8.
14. Ray BS, Wolff HG. Experimental studies on headache. Pain sensitive structures of the head and their significance in headache. Arch Surg 1940;41:813–56.
15. Russo AF. Calcitonin gene-related peptide (CGRP): a new target for migraine. Annu Rev Pharmacol Toxicol 2015;55:533–52.
16. Schuster NM, Rapoport AM. Calcitonin gene-related peptide-targeted therapies for migraine and cluster headache: a review. Clin Neuropharmacol 2017; 40(4):169–74.
17. Edvinsson L. Role of CGRP in migraine. Handb Exp Pharmacol 2019;255:121–30.
18. Guyuron B, Becker D. Surgical management of migraine headaches. In: Guyuron B, Kinney B, editors. Aesthetic plastic surgery video atlas. China: Elsevier Inc; 2012. p. 313–23.

19. Janis JE, Hatef DA, Hagan R, et al. Anatomy of the supratrochlear nerve: implications for the surgical treatment of migraine headaches. Plast Reconstr Surg 2013;131(4):743–50.

20. Guyuron B, Tucker T, Davis J. Surgical treatment of migraine headaches. Plast Reconstr Surg 2002; 109(7):2183–9.

21. Totonchi A, Pashmini N, Guyuron B. The zygomaticotemporal branch of the trigeminal nerve: an anatomical study. Plast Reconstr Surg 2005;115(1): 273–7.

22. Mosser SW, Guyuron B, Janis JE, et al. The anatomy of the greater occipital nerve: implications for the etiology of migraine headaches. Plast Reconstr Surg 2004;113(2):693–7 [discussion: 698–700].

23. Janis JE, Hatef DA, Ducic I, et al. The anatomy of the greater occipital nerve: Part II. compression point topography. Plast Reconstr Surg 2010;126(5): 1563–72.

24. Burstein R, Zhang X, Levy D, et al. Selective inhibition of meningeal nociceptors by botulinum neurotoxin type A: therapeutic implications for migraine and other pains. Cephalalgia 2014;34(11):853–69.

25. Janis JE, Hatef DA, Thakar H, et al. The zygomaticotemporal branch of the trigeminal nerve: Part II. Anatomic Variations. Plast Reconstr Surg 2010; 126(2):435–42.

26. Do TP, Hvedstrup J, Schytz HW. Botulinum toxin: a review of the mode of action in migraine. Acta Neurol Scand 2018;137(5):442–51.

27. Ramachandran R, Yaksh TL. Therapeutic use of botulinum toxin in migraine: mechanisms of action. Br J Pharmacol 2014;171(18):4177–92.

28. Binder WJ, Brin MF, Blitzer A, et al. Botulinum toxin type A (BOTOX) for treatment of migraine headaches: an open-label study. Otolaryngol Head Neck Surg 2000;123(6):669–76.

29. Silberstein S, Mathew N, Saper J, et al. Botulinum toxin type A as a migraine preventive treatment. for the BOTOX migraine clinical research group. Headache 2000;40(6):445–50.

30. Dodick DW, Turkel CC, DeGryse RE, et al. OnabotulinumtoxinA for treatment of chronic migraine: pooled results from the double-blind, randomized, placebo-controlled phases of the PREEMPT clinical program. Headache 2010;50(6):921–36.

31. Guyuron B, Rose K, Kriegler JS, et al. Hourglass deformity after botulinum toxin type A injection. Headache 2004;44(3):262–4.

32. Brin MF. Botulinum toxin: chemistry, pharmacology, toxicity, and immunology. Muscle Nerve Suppl 1997;6:S146–68.

33. Greene P, Fahn S, Diamond B. Development of resistance to botulinum toxin type A in patients with torticollis. Mov Disord 1994;9(2):213–7.

34. Dandy WE. Treatment of hemicrania (migraine) by removal of the inferior cervical and first thoracic sympathetic ganglion. Johns Hopkins University Bull 1931;48:357–61.

35. Guyuron B, Varghai A, Michelow BJ, et al. Corrugator supercilii muscle resection and migraine headaches. Plast Reconstr Surg 2000;106:429–34.

36. Guyuron B, Reed D, Kriegler JS, et al. A placebo-controlled surgical trial of the treatment of migraine headaches. Plast Reconstr Surg 2009;124(2):461–8.

37. Guyuron B, Kriegler JS, Davis J, et al. Comprehensive surgical treatment of migraine headaches. Plast Reconstr Surg 2005;115(1):1–9.

38. Janis JE, Barker JC, Javadi C, et al. A review of current evidence in the surgical treatment of migraine headaches. Plast Reconstr Surg 2014;134(4 Suppl 2):131S–41S.

39. Faber C, Garcia RM, Davis J, et al. A socioeconomic analysis of surgical treatment of migraine headaches. Plast Reconstr Surg 2012;129(4):871–7.

Complex Regional Pain Syndrome

Michael W. Neumeister, MD, FRCSC[a],*, Michael R. Romanelli, MD[b]

KEYWORDS

• Complex regional pain • CRPS • Causalgia • RSD

KEY POINTS

• Complex regional pain syndrome (CRPS) has been described as pain a patient feels that is disproportionate to the inciting event.
• The diagnosis and treatment of CRPS is challenged by the dynamic nature of its presentation and progression.
• The management that requires therapy and pain modulation is reviewed.

Complex regional pain syndrome (CRPS) has been described as pain a patient feels that is disproportionate to the inciting event. CRPS is, however, much more than pain because it is also associated with autonomic dysfunction, swelling, dystrophic skin changes, stiffness, functional impairment, and eventual atrophy. CRPS has a myriad of other synonyms, including but not limited to reflex sympathetic dystrophy, algoneurodystrophy, chronic traumatic edema, causalgia, neurodystrophy, and Sudeck atrophy. This hyperalgesic disease affects musculoskeletal, neural, and vascular structures more commonly in the upper extremity than the lower extremity.[1,2] The diagnosis and treatment of CRPS is challenged by the dynamic nature of its presentation and progression. The initial presentation may be confused with extraordinary postoperative pain and swelling. In a recent survey of 260 health professionals, half of respondents expressed difficulty in recognizing the symptoms of CRPS.[3] Acute presentation of CRPS pain can present as focal sympathetically maintained pain versus sympathetically independent pain (SMP vs SIP). Although patients with SMP may find initial relief with sympathetic blocks or medication, they may develop into SIP, thereby challenging treatment regimens.[4,5]

Early lack of consensus in diagnostic criteria for CRPS was clarified by the Budapest criteria in 2003. CRPS presentation was clarified as continuing pain, allodynia, or hyperalgesia, changes in skin perfusion, or abnormal sudomotor activity (edema and/or sweating) in the region of pain. These symptoms present with either an inciting noxious event to the nerve, CRPS type 1, or caused by other trauma, CRPS type 2. In 2007, given a tendency for overdiagnosis of CRPS, the Budapest criteria were refined to include the patient's report of at least 1 symptom in 3 of the 4 categories in their history, and display of at least 1 physical examination finding in 2 or more of the following categories: sensory, vasomotor, sudomotor/edema, or motor/trophic (**Table 1**).[6] Since 2007, the literature has recommended that additional efforts be made toward raising awareness surrounding the Budapest diagnostic criteria.[3] In 2010, Harden and colleagues[7] developed a CRPS severity score based on 17 different symptoms valued at 1 point each, which was validated most recently in 2017.

Patients with CRPS commonly describe hyperalgesia with characteristics of burning, searing, shooting, or aching pain. As expected, patients usually present with a greater physical disability

a Department of Surgery, Institute for Plastic Surgery, Southern Illinois University School of Medicine, Southern Illinois University, 747 North Rutledge Street, Suite 357, Baylis Building, Springfield, IL 62702, USA; b Institute for Plastic Surgery, Southern Illinois University School of Medicine, 747 North Rutledge Street, Suite 357, Baylis Building, Springfield, IL 62702, USA
* Corresponding author.
E-mail address: mneumeister@siumed.edu

Clin Plastic Surg 47 (2020) 305–310
https://doi.org/10.1016/j.cps.2019.12.009
0094-1298/20/Published by Elsevier Inc.

Table 1
Budapest criteria for complex regional pain syndrome

All of the following statements must be met:
- The patient has continuing pain disproportionate to any inciting event.
- The patient has 1 physical examination sign in 2 of the categories below.
- The patient reports 1 symptom in 3 of the categories below AND 1 sign in 2 of the categories below.
- No other diagnosis better explains the patient's presentation.

Category	Signs/Symptoms
Sensory	Symptoms: hyperesthesias and/or allodynia Signs: evidence of allodynia to light touch, deep pressure, or joint movement and/or hyperalgesia to pinprick
Vasomotor	Symptoms: reported temperature asymmetry and/or skin color changes and/or skin color asymmetry Signs: Evidence of the above symptoms
Sudomotor/Edema	Symptoms: reports of edema and/or sweating changes and/or sweating asymmetry Signs: Evidence of the above symptoms
Motor/Trophic	Symptoms: Decreased range of motion and/or motor dysfunction (weakness, tremor, dystonia) and/or trophic changes (hair, nail, skin) Signs: Evidence of the above symptoms

Adapted from Harden RN, Bruehl S, Stanton-Hicks M, et al: Proposed new diagnostic criteria for complex regional pain syndrome. Pain Med 2007; 8: pp. 326-331.

and have significantly more intense phenotype when compared with neuropathic pain of the extremities.[8] Innocuous stimuli frequently trigger allodynia caused by central pain sensitization of the neurons. Motor changes can include decreased range of motion, joint stiffness, weakness, tremor, and dystonia.

Thermoregulatory dysfunction seen in CRPS presents with distinct vascular dysregulation patterns. The body part in question has series of color and temperature changes. The skin can appear erythematous, hyperemic, blue, purple, pale, or mottled all within minutes of each other. Digit and hand swelling is accompanied with joint stiffness and disuse. Trophic skin and nail changes, including an increase or decrease in hair and nail growth with associated hyperkeratosis, are often seen within 10 days of onset in 30% of CRPS type 1 presentations.[9] In the first 6 months of the acute phase, patients will experience an increase in perfusion consistent with a warm regulation pattern. As the pathology continues to progress, patients may experience a cold regulation pattern, with intermittent changes of intermediate dysregulation throughout the course of disease.[10] Heat and cold aggravate the pain. Other trophic changes of the skin may be significant for discoloration, abnormal sweating, or thermoregulatory dysfunction.[11] The physical examination of a patient with concern for CRPS is often significant

for extensive sensory dysfunction, variable in both temporal progression and severity of symptoms.[11] Although focused examination may occasionally identify the etiology of an underlying disorder such as a compression neuropathy, the patients' presentations have many manifestations, which mask potential focal etiology. It is crucial to evaluate for compression neuropathies from cervical nerve compression and thoracic outlet syndrome to more distal peripheral nerve compression. In a recent review of sensory abnormalities using quantitative sensory testing methods, light touch correlated with pain outcomes in CRPS.[11] The Budapest criteria has actually published a template with a rating scale of 0 (not severe) to 4 (very severe) to aptly capture each clinical symptom as described by the patient, and physical examination findings as identified by the provider.[7]

Unfortunately, to date there are no serum markers or standard laboratory findings to help with the diagnosis of CRPS despite best attempts, which have included identifying experimental microRNA signatures that are significantly elevated in patients with CRPS.[1,12] Thermography is the most common imaging modality, although large thermal differences in measurement do not appear to correlate with the severity of pain.[13] Sudeck atrophy is a known historical description of plain film radiographic findings consistent with

CRPS that include diffuse osteopenia with juxta-cortical demineralization, and subchondral cystic changes that are actually determined to be commonly seen with any trauma.[14,15] Ultrasound has been used to characterize radiographic differences in muscle tissue and identify key areas of distortion in patients with CRPS. Ultrasound can identify focal or generalized muscle edema or dystrophic changes seen in CRPS. These findings are not present in neuropathic pain syndromes or in the normal resting muscle tone in asymptomatic patients.[16]

Although CRPS can occur following a variety of inciting events, fractures overall were the most common inciting event leading to CRPS type 1, specifically those of the distal radius and ulna.[2,17] Application of tight casts was also determined to be a secondary cause of type 2 CRPS.[18] Common hand and arm injuries or routine surgeries with no apparent complication can incite CRPS. CRPS affects female individuals at least 3 times more frequently than male individuals.[2] In the pediatric population, CRPS is most common in girls around the age of 12, and was found to be more frequently found in the lower extremity.[19] Any nerve irritation or injury can incite CRPS. The more common nerve injuries causing CRPS identified include injury to the palmar cutaneous branch of the median nerve during carpal tunnel release, injury to the superficial branch of the radial nerve during surgical approaches to the first and second extensor compartments, and trauma to the dorsal cutaneous branch of the ulnar nerve when approaching the distal ulna for fracture fixation.[20]

Although the etiology behind the pathophysiology of CRPS is unknown, the pain pathway extending from peripheral nociception to central nervous system modulation of stimuli is highly sensitized and overactive, disrupting the surrounding autonomic response.[21] Following an inciting disruption of the peripheral nervous system, it is hypothesized that neuropeptides, substance P, and calcitonin gene-related peptide, among other chemical modulators, evoke surrounding neurogenic inflammation and catechol-amine sensitization.[10,22] Following the persistent hyperactivation of the peripheral nervous system, it has been demonstrated in animal models that central nervous system sensitization decreases the threshold for response to stimuli.[21,23]

Although transient pain following any trauma or an inciting event is expected, the persistent and prolonged nature of the presentation of CRPS is abnormal.[24] An essential component of this particular pathogenesis is due to autonomic features of the sympathetic nerve system in which alterations of receptors, specifically an upregulation of adrenoceptors and reduced cutaneous nerve fiber density, appear to contribute to sympathetic maintained pain.[25] More extensive discussions of the physiology of pain are covered in Greg I. Lee and Michael W. Neumeister's article, "Pain: Pathways and Physiology," in this issue. It is important to note that there is not a distinct psychological component to CRPS, or associated personality disorder, and patients' symptoms should be addressed and worked up accordingly; however, the debilitating nature of the disease can lead to psychological comorbidities and significant psychological burden.

The treatment of patients with CRPS should be proactive in nature, patients should be seen frequently, and a multidisciplinary approach should be applied to the patient's management.[3] The management should be multidisciplinary, to include the involvement of physical and occupational therapists, pain clinic, primary care provider, psychological therapists, and case workers. Manual therapy has been shown to reduce oxidative stress and pain behavior in a murine model.[26] Acupuncture[27] and biofeedback[28] also may be useful to reduce pain, increase mobility, and ultimately improve functionality of the extremity. A Cochrane review in 2016 identified the greatest rehabilitation benefit from mirror therapy and graded motor imagery, which both significantly improved the patient's pain and quality of life.[29]

The treatment methodology can be divided into acute and chronic stages of CRPS (**Fig. 1**). Before the development of atrophy and contracture, acute treatment protocols should focus on alleviating pain, managing edema, and correcting any compressive or neuropathic abnormalities. Pain control should be prioritized starting with a focus on the peripheral nature of the disease, including local anesthetic blocks.[30,31] At early onset of symptoms, high-dose steroids coupled with a rapid taper have been shown to have good success; as an alternative for those not in the acute phase, a long-term low-dose course of steroids have also been considered beneficial.[32] Tramadol has been proven, given its dual action on mu opioid receptors and serotonin/norepinephrine reuptake.[33] Neuropathic medications, such as gabapentin, have shown evidence of pain reduction in patients with CRPS.[34,35] Medications commonly used in chronic pain management include antidepressants, such as selective serotonin reuptake inhibitors and tricyclic antidepressants.[36] In addition, ketamine gel application may play a role in pain relief. Similar to the treatment of chronic pain, management with intravenous ketamine has been associated with pain relief and

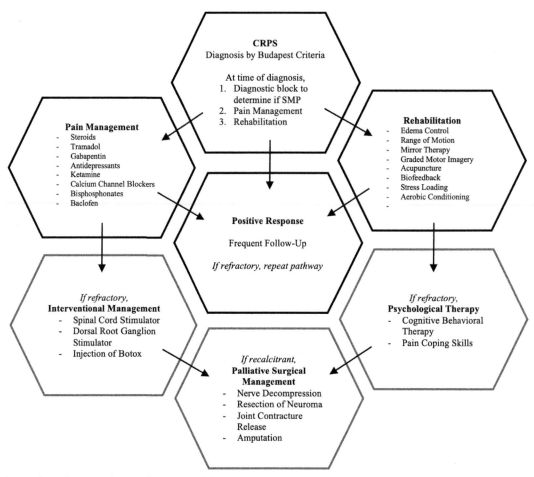

Fig. 1. Flow diagram of CRPS therapy guideline.

improvement of autonomic symptoms while under guidance of professionals.[37]

Other pain regimens directed at limiting the autonomic aspect of CRPS are commonly prescribed off-label. Adrenergics, such as phentolamine, have been shown to decrease pain for patients[38]; when patients experience relief after intravenous administration of phentolamine, it is pathognomonic for SMP.[4] In patients with edema and hyperalgesia, clonidine may provide patients with significant improvement.[39] Anticonvulsants, such as Dilantin, have been used to treat CRPS given their ability to stabilize hyperexcitable neurons.[34] Calcium channel blockers blockade of the sarcoplasmic reticulum and thus calcium, may also decrease sympathetic tone by stabilizing the cell membrane, which can result in pain relief.[39] Bisphosphonates may be used to prevent bone resorption and long-term effects of stiffness.[33,40] If patients experience significant autonomic effects, such as dystonia, baclofen may provide symptomatic relief.[41]

Interventional pain control has come to play a significant role in the management of CRPS. Sympathetic blockades, despite their short-term alleviation of symptoms, have been used as a diagnostic modality to determine whether CRPS is SMP or SIP (if it works, SMP) defined by temperature measurement or laser Doppler.[41] Spinal cord and dorsal root ganglion stimulators have been used and shown to provide some promise in the relief of pain.[42] Most recommendations suggest that stimulators should be considered earlier in the pain armamentarium.[43] As expected, further research must be performed to determine the safety and efficacy of use in the pregnant population.[44] One intriguing area of research includes proximal injection of Botox for patients with CRPS caused by myofascial pain syndromes.[45,46] Although most evidence in support of Botox are limited in levels of evidence, a recent study in a sample of 20 patients proved Botox effective in reducing self-assessed pain in refractory CRPS, and may be a promising new alternative for treatment.[47,48]

Following the late presentation of atrophy and contracture, a palliative approach may be tailored to the patient's needs for surgical correction of the contracture or deformity. Surgical intervention has historically been avoided unless clear indications such as mechanical or regenerative nerve pathology is identified. Examples of nerve-related pathology that may benefit from surgical intervention include resection of symptomatic neuromas or compression neuropathies.[49] As a last resort, amputation of the extremity with CRPS may be considered given the refractory nature of the symptoms. Amputations in patients with CRPS are controversial, however, and patients must be counseled on the risks of persistent symptoms and recurrence at the stump, and potential for phantom limb pain.[50] Ultimately, patients with amputations have shown consistently better results when compared with those who have not undergone amputation, and it should be considered given the difficult nature of this disease.[51]

DISCLOSURE

Nothing to disclose.

REFERENCES

1. Eisenberg E, Geller R, Brill S. Pharmacotherapy options for complex regional pain syndrome. Expert Rev Neurother 2007;7:521–31.
2. de Mos M, de Bruijn AG, Huygen FJ, et al. The incidence of complex regional pain syndrome: a population-based study. Pain 2007;129:12–20.
3. Grieve S, Llewellyn A, Jones L, et al. Complex regional pain syndrome: an international survey of clinical practice. Eur J Pain 2019;23:1890–903.
4. Raja SN, Treede RD, Davis KD, et al. Systemic alpha-adrenergic blockade with phentolamine: a diagnostic test for sympathetically maintained pain. Anesthesiology 1991;74:691–8.
5. Raja SN, Turnquist JL, Meleka S, et al. Monitoring adequacy of alpha-adrenoceptor blockade following systemic phentolamine administration. Pain 1996;64:197–204.
6. Harden RN, Bruehl S, Stanton-Hicks M, et al. Proposed new diagnostic criteria for complex regional pain syndrome. Pain Med 2007;8:326–31.
7. Harden RN, Bruehl S, Perez RS. Development of a severity score for CRPS. Pain 2010;151:870–6.
8. Palmer S, Bailey J, Brown C, et al. Sensory function and pain experience in arthritis, complex regional pain syndrome, fibromyalgia syndrome, and pain free volunteers: a cross-sectional study. Clin J Pain 2019;35:894–900.
9. Baron R, Maier C. Reflex sympathetic dystrophy: skin blood flow, sympathetic vasoconstrictor reflexes and pain before and after surgical sympathectomy. Pain 1996;67:317–26.
10. Stanton-Hicks M, Burton W, Bruel SP, et al. An updated interdisciplinary clinical pathway for CRPS: report of an expert panel. Pain Pract 2002;2(1):1–16.
11. Dietz C, Muller M, Reinhold AK, et al. What is normal trauma healing and what is complex regional pain syndrome I? An analysis of clinical and experimental biomarker. Pain 2019;160:2278–89.
12. Birklein F, Ajit SK, Goebel A, et al. Complex regional pain syndrome - phenotypic characteristics and potential biomarkers. Nat Rev Neurol 2018;14:272–84.
13. Shim H, Rose J, Halle S, et al. Complex regional pain syndrome: a narrative review for the practising clinician. Br J Anaesth 2019;123:424–33.
14. Bickerstaff DR, Charlesworth D, Kanis JA. Changes in cortical and trabecular bone in algodystrophy. Br J Rheumatol 1993;32:46–51.
15. Staunton H. Sudeck atrophy. Ir Med J 2006;10: 313–5.
16. Vas L, Pai R. Musculoskeletal ultrasonography to distinguish muscle changes in complex regional pain syndrome type 1 from those of neuropathic pain: an observational study. Pain Pract 2016;16: 1–13.
17. Bickerstaff DR, Kanis JA. Algodystrophy: an under-recognized complication of minor trauma. Br J Rheumatol 1994;33:240–8.
18. Field J, Protheroe DL, Atkins RM. Algodystrophy after Colles fractures is associated with secondary tightness of casts. J Bone Joint Surg Br 1994;76: 901–5.
19. Mesaroli G, Ruskin D, Campbell F, et al. Clinical features of pediatric complex regional pain syndrome: a 5-year retrospective chart review. Clin J Pain 2019;35:933–40.
20. Mitchell SW. Injuries of nerves and their consequences. Philadelphia: JB Lippincott; The Classics of Neurology & Neurosurgery Library; 1872.
21. Schwartzman RJ, Alexander GM, Grothusen J. Pathophysiology of complex regional pain syndrome. Expert Rev Neurother 2006;6:669–81.
22. Janig W, Baron R. Complex regional pain syndrome: mystery explained? Lancet Neurol 2003;2:687–97.
23. Guo TZ, Offley SC, Boyd EA, et al. Substance P signaling contributes to the vascular and nociceptive abnormalities observed in a tibial fracture rat model of complex regional pain syndrome type I. Pain 2004;108:95–107.
24. Koman LA, Smith TL, Smith BP, et al. The painful hand. Hand Clin 1996;12:757–64.
25. Knudsen LF, Terkelsen AJ, Drummond PD, et al. Complex regional pain syndrome: a focus on the autonomic nervous system. Clin Auton Res 2019;4: 457–67.

26. Salgado ASI, Stramosk J, Ludtke DD, et al. Manual therapy reduces pain behavior and oxidative stress in a murine model of complex regional pain syndrome type I. Brain Sci 2019;10:197.

27. Lee M, Ernst M. The sympatholytic effect of acupuncture as evidenced by thermography: a preliminary report. Orthop Rev 1983;12:67.

28. Grunert BK, Devine CA, Sanger JR, et al. Thermal self-regulation for pain control in reflex sympathetic dystrophy syndrome. J Hand Surg Am 1990;15:615–8.

29. Smart KM, Wand BM, O'Connell NE. Physiotherapy for pain and disability in adults with complex regional pain syndrome (CRPS) types I and II. Cochrane Database Syst Rev 2016;(2):CD010853.

30. Iolascon G, Moretti A. Pharmacotherapeutic options for complex regional pain. Expert Opin Pharmacother 2019;20:1377–86.

31. O'Connell NE, Wand BM, Gibson W, et al. Local anaesthetic sympathetic blockade for complex regional pain syndrome. Cochrane Database Syst Rev 2016;(7):CD004598.

32. Grundberg A. Reflex sympathetic dystrophy: treatment with long-acting intramuscular corticosteroids. J Hand Surg Am 1996;21:667–70.

33. Rowbotham MC. Pharmacologic management of complex regional pain syndrome. Clin J Pain 2006;22:425–9.

34. Mellick G, Mellicy L. Gabapentin in the management of reflex sympathetic dystrophy. J Pain Symptom Manage 1995;10:265–6.

35. van de Vusse AC, Stomp-van den Berg SG, Kessels AH, et al. Randomised controlled trial of gabapentin in complex regional pain syndrome type 1. BMC Neurol 2004;4:13.

36. Magni G. The use of antidepressants in the treatment of chronic pain. Drugs 1991;42:730–48.

37. Gammaitoni A, Gallagher RM, Welz-Bosna M. Topical ketamine gel: possible role in treating neuropathic pain. Pain Med 2000;1:97–100.

38. Arner S. Intravenous phentolamine test: diagnostic and prognostic use in reflex sympathetic dystrophy. Pain 1991;46:17–22.

39. Czop C, Smith TL, Koman LA. The pharmacologic approach to the painful hand. Hand Clin 1996;12:633–42.

40. Varenna M, Adami S, Rossini M, et al. Treatment of complex regional pain syndrome type I with neridronate: a randomized, double-blind, placebo-controlled study. Rheumatology (Oxford) 2013;52:534–42.

41. Cepeda MS, Lau J, Carr DB. Defining the therapeutic role of local anesthetic sympathetic blockade in complex regional pain syndrome: a narrative and systematic review. Clin J Pain 2002;18:216–33.

42. Harke H, Gretenkort P, Ladleif HU, et al. Spinal cord stimulation in sympathetically maintained complex regional pain syndrome type I with severe disability. A prospective clinical study. Eur J Pain 2005;9(4):363–73.

43. Poree L, Krames E, Pope J, et al. Spinal cord stimulation as treatment for complex regional pain syndrome should be considered earlier than last resort therapy. Neuromodulation 2013;16:125–41.

44. Jozwiak MJ, Wu H. Complex regional pain syndrome management: an evaluation of the risks and benefits of spinal cord stimulator use in pregnancy. Pain Pract 2019. https://doi.org/10.1111/papr.12825.

45. Safarpour D, Jabbari B. Botulinum toxin A (Botox) for treatment of proximal myofascial pain in complex regional pain syndrome: two cases. Pain Med 2010;11:1415–8.

46. Argoff CE. A focused review on the use of botulinum toxins for neuropathic pain. Clin J Pain 2002;18:177–81.

47. Birthi P, Sloan P, Salles S. Subcutaneous botulinum toxin A for the treatment of refractory complex regional pain syndrome. PM R 2012;4:446–9.

48. Lessard L, Bartow MJ, Jee J, et al. Botulinum toxin A: a novel therapeutic modality for upper extremity complex regional pain syndrome. Plast Reconstr Surg Glob Open 2018;6:e1847.

49. Placzek JD, Boyer MI, Gelberman RH, et al. Nerve decompression for complex regional pain syndrome type II following upper extremity surgery. J Hand Surg Am 2005;30(1):69–74.

50. Bodde MI, Dijkstra PU, den Dunnen WF, et al. Therapy-resistant complex regional pain syndrome type I: to amputate or not? J Bone Joint Surg Am 2011;93:1799–805.

51. Midbari A, Suzan E, Adler T, et al. Amputation in patients with complex regional pain syndrome: a comparative study between amputees and non-amputees with intractable disease. Bone Joint J 2016;98:548–54.

Regenerative Peripheral Nerve Interfaces for Prevention and Management of Neuromas

Katherine B. Santosa, MD, MS[a], Jeremie D. Oliver, BS, BA[b],
Paul S. Cederna, MD[a], Theodore A. Kung, MD[a],*

KEYWORDS

- Peripheral nerve • Pain • Amputation • Regenerative peripheral nerve interface • RPNI
- Neuroma pain • Phantom limb pain

KEY POINTS

- Painful neuromas are a substantial cause of morbidity in people with limb loss.
- Regenerative peripheral nerve interfaces may benefit patients with symptomatic postamputation neuromas through the use of free muscle grafts as physiologic targets for peripheral nerve reinnervation.
- Regenerative peripheral nerve interfaces should also be considered prior to amputation in order to prevent the development of symptomatic neuromas.
- Regenerative peripheral nerve interface surgery is a straightforward, reproducible procedure that can be effective in the prevention and management of symptomatic neuromas.

INTRODUCTION

In the United States alone, an estimated 2 million people live with the devastating consequences of major limb loss. Worldwide, more than 1 million extremity amputations are performed every year.[1] Major lower extremity amputation is more commonly performed than major upper extremity amputation[2] and indications for major limb amputation include vascular disease (54%), trauma (45%), and cancer (<2%).[3] In elderly patients, the indication for major limb amputation is commonly vascular disease relating to peripheral vascular occlusive disease or diabetes.[2] However, 80% of major amputations after severe limb trauma occur before the age of 40.[4] Combat-related major limb amputations occur primarily in younger individuals and lead to long-term functional and psychosocial deficits. For example, during the recent American military operations in the Middle East, nearly 10% of the medically evacuated personnel suffered from injuries that resulted in major limb amputation.[5] Regardless of the reason for major limb loss, all patients sustaining limb loss will contend with postamputation pain and a considerable number of them will develop debilitating chronic pain.

Postamputation pain is a general term that encompasses various unpleasant sensations experienced by patients with limb loss after the acute postoperative period. Postamputation pain can affect up to 95% of all patients with limb loss[6] and is generally categorized into several categories: (1) phantom sensations, (2) phantom limb pain, and (3) residual limb pain.[7–9] Despite being commonly designated as a type of postamputation pain, phantom sensations are nonpainful perceptions of their absent limb that can be kinetic

[a] Section of Plastic Surgery, Department of Surgery, University of Michigan, 1500 East Medical Center Drive, Ann Arbor, MI 48109, USA; [b] Mayo Clinic School of Medicine, 200 First Street Southwest, Rochester, MN 55905, USA
* Corresponding author.
E-mail address: thekung@med.umich.edu

Clin Plastic Surg 47 (2020) 311–321
https://doi.org/10.1016/j.cps.2020.01.004

(ie, perceived movements of the amputated part),[10] kinesthetic (ie, perceived shape or position of the amputated part), or exteroceptive (ie, perceived touch, pressure, itching, vibration, etc, in the phantom limb).[6] Studies demonstrate that up to 90% of patients will experience some sort of phantom sensation within 6 months of amputation.[11] Distinct from phantom sensations, phantom limb pain is a pathologic, painful condition impacting the phantom limb.[8,12,13] Phantom limb pain is thought to be due to functional reorganization of the somatosensory cortex, leading to chronic perceptions of pain in the portion of the limb that has been amputated.[14,15] Studies demonstrate that up to 85% of patients with limb loss suffer from phantom limb pain.[15,16]

In contrast with the phenomena of phantom sensations and phantom limb pain, both mediated by mechanisms involving the central nervous system, residual limb pain (also known as stump pain) is defined as pain that is localized within the residual limb and caused by a variety of local factors, such as peripheral nerve neuromas, wounds, heterotopic ossification, osteophytes, bursa, and poorly fitting prosthetic devices.[7,8,15,17] Symptomatic neuroma formation can be common in patients with limb loss, and existing strategies for addressing this condition are largely ineffective. This article focuses on a novel surgical technique that uses regenerative peripheral nerve interfaces (RPNIs) to treat and prevent neuroma formation. Additionally, this review discusses the potential for RPNI surgery to modulate the experience of phantom limb pain in patients with limb loss.

SYMPTOMATIC NEUROMAS

A transected peripheral nerve will attempt to regenerate to reestablish contact with motor or sensory end organs; however, in the setting of amputation, the regenerating axons are prone to forming an end neuroma consisting of a painful mass of axonal sprouts, connective tissue, and blood vessels.[17] Ectopic activity, mechanical sensitivity, and chemosensitivity to catecholamines within the microenvironment of the neuroma creates discomfort for the patient.[8] Within a neuroma, there is altered expression of transduction molecules, upregulation of sodium channels, downregulation of potassium channels, and development of nonfunctional connections between axons. This series of unfavorable events exacerbates neural hyperexcitability and spontaneous discharge seen within symptomatic painful neuromas.[18] Although every transected peripheral nerve is expected to form a terminal neuroma, 50% to 70% of these neuromas will be

symptomatic for patients with limb loss.[19–21] Symptomatic neuromas are frequently the cause of residual limb pain and are known to compromise prosthetic rehabilitation and diminish the quality of life after amputation.[22] In fact, painful neuromas have been cited to be a key factor driving patient abandonment of a prosthetic limb in up to 30% of cases.[23]

Although neuroma pain is a separate entity from phantom limb pain, a growing body of evidence demonstrates that pain derived from the peripheral nervous system influences central nervous system pain mechanisms and vice versa. Specifically, ongoing neuropathic pain originating from symptomatic neuromas can lead to imbalances between excitatory and inhibitory signaling in the central nervous system, a phenomenon known as central sensitization.[24] Alterations in ion channel function in sensory fibers (such as Aβ, Aδ, and C) in the peripheral nervous system affect spinal cord activity, leading to an excess of excitation and loss of inhibition. Perceptions of pain then travel via the spinothalamic pathway and are projected to the somatosensory cortex, where the location and intensity of the pain is registered.[25] Eventually, this feedback of chronic nociceptive input results in a variety of maladaptive functional changes to the central nervous system. Ultimately, these changes contribute to a vicious cycle where central sensitization stemming from peripheral pain then further amplifies the experience of peripheral pain. Accordingly, in the setting of amputation, effective treatment of symptomatic neuromas will not only alleviate pain within the residual limb, but also interrupt the pathway of noxious afferent signals sensitizing central structures and furthermore may modulate centrally mediated pain, such as phantom limb pain.[26,27]

Surgical Treatment of Symptomatic Neuromas

Although many treatment modalities have been explored for symptomatic neuromas, none are universally accepted.[28] Nonsurgical treatment attempts have included desensitization, work hardening, biofeedback, chemical or anesthetic injections, transcutaneous electrical nerve stimulation, topical lidocaine, pain catheters administering local anesthetics, and medications (antidepressants, anticonvulsants, and opioids).[17] However, symptomatic neuromas are most definitively treated with surgical techniques. A recent meta-analysis suggests that surgical treatment of symptomatic neuromas can be effective in more than 75% of patients[29] and significantly improves patient-reported outcomes such as pain, depression, and quality of life.[30,31] Many surgical treatments for symptomatic neuromas have been described, such as simple neuroma excision alone[22]; nerve capping[32–34]; excision with transposition into bone,[35] vein,[17] or muscle[35,36]; and nerve grafting.[30] Although surgery has been shown to be beneficial in treating symptomatic neuroma, there is no consensus on which technique is superior for long-term outcomes.

The most common technique for the treatment of a symptomatic end neuroma involves resection of the terminal bulb and implantation of the residual peripheral nerve into a nearby muscle belly. On the basis of neurophysiology, the freshly cut peripheral nerve will undergo a process of axonal sprouting and elongation; however, this process will undoubtedly lead to a recurrence of the neuroma because the muscle belly is already fully innervated by its native motor nerve and thus the regenerating axons of the transected peripheral nerve will not be presented with any targets to reinnervate. Nonetheless, the recurrent neuroma will be cushioned within the recipient muscle belly and better protected from external stimuli such as pressure from the socket of a prosthetic device. Therefore, any alleviation of pain from application of this strategy is likely the result of simple transposition of the recurrent neuroma to a somewhat more favorable location. For this reason, a superior surgical strategy to treat symptomatic neuromas would capitalize on the physiologic process of nerve regeneration to actually prevent the reformation of a neuroma. In turn, such a technique would also serve to diminish the noxious afferent feedback contributing to central sensitization and possibly mitigate the experience of phantom limb pain.

The Regenerative Peripheral Nerve Interface

The RPNI is a simple and reproducible surgical solution to prevent neuroma formation that leverages several biologic processes and addresses many of the limitations of existing neuroma treatment strategies. An RPNI is constructed by implanting the distal end of a transected peripheral nerve into a free skeletal muscle graft[37] (**Figs. 1–3**). Because the denervated muscle graft is initially devascularized at the time of harvest, it will undergo a well-described process of degeneration followed by regeneration.[38,39] Early in this process, the graft is supported by imbibition; however, after regeneration the muscle graft becomes revascularized just as any free tissue graft would be after nonvascularized autologous transfer (ie, a full-thickness or split thickness skin graft).[39] These regenerating muscle fibers concomitantly serve as denervated targets for regenerating axons sprouting from the

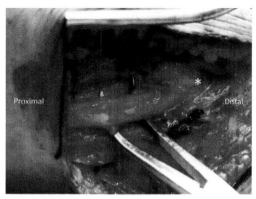

Fig. 1. Treatment of symptomatic common peroneal nerve neuroma with RPNI surgery. This patient with a lower extremity traumatic amputation injury presented with a painful neuroma of the common peroneal nerve just distal to the knee. The common peroneal nerve was exposed and a healthy portion of the nerve was identified and divided to separate it from the end neuroma, which remained buried distally in scar (marked with an *asterisk*). Note the visible division of the common peroneal nerve into superficial and deep branches at the level of the knee. These branches are separated to form 2 individual RPNIs.

end of the peripheral nerve. As a result of these functional connections, substantially fewer regenerating axons will be available to form a problematic neuroma. Through the processes of muscle revascularization and regeneration, and nerve regeneration and reinnervation, with formation of new neuromuscular junctions within the muscle graft (synaptogensis),[40] a mature RPNI is a stable biologic structure that naturally minimizes neuroma formation.[41–47] The RPNI was originally conceived of as a means to transduce and amplify neural signals for the purpose of controlling a neuroprosthetic limb.[48] Many preliminary studies regarding RPNI use in prosthetic control in animal models and human subjects have also demonstrated the biologic stability, longevity, and functional capabilities of RPNI and its potential to reduce neuroma formation.[37,49]

Synaptogenesis Mitigates Neuroma Formation

After peripheral nerve transection injury, the nerve undergoes 3 biologic processes: Wallerian degeneration, axonal sprouting/regeneration, and muscle reinnervation if end organs are present.[50] When the distal end of a nerve is in proximity to the proximal end of the nerve (ie, end-to-end neurorrhaphy) axons will regenerate into distal endoneurial tubes and elongate until they reinnervate the end organ, achieving maximal functional

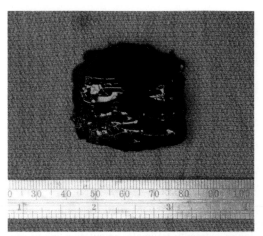

Fig. 2. Free muscle graft harvested from donor thigh muscle. The grafts are trimmed of connective tissue such as fat and tendon. For most peripheral nerves, the free muscle grafts are approximately 3 cm long, 2 cm wide, and 0.5 cm in thickness. Small caliber peripheral nerves will receive smaller free muscle grafts. Because the free muscle graft survives through imbibition and muscle regeneration, there is a limit to the size of the muscle graft that can be used for each RPNI. Therefore, large caliber nerves (eg, common peroneal, sciatic) can be separated into component branches to create multiple RPNIs. This modification also serves to optimize the ratio between the number of regenerating axons within the RPNI and the number of available denervated muscle fibers in the graft.

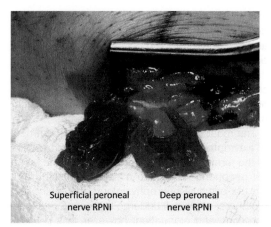

Superficial peroneal nerve RPNI

Deep peroneal nerve RPNI

Fig. 3. Creation of superficial peroneal nerve RPNI (complete) and deep peroneal nerve RPNI (in progress). The distal end of the transected nerve is implanted into the center of the free muscle graft. The epineurium is secured to the muscle graft and the free muscle graft is then wrapped around the nerve with 6-0 nonabsorbable sutures. Each RPNI is then positioned within the wound in a relatively protected and well-vascularized location.

recovery. However, in the context of amputation, the end organs are missing and therefore all of the peripheral nerves in the residual limb continue to sprout and regenerate until they form a neuroma. The use of free muscle grafts during RPNI surgery offers of a vast supply of denervated muscle targets for the regenerating axons. This distinguishing characteristic of RPNI surgery wholly differentiates it from the conventional technique of implanting a peripheral nerve into an already innervated local muscle belly. For regenerating efferent motor neurons, RPNIs provide ample denervated muscle fibers to facilitate the reestablishment of neuromuscular junctions.[48] Denervated muscle fibers atrophy unless axonal input is reinstated within a finite period of time.[51] In response to loss of innervation, these muscle fibers display dispersion of acetylcholine receptors along the sarcolemma and express of a variety of neurotrophic factors,[52] events that foster an environment conducive to reinnervation. A regenerating axon that then makes contact with a denervated muscle fiber provides necessary trophic support to prevent atrophy,[53] induces congregation of acetylcholine receptors to reform a neuromuscular junction, and initiates reconstitution of a motor unit.[54] This innately orchestrated

process of reinnervation has been observed with the RPNI. Early immunohistochemical studies in animal models revealed extensive colocalization of motor end plates and terminal axons within the free muscle graft of an RPNI. Electrophysiologic experiments confirmed that these new neuromuscular junctions were functional and capable of transducing nerve signals to muscle action potentials.[48] More recent studies investigating the potential of RPNIs to facilitate control of an artificial limb in human subjects have also corroborated the fact that functional neuromuscular junctions develop within RPNIs.[55,56] These findings are compelling evidence that RPNIs can reduce neuroma formation in transected peripheral nerves containing motor axons by giving these axons targets to form neuromuscular junctions. As a result of this extensive research, RPNIs have been increasingly performed in human patients both to treat symptomatic neuromas and to prevent neuromas at the time of amputation.

Although efferent motor neurons can be expected to form new neuromuscular junctions within RPNIs, the fate of regenerating afferent sensory axons (eg, digital nerves) within a free muscle graft remain unclear. However, preliminary clinical experience suggests that RPNIs may be quite effective in preventing neuroma formation in sensory nerves as well. Although the exact mechanism of how free muscle grafts mitigate neuroma pain stemming from regenerating sensory axons is currently under investigation, studies that have investigated the possibility of sensory-to-motor crossover provide potential explanations for this effect. Previous studies have demonstrated the ability of sensory axons to provide trophic support of denervated muscle tissue, a phenomenon known as sensory protection.[57–62] In these experiments, a donor sensory nerve is coapted to a motor nerve after denervation of a skeletal muscle. In this case, the sensory protected skeletal muscle demonstrates significantly preserved structure and function compared with controls. Notably, although neuroma formation was not a primary end point in these studies, none of these reports include a description of neuromas in the histologic or immunohistochemical analyses. Therefore, it is probable that, when regenerating sensory axons reach the denervated muscle distal to the site of nerve coaptation, neuroma formation does not occur as a result of the neurotrophic and myotrophic milieu characteristic of sensory protection.[61] Furthermore, there is strong evidence that, although functional neuromuscular junctions may not be expected to form, sensory receptors (Golgi tendon organs and spindle cells) within the skeletal muscle can be readily reinnervated by donor sensory axons.[63] These collective findings, along with preliminary experience with sensory protection in the clinical setting,[57,59] suggest that, when a donor sensory nerve is introduced to a denervated muscle, the regenerating axons are engaged in physiologically trophic processes that in turn diminishes the number of axons available for symptomatic neuroma formation. Based on this premise, symptomatic neuromas may be treated or even prevented by implanting a transected sensory nerve into a free muscle graft to create an RPNI.

Outcomes of Regenerative Peripheral Nerve Interface Surgery to Treat and Prevent Neuroma Pain

Studies examining the efficacy of RPNI surgery to treat symptomatic neuromas were inspired by enormously positive feedback from patients and their physiatrists during the course of rehabilitation after limb amputation. Among patients with limb loss who underwent RPNI surgery for the purpose of treating symptomatic neuromas, 71% of patients reported a decrease in neuroma pain within the residual limb.[37] Remarkably, there was also a 53% decrease in phantom limb pain, a finding that supports the concept of peripheral nerve treatments favorably influencing centrally mediated pain. These patients also reported significantly decreased pain interference, high satisfaction levels, and more than one-half were using fewer pain medications after RPNI surgery.

Additionally, more patients were also able to use their prosthetic limb after RPNI surgery, indicating that improved management of postamputation pain also translates to better function. These patient-reported outcomes highlight the potential that RPNIs have in treating symptomatic neuromas in amputation patients.

Symptomatic neuromas and phantom limb pain can also be mitigated by performing RPNI surgery at the time of limb amputation. A recent retrospective investigation compared postamputation pain outcomes between patients who underwent RPNI surgery prophylactically at the time of amputation and control patients who underwent standard limb amputation without RPNI surgery.[64] Control patients were matched for age, gender, level of amputation, and mean duration of follow-up. RPNI patients experienced a substantially lower incidence of symptomatic neuromas within the residual limb compared with control patients (0% vs 13.3%). Moreover, at a mean follow-up time of almost 1 year, RPNI patients reported a significantly lower rate of phantom limb pain (51.1% vs 91.1%). Although the control group was overrepresented by vascular patients with ischemic disease, an examination of major and minor complications between groups suggests that the addition of RPNI surgery performed at the time of major limb amputation does not increase the overall complication rate. Given this encouraging preliminary experience, RPNI surgery is being performed prophylactically in a variety of clinical settings, such as hand and digit amputations, large soft tissue tumor resections, and major limb amputations at all levels, including hip and shoulder disarticulations. As the indications for RPNI surgery expand, ongoing prospective studies are being conducted to elucidate the efficacy of RPNI surgery to treat and prevent postamputation pain.

Regenerative Peripheral Nerve Interface Surgery and Targeted Muscle Reinnervation for Symptomatic Neuromas

Given the understanding that neuromas will form when regenerating axons are not presented with end organs for reinnervation, any strategy that reduces the number of aimless axons within a residual limb will serve to reduce symptomatic neuromas. In recent years, both RPNI surgery and targeted muscle reinnervation (TMR) have been developed as innovative methods to facilitate prosthetic control as well as neuroma prevention.[65] TMR is a prosthetic control strategy that involves multiple nerve transfers to reroute transected peripheral nerves from an amputated limb to motor nerve branches of donor muscles. For example, in the setting of a transhumeral amputation, the median nerve can be coapted to small musculocutaneous nerve branches that innervate the short head of the biceps. After coaptation, axons from the median nerve will innervate a discrete portion of the biceps muscle, allowing this area of the muscle to generate electromyographic (EMG) signals representing median nerve information that can be recorded from a transcutaneous electrode. In regards to the potential of providing multiple independent signals for operating a prosthetic device with a high number of degrees of freedom, there are fundamental differences between RPNI surgery and TMR that are beyond the scope of this discussion. Regardless of these differences, like RPNI surgery, TMR may decrease neuroma formation by capitalizing on biologic processes characteristic of regenerating peripheral nerves. Both techniques involve reinnervation of denervated muscle and in doing so both strategies foster the formation of functional connections for regenerating axons. This in turn will minimize the number of axons available to contribute to symptomatic neuromas. As a method for managing postamputation pain, both RPNI surgery and TMR are increasingly performed in human patients to treat or prevent symptomatic neuromas.

However, it is important to note that with TMR there is an inherent need to sacrifice donor nerves and partially denervate muscles that might otherwise still be useful during prosthetic rehabilitation, such as with a myoelectric prosthesis. Myoelectric artificial limbs are commercially available devices that detect EMG signals produced by residual muscles in the residual limb.[66] For example, EMG signals from the biceps and triceps muscles in a transhumeral amputation patient could be harnessed by transcutaneous electrodes to control the opening and closing of a myoelectric robotic hand. It is, therefore, possible that partial denervation of these residual muscles for TMR may complicate the acquisition of discrete high-fidelity EMG signals and ultimately compromise the reliability of myoelectric device use. Another important consideration is that the nerve transfers in TMR usually involve very large size mismatches at the site of nerve coaptation. Although the discrepancies in nerve sizes between the donor nerves and the recipient nerves used for TMR have not been quantified, in some cases the axon count for the donor nerve (eg, median nerve at the level of the upper arm) may approach an order of magnitude higher than the axon counts of the recipient motor branches (eg, branches to the short head of the biceps).[67] Size mismatch is

a known risk factor for formation of a neuroma in continuity.[68] Furthermore, the proximal end of the sacrificed motor nerve in TMR is shortened and relocated away from the coaptation site because otherwise it may reinnervate its native muscle and interfere with the nerve transfer.[67] However, it is precisely this natural propensity for the donor nerve to regenerate and attempt reinnervation of its original muscle that conceivably could lead to neuroma formation of the sacrificed nerve. These additional neuromas resulting from TMR could potentially contribute to residual limb pain and central sensitization.

In contrast, RPNI surgery does not involve denervation of any residual muscles, leaving their EMG signals intact and fully accessible for capture of EMG signals to control a prosthetic device.[69] RPNI surgery is efficient and does not require tedious dissection to isolate small motor branches to muscle within the residual limb. Furthermore, because no nerve transfers are involved and no intact native nerves are cut, there is not the potential of forming neuromas in continuity or end neuromas. Despite these differences, as continued research elucidates the merits of RPNI surgery and TMR, the 2 techniques may have complimentary roles depending on the rehabilitative goals of a patient with limb amputation. Ultimately, both RNPI surgery and TMR have been shown to decrease postamputation pain,[31,64] and the mechanisms by which they do so are rooted in the fact that both methods leverage principles of neurobiology to minimize the number of aimless regenerating axons forming neuromas.

Indications for Regenerative Peripheral Nerve Interface Surgery for Symptomatic Neuromas

RPNI surgery is indicated for the treatment of all symptomatic neuromas and is commonly performed after major limb amputation. All patients who have had major limb amputation without any effort to provide new targets for reinnervation can be expected to have multiple neuromas, many of which will be symptomatic. Patients will report localized tenderness caused by a neuroma that is epitomized by neuropathic qualities, such as zinging, shooting, stabbing, or electrical shock pains. Usually, patients can point to the exact location where the neuroma pain originates. Tinel's sign is positive when neuropathic pain is elicited by robust tapping precisely over the location of the symptomatic neuroma. The presence of a symptomatic neuroma can be confirmed by demonstrating alleviation of the pain after injection of local anesthetic solution into the area. Further confirmation and documentation of the neuroma can be achieved through ultrasound imaging. Ul-trasound imaging may also be useful in diagnosing other symptomatic neuromas or other anomalies that may be contributing to residual limb pain. For example, if several symptomatic neuromas exist within the residual limb along with bone spurs or heterotopic ossification, treatment of just the most painful neuroma with RPNI surgery may not lead to a satisfactory decrease in residual limb pain. In these instances, patients may report allevi-ation of neuroma pain at one site, but will notice more predominant pain in the other areas owing to an unmasking effect of only removing the most noxious cause of pain. This unmasking effect has been demonstrated in other realms such as nerve compression surgery and migraine sur-gery.[70] Notably, some neuromas identified by ul-trasound imaging may not be symptomatic. RPNI surgery on nonpainful neuromas should be considered on a case-by-case basis. Although surgical intervention may reduce unfavorable neu-ral feedback from the neuroma and help to diminish centrally mediated phenomena such as phantom limb pain, traumatic disruption of a non-symptomatic neuroma may in itself cause addi-tional pain.

In addition to a full workup of all potential causes of residual limb pain, preoperative consultation should involve a disclosure of any other painful conditions, such as chronic back pain, and long-standing pain medications. Both can affect central sensitization and therefore obfuscate the efficacy of RPNI surgery. Additionally, a thorough discus-sion of the risks and benefits of RPNI surgery must include a discussion regarding the donor site for muscle grafts. When RPNI surgery is per-formed after major upper or lower limb amputa-tion, the most common donor site is the vastus lateralis through a separate thigh incision. Multiple small muscle grafts can be harvested without significantly affecting the function of the vastus lat-eralis muscle and the donor site morbidity is mini-mal. Alternative donor sites include distal residual muscles at the site of major limb amputation or muscle that are considered expendable depend-ing on the level of amputation (eg, gracilis, bra-chioradialis). Another important goal of the preoperative visit is to set expectations about pain relief. Although RPNI surgery offers a physio-logic means of decreasing neuroma pain by providing peripheral nerve axons targets for rein-nervation, incomplete pain relief is a possibility. Although this may be due to untreated cases of pain within the residual limb, patients with chronic pain often experience remodeling of the central nervous system that impedes resolution of pain, even when the peripheral trigger is treated. For

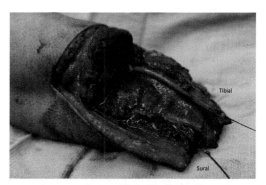

Fig. 4. RPNIs can be prophylactically performed at the time of amputation surgery. Here, a patient has un-dergone below-knee amputation with identification and preservation of the tibial nerve and sural nerve.

this reason, a multidisciplinary approach to pain control after RPNI surgery is recommended involving providers from various fields such as physical medicine and rehabilitation, physical ther-apy, occupational therapy, and primary care.

RPNI surgery can also be performed to prevent neuroma formation at the time of amputation (**Figs. 4–6**). Free muscle grafts can be harvested to created RPNIs involving any transected periph-eral nerves, including large mixed nerves (eg, sciatic nerve, tibial nerve, median nerve) and purely sensory nerves (eg, radial sensory nerve, digital nerve, intercostal nerve). The principal goal of performing RPNIs concurrently with ampu-tation surgery is to minimize the formation of pain-ful neuromas at the ends of transected peripheral nerves. In turn, this will decrease the need for pain medications postoperatively and facilitate prosthetic rehabilitation. Furthermore, prevention of peripheral nerve pain is likely to mitigate the

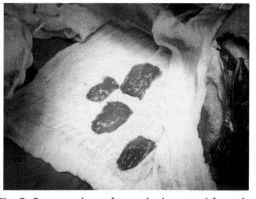

Fig. 5. Free muscle grafts can be harvested from the amputated extremity or from a remote donor muscle. In this case, multiple free muscle grafts were har-vested from the amputated lower extremity after below-knee amputation. The grafts are sharply cut to the necessary size for each RPNI and cleaned on a back table.

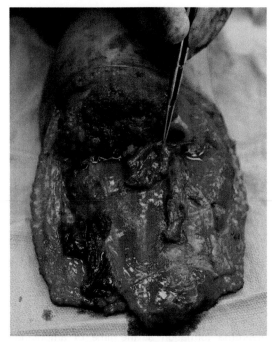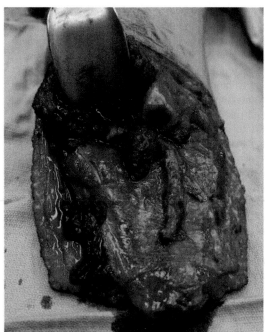

Fig. 6. Creation of a tibial nerve RPNI with a free muscle graft. The tibial nerve is shortened and the RPNI is created. The tibial nerve RPNI is then positioned proximal to the cut edge of the tibia to protect it from external forces, such as regular use of a prosthetic device.

experience of phantom limb pain and avert the maladaptive feedback to the central nervous system that is known to contribute to chronic pain syndromes.

Postoperatively, patients are followed regularly for at least 1 year to ascertain reported levels of residual limb pain and phantom limb pain as well as other quality-of-life measures through the use of various validated patient-reported outcomes instruments. At each follow-up visit, the number of pain medications being taken by the patient for amputation-related pain are thoroughly documented. The residual limb is carefully evaluated to identify any pain-related obstacles to using a prosthetic device. These may include recurrent neuromas, symptomatic neuromas that were not previously addressed with RPNIs, the development of bony spurs or heterotopic ossification, and excess soft tissue causing a poor prosthetic fit. Patients should be counseled that additional operations may be recommended to further decrease their pain and that surgical intervention may interfere with or delay prosthetic rehabilitation.

SUMMARY

RPNI surgery has enormous potential to transform the care of amputation patients. Although exciting research is being conducted to develop the RPNI as a novel interface for prosthetic control in the near future, RPNIs can be performed now for postamputation pain and represents a substantial advancement in the treatment of both symptomatic neuromas and phantom limb pain. The mechanisms of how RPNIs can affect postamputation pain are based upon the fundamental biologic principles of peripheral nerve regeneration, muscle reinnervation, and cessation of noxious afferent feedback to the central nervous system. The indications for RPNI surgery are expanding and this technique can be applied to any transected peripheral nerve to provide denervated target organs for reinnervation. This straightforward and reproducible surgical technique can be used not only to treat symptomatic neuromas, but also performed at the time of amputation to mitigate neuroma formation.

DISCLOSURE

The authors have nothing to disclose.

REFERENCES

1. Owings MF, Kozak LJ. Ambulatory and inpatient procedures in the United States, 1996. Vital Health Stat 13 1998;(139):1–119.
2. Chalya PL, Mabula JB, Dass RM, et al. Major limb amputations: a tertiary hospital experience in northwestern Tanzania. J Orthop Surg Res 2012;7:18.

3. Pinzur MS, Gottschalk FA, Pinto MA, et al. Controversies in lower-extremity amputation. J Bone Joint Surg Am 2007;89:1118–27.

4. Dillingham TR, Pezzin LE, MacKenzie EJ. Incidence, acute care length of stay, and discharge to rehabilitation of traumatic amputee patients: an epidemiologic study. Arch Phys Med Rehabil 1998;79: 279–87.

5. Goldberg M. Updated death and injury rates of U.S. Military personnel during the conflicts in Iraq and Afghanistan. Working Paper Series of the Congressional Budget Office; 2014.

6. Ephraim PL, Wegener ST, MacKenzie EJ, et al. Phantom pain, residual limb pain, and back pain in amputees: results of a national survey. Arch Phys Med Rehabil 2005;86:1910–9.

7. Neil M. Pain after amputation. BJA Educ 2015;16: 107–12.

8. Hsu E, Cohen SP. Postamputation pain: epidemiology, mechanisms, and treatment. J Pain Res 2013;6:121–36.

9. Clarke C, Lindsay DR, Pyati S, et al. Residual limb pain is not a diagnosis: a proposed algorithm to classify postamputation pain. Clin J Pain 2013;29: 551–62.

10. Bjorkman B, Arner S, Lund I, et al. Adult limb and breast amputees' experience and descriptions of phantom phenomena-A qualitative study. Scand J Pain 2010;1:43–9.

11. Jensen TS, Krebs B, Nielsen J, et al. Phantom limb, phantom pain and stump pain in amputees during the first 6 months following limb amputation. Pain 1983;17:243–56.

12. Kooijman CM, Dijkstra PU, Geertzen JH, et al. Phantom pain and phantom sensations in upper limb amputees: an epidemiological study. Pain 2000;87: 33–41.

13. Parkes CM. Factors determining the persistence of phantom pain in the amputee. J Psychosom Res 1973;17:97–108.

14. Karl A, Birbaumer N, Lutzenberger W, et al. Reorganization of motor and somatosensory cortex in upper extremity amputees with phantom limb pain. J Neurosci 2001;21:3609–18.

15. Davis RW. Phantom sensation, phantom pain, and stump pain. Arch Phys Med Rehabil 1993;74: 79–91.

16. Jensen TS, Krebs B, Nielsen J, et al. Immediate and long-term phantom limb pain in amputees: incidence, clinical characteristics and relationship to pre-amputation limb pain. Pain 1985;21:267–78.

17. Stokvis A, van der Avoort DJ, van Neck JW, et al. Surgical management of neuroma pain: a prospective follow-up study. Pain 2010;151:862–9.

18. Nikolajsen L. Postamputation pain: studies on mechanisms. Dan Med J 2012;59:B4527.

19. Soroush M, Modirian E, Soroush M, et al. Neuroma in bilateral upper limb amputation. Orthopedics 2008; 31 [pii:orthosupersite.com/view.asp?rID=32929].

20. Buchheit T, Van de Ven T, Hsia HL, et al. Pain phenotypes and associated clinical risk factors following traumatic amputation: results from veterans integrated pain evaluation research (VIPER). Pain Med 2016;17:149–61.

21. Hanley MA, Ehde DM, Jensen M, et al. Chronic pain associated with upper-limb loss. Am J Phys Med Rehabil 2009;88:742–51 [quiz: 752, 779].

22. Sehirlioglu A, Ozturk C, Yazicioglu K, et al. Painful neuroma requiring surgical excision after lower limb amputation caused by landmine explosions. Int Orthop 2009;33:533–6.

23. McFarland LV, Hubbard Winkler SL, Heinemann AW, et al. Unilateral upper-limb loss: satisfaction and prosthetic-device use in veterans and servicemembers from Vietnam and OIF/OEF conflicts. J Rehabil Res Dev 2010;47:299–316.

24. Harte SE, Harris RE, Clauw DJ. The neurobiology of central sensitization. J Appl Biobehav Res 2018;23: e12137.

25. Colloca L, Ludman T, Bouhassira D, et al. Neuropathic pain. Nat Rev Dis Primers 2017;3:17002.

26. Prantl L, Schreml S, Heine N, et al. Surgical treatment of chronic phantom limb sensation and limb pain after lower limb amputation. Plast Reconstr Surg 2006;118:1562–72.

27. Economides JM, DeFazio MV, Attinger CE, et al. Prevention of painful neuroma and phantom limb pain after transfemoral amputations through concomitant nerve coaptation and collagen nerve wrapping. Neurosurgery 2016;79:508–13.

28. Elliot D. Surgical management of painful peripheral nerves. Clin Plast Surg 2014;41:589–613.

29. Poppler LH, Parikh RP, Bichanich MJ, et al. Surgical interventions for the treatment of painful neuroma: a comparative meta-analysis. Pain 2018; 159:214–23.

30. Domeshek LF, Krauss EM, Snyder-Warwick AK, et al. Surgical treatment of neuromas improves patient-reported pain, depression, and quality of life. Plast Reconstr Surg 2017;139:407–18.

31. Dumanian GA, Potter BK, Mioton LM, et al. Targeted muscle reinnervation treats neuroma and phantom pain in major limb amputees: a randomized clinical trial. Ann Surg 2019;270(2):238–46.

32. Swanson AB, Boeve NR, Lumsden RM. The prevention and treatment of amputation neuromata by silicone capping. J Hand Surg 1977;2:70–8.

33. Sosin M, Weiner LA, Robertson BC, et al. Treatment of a recurrent neuroma within nerve allograft with autologous nerve reconstruction. Hand (N Y) 2016; 11:Np5–9.

34. Hong T, Wood I, Hunter DA, et al. Neuroma management: capping nerve injuries with an acellular nerve

allograft can limit axon regeneration. Hand (N Y) 2019. https://doi.org/10.1177/1558944719849115. 1558944719849115.

35. Burchiel KJ, Johans TJ, Ochoa J. The surgical treatment of painful traumatic neuromas. J Neurosurg 1993;78:714–9.

36. Dellon AL, Mackinnon SE. Treatment of the painful neuroma by neuroma resection and muscle implantation. Plast Reconstr Surg 1986;77:427–38.

37. Woo SL, Urbanchek MG, Cederna PS, et al. Revisiting nonvascularized partial muscle grafts: a novel use for prosthetic control. Plast Reconstr Surg 2014;134:344e–6e.

38. Dumont NA, Bentzinger CF, Sincennes MC, et al. Satellite cells and skeletal muscle regeneration. Compr Physiol 2015;5:1027–59.

39. White TP, Devor ST. Skeletal muscle regeneration and plasticity of grafts. Exerc Sport Sci Rev 1993; 21:263–95.

40. Wu H, Xiong WC, Mei L. To build a synapse: signaling pathways in neuromuscular junction assembly. Development 2010;137:1017–33.

41. Gutmann E, Carlson BM. A comparison between the free grafting of sliced and intact muscles in the rat-1. Experientia 1975;31:848–50.

42. Mong FF. Histological and histochemical studies on the nervous influence on minced muscle regeneration of triceps surae of the rat. J Morphol 1977;151:451–62.

43. Bader D. Reinnervation of motor endplate-containing and motor endplate-less muscle grafts. Dev Biol 1980;77:315–27.

44. Hakelius L, Nystrom B, Stalberg E. Histochemical and neurophysiological studies of autotransplanted cat muscle. Scand J Plast Reconstr Surg 1975;9:15–24.

45. Killer H, Muntener M. Time course of the regeneration of the endplate zone after autologous muscle transplantation. Experientia 1986;42:301–2.

46. Carlson BM, Faulkner JA. The regeneration of skeletal muscle fibers following injury: a review. Med Sci Sports Exerc 1983;15:187–98.

47. Carlson BM, Gutmann E. Contractile and histochemical properties of sliced muscle grafts regenerating in normal and denervated rat limbs. Exp Neurol 1976;50:319–29.

48. Kung TA, Langhals NB, Martin DC, et al. Regenerative peripheral nerve interface viability and signal transduction with an implanted electrode. Plast Reconstr Surg 2014;133:1380–94.

49. Kung TA, Bueno RA, Alkhalefah GK, et al. Innovations in prosthetic interfaces for the upper extremity. Plast Reconstr Surg 2013;132:1515–23.

50. Menorca RM, Fussell TS, Elfar JC. Nerve physiology: mechanisms of injury and recovery. Hand Clin 2013; 29:317–30.

51. Fu SY, Gordon T. Contributing factors to poor functional recovery after delayed nerve repair: prolonged axotomy. J Neurosci 1995;15:3876–85.

52. Kuromi H, Kidokoro Y. Nerve disperses preexisting acetylcholine receptor clusters prior to induction of receptor accumulation in Xenopus muscle cultures. Dev Biol 1984;103:53–61.

53. Borisov AB, Dedkov EI, Carlson BM. Interrelations of myogenic response, progressive atrophy of muscle fibers, and cell death in denervated skeletal muscle. Anat Rec 2001;264:203–18.

54. Grumbles RM, Almeida VW, Casella GT, et al. Motoneuron replacement for reinnervation of skeletal muscle in adult rats. J Neuropathol Exp Neurol 2012; 71:921–30.

55. Ursu DC, Urbanchek MG, Nedic A, et al. In vivo characterization of regenerative peripheral nerve interface function. J Neural Eng 2016;13:026012.

56. Frost CM, Ursu DC, Flattery SM, et al. Regenerative peripheral nerve interfaces for real-time, proportional control of a Neuroprosthetic hand. J Neuroeng Rehabil 2018;15:108.

57. Placheta E, Wood MD, Lafontaine C, et al. Enhancement of facial nerve motoneuron regeneration through cross-face nerve grafts by adding end-to-side sensory axons. Plast Reconstr Surg 2015;135:460–71.

58. Bain JR, Veltri KL, Chamberlain D, et al. Improved functional recovery of denervated skeletal muscle after temporary sensory nerve innervation. Neuroscience 2001;103:503–10.

59. Bain JR, Hason Y, Veltri K, et al. Clinical application of sensory protection of denervated muscle. J Neurosurg 2008;109:955–61.

60. Hynes NM, Bain JR, Thoma A, et al. Preservation of denervated muscle by sensory protection in rats. J Reconstr Microsurg 1997;13:337–43.

61. Papakonstantinou KC, Kamin E, Terzis JK. Muscle preservation by prolonged sensory protection. J Reconstr Microsurg 2002;18:173–82 [discussion: 183–4].

62. Wang H, Gu Y, Xu J, et al. Comparative study of different surgical procedures using sensory nerves or neurons for delaying atrophy of denervated skeletal muscle. J Hand Surg 2001;26:326–31.

63. Elsohemy A, Butler R, Bain JR, et al. Sensory protection of rat muscle spindles following peripheral nerve injury and reinnervation. Plast Reconstr Surg 2009;124: 1860–8.

64. Kubiak CA, Kemp SWP, Cederna PS, et al. Prophylactic regenerative peripheral nerve interfaces to prevent postamputation pain. Plast Reconstr Surg 2019;144(3):421e–30e.

65. Souza JM, Cheesborough JE, Ko JH, et al. Targeted muscle reinnervation: a novel approach to postamputation neuroma pain. Clin Orthop Relat Res 2014; 472:2984–90.

66. Peerdeman B, Boere D, Witteveen H, et al. Myoelectric forearm prostheses: state of the art from a user-centered perspective. J Rehabil Res Dev 2011;48: 719–37.

67. Gart MS, Souza JM, Dumanian GA. Targeted muscle reinnervation in the upper extremity amputee: a technical roadmap. J Hand Surg 2015;40:1877–88.

68. Mavrogenis AF, Pavlakis K, Stamatoukou A, et al. Current treatment concepts for neuromas-in-continuity. Injury 2008;39(Suppl 3):S43–8.

69. Vu PP, Irwin ZT, Bullard AJ, et al. Closed-loop continuous hand control via chronic recording of regenerative peripheral nerve interfaces. IEEE Trans Neural Syst Rehabil Eng 2018;26:515–26.

70. Fitzgerald M, McKelvey R. Nerve injury and neuropathic pain - a question of age. Exp Neurol 2016; 275 Pt 2:296–302.

Perioperative Pain Management in Hand and Upper Extremity Surgery

Evyn L. Neumeister, MD, MPH[a], Austin M. Beason, MD[b],
Jacob A. Thayer, MD[a], Youssef El Bitar, MD[b],*

KEYWORDS

- Perioperative pain management • Upper extremity surgery • Multimodal therapy
- Preoperative education • Upper extremity pain

KEY POINTS

- A multimodal analgesia approach including oral and intravenous therapies is the most effective means of managing perioperative pain of patients undergoing surgery of the hand and upper extremity.
- Regional anesthesia for upper extremity surgery is effective for procedures involving distinct anatomic regions and is augmented with continuous infusions to reduce postoperative pain and opioid requirements.
- Preoperative pain science education and pain management education can decrease postoperative opioid use and increase patient satisfaction.

INTRODUCTION

Outpatient surgeries have become increasingly popular over the past few decades, in line with the significant advances in surgical techniques, improving technology, availability of more efficient anesthetic medications, and evolving pain management strategies.[1] In 2010, there were an estimated 48.3 million ambulatory surgery procedures performed in the United States,[2] which is estimated to keep rising with the current shift away from inpatient surgery to improve efficiency and reduce cost.[3]

Hand and upper extremity surgeries are among the most common procedures performed in an outpatient setting, and patients are commonly prescribed opioid medications for postoperative pain management.[4] Approximately one-third of patients complain of moderate to severe pain after surgery[5] and adequate pain management allows patients to progress more comfortably and efficiently through rehabilitation and to improve patient satisfaction and surgical outcomes.[6] Additionally, postoperative pain complaints are the most common causes for unanticipated inpatient admissions,[7] and severe acute postoperative pain is associated with the development of chronic pain[8] and frequent visits to the outpatient clinic and emergency department.[9] Persistent pain in elderly patients has been associated with cognitive decline, increased risk for dementia, memory loss, and loss of executive function.[7] Given these known associations stemming from postoperative pain and the potential effect on patients' quality of life, surgeons should be thoughtful in their perioperative pain management practices.

[a] Department of Surgery, Institute for Plastic Surgery, Southern Illinois University School of Medicine, 747 North Rutledge Street, Springfield, IL 62794-9653, USA; [b] Department of Surgery, Division of Orthopaedic Surgery, Southern Illinois University School of Medicine, 701 North 1st Street, Suite D-306, Springfield, IL 62794-9638, USA
* Corresponding author.
E-mail address: yelbitar65@siumed.edu

Clin Plastic Surg 47 (2020) 323–334
https://doi.org/10.1016/j.cps.2019.12.004

There are several strategies implemented to offer patients proper pain control, which is most efficiently achieved by a multimodal approach.[10] Pain management starts in the preoperative setting with patient education, establishing proper expectations, psychosocial therapies, and addressing opioid medication habits especially in opioid-tolerant patients. Intraoperative analgesia and anesthesia usually set the tone for the postoperative pain management phase and includes peripheral regional blocks, intravenous (IV) regional anesthesia (RA), continuous infusion pumps, periarticular infiltration, local infiltration, and wide-awake surgery. Postoperative analgesia starts in the postanesthesia care unit including cryotherapy, injectable and oral medications, transdermal patches, and selective regional blocks. Home analgesia involves multiple different medications with different efficiencies and modes of action, such as acetaminophen, nonsteroidal anti-inflammatory drugs (NSAIDs), muscle relaxers, gabapentinoids, ketorolac, and opioids.[4]

Opioid pharmacotherapy has long been the mainstay for postoperative pain control following surgeries of the hand and upper extremity, but in the face of the opioid epidemic[11] there has been a great deal of attention directed at ways to reduce opioid prescriptions and reduce the rates of substance-related deaths in the United States. The annual opioid-related economic burden is $78.5 billion, and this is mostly because of health care cost, treatment of substance abuse and dependence, and lost productivity and incarceration.[12]

The Centers for Disease Control and Prevention has reported more than 400,000 opioid-related deaths from 1999 to 2017, and the numbers keep rising.[11] There were around 48,000 deaths in 2017 alone related to opioid overdose including prescription and illegal drugs, a staggering 130 mortalities per day, six times higher than in 1999.[11] There are increasing efforts to finding alternative ways to provide proper pain management for all patients, especially orthopedic surgery patients, the third highest recipients of opioid prescriptions in all medical and surgical specialties.[13]

This review discusses the different pain management modalities used in surgeries of the hand and upper extremity, describing the mode of action of each modality, the effectiveness of each pain management option, and the risks and potential complications.

PAIN PATHWAYS AND MODULATION

The pain pathway is broken down into two different categories: the central and peripheral nervous systems (CNS and PNS). Each system has several modulators, which are the targets of perioperative pain control. Therefore, a basic understanding of the pain pathway is helpful in understanding and providing effective perioperative pain management.

Surgery is a trauma that stimulates nociceptors in the PNS. The resulting inflammatory reaction at the site of injury initiates a cascade of locally released inflammatory mediators,[14] among which are cyclooxygenase (COX) and prostaglandins,[8] the targets of acetaminophen, NSAIDs, and other common perioperative medications. Inflammatory mediators sensitize nociceptors, decreasing their excitability threshold.[14]

Nociceptors carry signals to the dorsal horn of the spinal cord, part of the CNS, where inhibitory neuronal pathways can modulate pain.[14] Psychological factors can play a role in these inhibitory neuronal pathways,[14] with the signal ultimately carried to the brain where sensations are perceived. Neurons in the CNS, in the brain and spinal cord, have excitatory and inhibitory receptors, including the N-methyl-D-aspartate (NMDA) receptors and α_2-adrenergic receptors, respectively, which can be targeted by pharmacotherapy. In response to inflammation and nociceptor stimulation, expression of receptors and channels on neurons in the CNS undergo modulation (reversible changes) and modification (long-lasting changes) of these neurons.[8,15] These changes result in short-lived or long-lasting changes in excitability, changes that are the basis of hyperalgesia, chronic pain, and pathologic pain.[8,15,16]

PHARMACOTHERAPY AND MULTIMODAL ANALGESIA
Inhibition of Inflammation and Prostaglandins

Prostaglandins are found in the pain pathway in the PNS and CNS, inflammatory mediators that sensitize nociceptors in the setting of injury. Therefore, modulation of the inflammatory pathway is an important target for postoperative pain control. Acetaminophen and ibuprofen reduce inflammation and prostaglandin production.[17]

Acetaminophen (Tylenol) is the most widely used medication in multimodal therapy with its low side-effect profile and minimal contraindications compared with other medications.[18] Acetaminophen given 24 hours before surgery has been shown to reduce morphine intake by up to 20%.[7] Hepatotoxicity is a side effect of acetaminophen that should be considered, especially in patients with cirrhosis of the liver or liver injury.

NSAIDs exert their effects either through nonselective inhibition of the COX-1 and -2 enzymes (ketorolac, ibuprofen, meloxicam),[19] or selective COX-2 inhibition (celecoxib).[20] Preoperative and postoperative NSAIDs including ketorolac (Toradol), ibuprofen, and celecoxib, have all been shown to significantly reduce postoperative pain.[16,20,21] These have increased anti-inflammatory properties when compared with acetaminophen alone. The side effects of NSAIDs (gastric irritation, cardiovascular events, and renal toxicity) must be considered in each patient individually to ensure safety. Selective COX-2 inhibitors are considered for their reduced gastrointestinal and renal risk profile. A theoretic risk of bone healing problems is associated with NSAID use, but evidence to this effect has not been strong enough to preclude its use in this setting.[22]

Gabapentinoids

Gabapentinoids, such as gabapentin and pregabalin, are associated with reduced opioid requirements, reduced postoperative pain,[23,24] and decreased risk of progression to chronic pain by mitigating central and peripheral sensitization.[15] Both medications are effective when dosed preoperatively and exert their effects by blocking voltage-dependent calcium channels and modulating excitatory neurotransmitter release[16,25] thereby reducing hypersensitivity in spinal cord dorsal horn neurons.[22] There has been no consensus on recommended perioperative dosing; studies have recommended anywhere from a 2-week preoperative course[23] to a high-dose bolus 1 to 2 hours before surgery, to simply starting a course of gabapentinoids postoperatively.[26] Caution should be used in patients with contraindications, such as renal dysfunction, or those with higher risk of sedation and dizziness because these are side effects of gabapentinoids.[16]

N-Methyl-D-Aspartate Receptor Antagonists

Ketamine is well-known for its action as an NDMA receptor antagonist, with a complex mechanism of action, acting peripherally and centrally[27] on multiple other binding sites including nicotinic, muscarinic, monoaminergic, and opioid receptors. Ketamine also decreases proinflammatory cytokine formation.[18] Intraoperative ketamine has been shown to decrease central pain sensitization,[23] opioid requirements postoperatively, and persistent postoperative pain[16,28] at subanesthetic doses.[17] Risks of administration including hallucinations and nightmares have become less frequent with modern reduced doses of ketamine used perioperatively.[27] Still,

the American Pain Society recommends that ketamine be used for major surgeries given its known side effects.[26]

IV and intra-articular magnesium[18] and nitric oxide[8] have NMDA receptor antagonistic effects and have been considered for use to control postoperative pain, although none of these have received a significant amount of attention in the literature.

Other Nonopioid Pain Medications

α_2-Adrenergic receptor agonists, such as dexmedetomidine and clonidine, have shown promising effects on decreasing perioperative pain and hyperalgesia[15,17,23] by acting centrally and increasing the effects of inhibitory γ-aminobutyric acid neurons. Intraoperative corticosteroids have also demonstrated decreased postoperative pain and opioid consumption, with prolonged RA.[29]

Lidocaine, typically known for its action on sodium channels providing local anesthesia, also demonstrates action on other familiar receptors within the pain pathway. IV lidocaine has been shown to have anti-inflammatory properties and central NMDA receptor antagonism.[30] IV lidocaine has demonstrated decreased postoperative pain scores and opioid consumption.[15,18]

Opioids

Opioids mimic endogenous opioid proteins and bind to mu, delta, and kappa receptors thereby reducing neuronal excitability and decreasing the release of the nociceptive neurotransmitter, substance P.[31] Oral opioids have been shown to be equally effective for postoperative pain control as IV.[32] The cautions of opioid medication include addiction potential; nausea; vomiting; ileus; constipation; urinary retention; sleep disturbance; delirium; and, most significantly, sedation, respiratory depression; and tolerance.[26,33] Opioids have been shown to cause opioid-induced hypersensitivity, a paradox in which opioids lead to increased pain perception. Some opioids activate NMDA receptors, activating central excitatory neurons, leading to increased perceptions of pain.[27] Short-acting opioids, such as fentanyl, used intraoperatively have been shown to be clinically associated with higher opioid requirements postoperatively after the infusion had been stopped.[8]

Multimodal Analgesia

Multimodal pain therapy takes advantage of the science behind pain perception by targeting different receptors involved in modulation of pain perception.[27] Studies have demonstrated that, compared with narcotic-only management, multimodal therapy provides as effective or superior pain management, in addition to reducing the amount of opioids used.[18,34,35] Additionally, enhanced recovery protocols have been developed on the idea that reducing metabolic stress with multimodal therapy leads not only to improved pain management but also to decreased catabolism and perioperative insulin resistance, thereby reducing poor surgical outcomes.[18] Multimodal therapy is an especially important concept to use when operating on patients with risk factors associated with increased postoperative pain. These risk factors include preoperative opioid use/substance abuse, morbid obesity, anxiety and depression, younger patients, female patients, preexisting pain syndromes, and lower education.[5,15,36]

Preventative and preemptive pain management are other important considerations in perioperative pain management in terms of medication timing. The role of preventative analgesia is reducing CNS sensitization, and improving postoperative pain control.[37] Preemptive analgesia (eg, local/regional anesthetic before the incision) aims to mitigate the afferent nociceptive pathway, the first step in pain perception.[37] Although preemptive analgesia helps with immediate postoperative pain control, it has not consistently been shown to be as effective as preventative analgesia in reducing surgery-related opioid use.[7,38]

There is a paucity of publications regarding multimodal therapy in upper extremity surgery specifically, but there is evidence that upper extremity surgeons have room to improve routine multimodal analgesia practices. In a study evaluating 170 shoulder surgeons,[39] more than 90% reported that they had a pain management regimen, but less than 50% regularly gave acetaminophen or ibuprofen, less than 15% regularly gave gabapentin, and more than 75% gave short-acting narcotics. There is also evidence of overprescribing opioids up to five times what patients consume,[36] in orthopedic literature. In one study of 1199 procedures including shoulder arthroscopy, endoscopic carpal tunnel release, hip, and total knee surgeries, patients reported unused opioids in 61% of procedures.[40] Even after one institution used an early recovery protocol, the rate of opioid prescriptions was still 72% for patients with low opioid consumption before discharge and low pain scores.[41] Increased mindfulness regarding opioid requirements can mitigate this discrepancy. Kim and colleagues[42] documented the number of opioid pills patients consumed among several upper extremity surgeries, and created a helpful template (**Table 1**).

REGIONAL ANESTHESIA

RA is a means of achieving a combination of motor and sensory blockade via targeted administration of anesthetic agents and adjuvants into a specific anatomic region.[43] In upper extremity surgery, RA is often a peripheral block of the brachial plexus, which can be anesthetized in various anatomic regions to achieve the desired anesthetic effect. Commonly, RA of the brachial plexus is aimed at the interscalene, supraclavicular, infraclavicular, or axillary regions (**Fig. 1**).[44] The advent of ultrasound and neurostimulation as a means of localizing these regions has increased the adoption, safety, and efficacy of RA as an alternative to general anesthesia.[45–47] Long- and short-acting local agents for RA are available and the dose required is dependent on agent used, technique (eg, ultrasound guided), and physician preference. Bupivacaine is a long-acting agent that has been shown effective for interscalene brachial plexus blocks (ISB). Its association with cardiotoxicity and neurotoxicity led to the development of levobupivacaine and ropivacaine, which have been shown to have improved side effect profiles.[48] Adjuvants to RA including epinephrine, clonidine, and dexamethasone are used to improve local absorption and prolong duration of analgesia; however, those benefits must be weighed against their known associations with intraoperative bradycardia, hypotension, and sedation.[43]

The ISB is commonly used in upper extremity surgery and is most ideally suited for shoulder surgery.[6,43] The ISB covers the supraclavicular nerves and provides sensory blockade to the skin overlying the shoulder. However, it is considered "ulnar sparing" because its blockade of the C8 and T1 ventral rami are poor. This incomplete anesthetic effect makes the ISB poorly suited for forearm and hand surgery, but it is used in elbow surgery with the understanding that it has incomplete sensory block.

RA for procedures distal to the midhumerus is better achieved by a supraclavicular block. This anesthetizes the entire brachial plexus distal to the site of injection because all the trunks traverse this narrow anatomic space within the compact fascial sheath.[44] Relative contraindications for supraclavicular blocks include enlarged lung volumes (eg, chronic obstructive pulmonary disease) and shoulder surgery because the sensory block of the superficial shoulder is inadequate.

The infraclavicular brachial plexus block is an effective RA technique for surgery of the elbow, forearm, wrist, and hand.[44] Moreover, the infraclavicular block carries a lower risk of pneumothorax than the supraclavicular technique and it has been

Table 1
Opioid recommendations for upper extremity procedures

Operation	Typical Volume of 1% Lidocaine with 1:100,000 Epinephrine and 8.4% Bicarbonate (Mixed 10 mL:1 mL)	Location of Injection
Carpal tunnel	20 mL	10 mL between ulnar and median nerves (5 mm proximal to wrist crease and 5 mm ulnar to median nerve); another 10 mL under incision
Trigger finger	4 mL	Subcutaneously beneath the center of the incision
Finger sensory block (SIMPLE)[5]	2 mL	Volar middle of proximal phalanx just past palmar-finger crease
Finger soft tissue lesions or other surgery when finger base tourniquet is not desirable and finger epinephrine is used for hemostasis	5 mL volar distributed among 3 phalanges, 4 mL dorsal split between 2 phalanges	2 mL volar and 2 mL dorsal subcutaneous midline fat, in proximal and middle phalanges The distal phalanx gets only 1 mL midline volar, just past the DIP crease
PIP arthrodesis	8 mL total, 4 mL volar (2 in each phalanx), and 4 mL dorsal (2 in each phalanx)	2 mL midvolar and another 2 mL middorsal of proximal and middle phalanges
Thumb MCP arthrodesis and collateral ligament tears of the MCP joint	15 mL	2 mL on each of volar and dorsal aspects of proximal phalanx and the rest all around the metacarpal head
Dupuytren contracture or zone II flexor tendon repair	15 mL/ray	10 mL (or more) in the palm, then 2 mL in the proximal and middle phalanges and 1 mL in the distal phalanx (if required)
Trapeziectomy or Bennet fracture	40 mL	Radial side of the hand under the skin and all around the joint, including the median nerve If LRTI is performed, decrease concentration to 0.5% lidocaine with 1:200,000 epinephrine, and also inject all around where FCR or APL will be dissected
Metacarpal fractures	40 mL	All around the metacarpal where dissection or K-wires will occur

Abbreviations: APL, abductor pollicis longus; DIP, distal interphalangeal joint; FCR, flexor carpi radialis; LRTI, ligament reconstruction and tendon interposition; MCP, metacarpophalangeal joint; PIP, proximal interphalangeal joint; SIMPLE, single subcutaneous injection in the middle of the proximal phalanx with lidocaine and epinephrine.
Modified from Lalonde DH, Wong A. Dosage of local anesthesia in wide awake hand surgery. J Hand Surg Am. 2013;38(10):2025-2028; with permission.

shown to effectively alleviate forearm tourniquet pain.[49]

The axillary brachial plexus block is used frequently in outpatient surgery clinics for procedures isolated to the forearm and hand. However, it does not anesthetize the musculocutaneous nerve because it exits the plexus sheath proximal to the injection site. The axillary technique is distant from the pleura and other at-risk neurologic structures (ie, phrenic nerve and stellate ganglion), which significantly reduces the risk for pneumothorax and neurologic injury.[44]

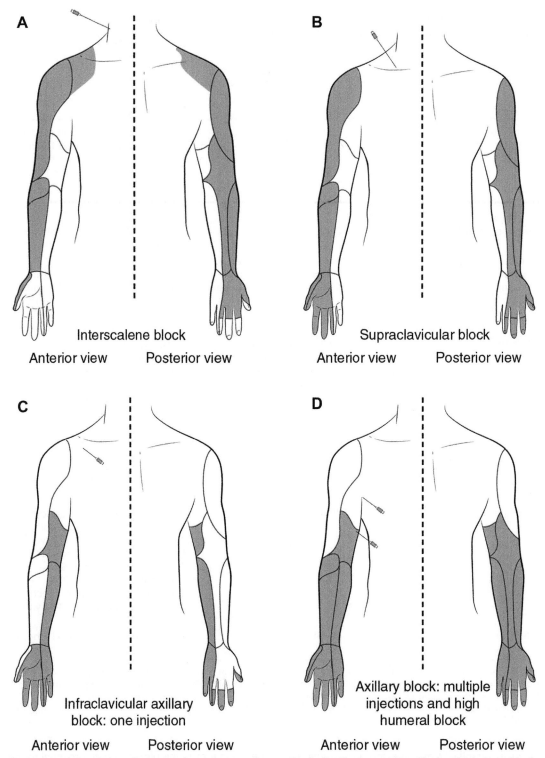

Fig. 1. Anterior and posterior views of upper extremity anesthetic distribution achieved by brachial plexus blocks. (*A*) Interscalene block. (*B*) Supraclavicular block. (*C*) Infraclavicular block. (*D*) Axillary block. (*From* Bruce BG, Green A, Blaine TA, et al. Brachial plexus blocks for upper extremity orthopaedic surgery. J Am Acad Orthop Surg. 2012;20(1):38-47; with permission.)

Safe administration of RA in the upper extremity requires a complete understanding of the anatomic landmarks and neurovascular structures. Risks involved with RA of the brachial plexus include nerve injury (mechanical trauma, drug neurotoxicity, compression, or stretch), pneumothorax, vascular injury, and systemic complications (seizures, respiratory failure secondary to phrenic nerve blockade).[43,50] Despite these risks, RA is associated with fewer systemic adverse effects than general anesthesia,[51] and RA for upper extremity surgery has been reported to decrease postoperative pain and opioid requirements, decrease duration of stay in the postanesthesia care unit, and facilitate outpatient procedures by reducing the number of overnight hospitalizations.[43,52–54] RA as part of a multimodal oral analgesic regimen including opioids, NSAIDs, and gabapentinoids is recommended for patients undergoing surgery of the upper extremity.[55]

INTRAVENOUS REGIONAL ANESTHESIA

IVRA is an effective means of anesthesia for short procedures and its success relies on appropriate patient selection and tolerance of a tourniquet while providing a bloodless surgical field.[56,57] IVRA was first described by German surgeon August Bier in 1908 and involves the use of a single- or double-lumen tourniquet applied to the proximal arm.[58] A single-lumen tourniquet is ideal for surgeries less than 20 minutes, whereas the double-lumen tourniquet is preferable in cases that may extend up to 60 minutes.[56] Regardless of procedure time, the tourniquet is usually left inflated for a minimum of 30 minutes to reduce the risk of systemic local anesthetic toxicity, and a dose of 3 mg/kg 0.5% lidocaine is used most frequently.[56,57]

Anxious patients tend to not tolerate the tourniquet pain often associated with the Bier block, therefore identifying these patients early can allow for plans to use IV anxiolytics and sedatives. However, this may defeat the primary purposes of using the Bier block, which are decreased recovery time and cost reductions.[56,59] Procedure duration is another limiting factor in deciding to use the Bier block; any procedure longer than 60 minutes is less than ideal for IVRA because tourniquet pain is common. The use of IVRA adjuvants has been studied and despite the accepted benefit of ketamine as a systemic pharmacologic therapy, it has been shown to have no additional effect when injected in combination with IVRA lidocaine.[60] Conversely, the addition of 300 mg of acetaminophen to the IVRA injection has been shown to significantly reduce intraoperative pain, which supports its use as an IVRA adjuvant.[61]

The forearm Bier block has been developed as a safe and efficient alternative to the traditional Bier block that requires only a single tourniquet just distal to the elbow and a lesser amount of lidocaine.[57] Although the Bier block offers a simple and efficient means of anesthesia, the use of lidocaine and a tourniquet increase the risk of systemic local anesthetic toxicity and postoperative tourniquet pain, respectively, and many surgeons have transitioned to brachial plexus blocks for RA in upper extremity surgery.

CONTINUOUS INFUSIONS

A single-injection ISB has been reported to provide effective dynamic pain relief for up to 6 hours after surgery and pain relief at rest for 8 hours. However, postoperative rebound pain at 24 hours is a concern.[62] Duration of analgesia for single-injection RA is often reported to be approximately 12 hours,[43] therefore continuous infusion modalities involving indwelling catheters have been developed to prolong pain relief. Bupivacaine continuous infusions via catheter has been shown to significantly reduce postoperative pain scores, decrease opioid use and opioid-related side effects, and improve sleep patterns.[63] There are concerns with catheter dislodgement and premature removal of the catheter, and catheter site infections. Catheters placed using the infraclavicular approach have been reported to have a regional anatomy that allows for quicker and more stable placement, permitting easy access for postoperative catheter care, and having a more pronounced blockade than supraclavicular continuous infusions.[44,64] Although continuous infusions can prolong the effects of analgesia, they require patient-physician cooperation and coordination after discharge, and is technically challenging to implement.[65] The development of daily bupivacaine dose limitations, disposable and tamper-resistant infusion pumps, and the recommendation for an at-home patient caretaker to assist with catheter care has improved the safety profile of this postoperative pain management modality.[43,64,66]

LOCAL ANESTHESIA
Periarticular Infiltration

Periarticular infiltration for shoulder surgery with liposomal bupivacaine as a component of multimodal analgesia is an increasingly accepted means of reducing postoperative pain, but the risk of chondrolysis still exists.[67,68]

Local Infiltration and Wide-Awake Hand Surgery with No Tourniquet

An entire paradigm shift in upper extremity surgery was based on soft tissue infiltration of local anesthesia. Local infiltration and wide-awake hand surgery with no tourniquet (WALANT) techniques have provided an alternative analgesic regimen rendering perioperative anesthesia unnecessary in many upper extremity procedures. It uses lidocaine with epinephrine in field and nerve block fashion to provide complete anesthesia to allow for upper extremity procedures to be performed while the patient is awake and able to follow instructions during surgery. Up to 7 mg/kg of lidocaine with epinephrine are used[69] at varying concentrations depending on the size of the field. Lalonde and Martin[70,71] recommend the use of 1% lidocaine with epinephrine if less than 50 mL are required and 0.25% lidocaine with epinephrine if more than 100 to 200 mL of lidocaine are required. The addition of 0.5% bupivacaine is used when the procedure is planned to take longer than 2.5 hours.[69] Lalonde and Martin[71] provide tips to decrease injection pain including using a 27-gauge or 30-gauge needle, buffering lidocaine with 8.4% bicarbonate in 1:10 ratio, injecting perpendicular to the skin, injecting slowly, and injecting lidocaine continuously while advancing the needle. The dose of lidocaine injection needed for common anatomic locations can vary (**Table 2**).[69] Of note, it is now well documented that lidocaine with epinephrine does not cause finger necrosis.[71]

WALANT has allowed for optimal clinical results in hand tendon transfers and flexor tendon repairs because the patient's participation allows surgeons to identify tendon repair gapping, catching on pulleys, and mismatched tendon tension in surgery, making corrections immediately to prevent postoperative complications.[71,72]

In a study evaluating distal radius fracture fixations using WALANT, there were no differences in clinical outcomes in range of motion or time to bony union, and patients' visual analogue scale on postoperative day 1 was significantly lower in patients who underwent WALANT rather than traditional anesthesia.[73] This could perhaps be caused by the extensive use of preemptive analgesia or the feeling of control that the patients have when able to observe and participate in their own surgeries.

CRYOTHERAPY AND TRANSCUTANEOUS ELECTRICAL NERVE STIMULATION

In addition to pharmacologic measures, surgeons should consider physical modalities when addressing postoperative pain. This includes cryotherapy, transcutaneous electrical nerve stimulation (TENS), acupuncture, massage, and localized heat. Physical modalities are safe and carry virtually no risk to the patient. TENS involves the use of low-voltage electrical current delivered through a portable hand-held device for the treatment of pain. Electrodes are selectively placed throughout the body and are believed to activate inhibitory descending pain pathways thereby reducing the pain response via large afferent fibers.[74] These electrodes are most commonly placed directly at the surgical site but others have reported utility in placing them also at distant acupoints. TENS has been reported to decrease postoperative analgesia by 25% by a systematic review of more than 20 randomized trials.[75]

Cooling techniques involve surrounding the affected surgical site with cold compresses, cooled air, or fluid circulation devices. This theoretically leads to reduced tissue temperature, edema, and resulting pain. Studies have reported varying outcomes with no pointed consensus backing the utility of this therapy as compared with no cold therapy in terms of postoperative pain or total analgesic use.[76–78]

There is conflicting evidence regarding the utility of acupuncture and massage on the reduction of postoperative pain in adults or its effect on overall analgesic use.[79–83] Acupuncture originated from Chinese medicine practices and involves the use of needle placement into differing soft tissue points throughout the body.[84,85] This is combined with electric current (electroacupuncture)[86,87] or can involve the use of pressure at the selected locations instead of needles (acupressure).[88]

Table 2
Typical (local anesthetic) volumes used for common operations

Surgery Type	Number of Opioid Pain Pills Dispensed
Hand or wrist soft tissue	≤10
Hand or wrist fractures	≤20
Elbow or forearm soft tissue	≤15
Elbow or forearm fractures	≤20
Upper arm or shoulder soft tissue or fractures	≤30

Data from Kim N, Matzon JL, Abboudi J, et al. A Prospective Evaluation of Opioid Utilization After Upper-Extremity Surgical Procedures: Identifying Consumption Patterns and Determining Prescribing Guidelines. J Bone Joint Surg Am. 2016;98(20):e8.

PERIOPERATIVE PAIN EDUCATION

Perioperative pain education should be considered part of multimodal therapy.[22] Psychological factors can play a role in the inhibitory neuronal pathways,[14] and are therefore a necessary consideration in perioperative pain management. Mood disorders, specifically anxiety and depression, and pain catastrophizing have been associated with increased postoperative pain.[7,15,17,22,36,37,89–91] Specifically in hand surgery, depression has been shown to be a predictor of postoperative pain severity because of catastrophizing and maladaptive coping mechanisms.[22] Studies have suggested targeting pain catastrophizing with preoperative education as a way to decrease postoperative pain.[37] Results of studies on the efficacy of preoperative education on postoperative pain have had mixed results. A Cochrane Review showed low quality evidence that these techniques have a beneficial effect on postoperative pain.[91] Other studies found no change in postoperative pain but a decrease in opioid use and high patient satisfaction rates in patients who received prescription guidelines before surgery.[22] The content of preoperative education and consideration of patients' health literacy[5,92,93] play a role in its efficacy. In a systematic review of preoperative pain education in 1021 patients receiving total knee and total hip surgeries, only one study showed a decrease in postoperative pain with the use of preoperative pain education.[92] This review concluded that the unique aspect of this study was its inclusion of pain science education, which may be the key to successful results with preoperative pain education.[92] The American Pain Society Guidelines on Management of Postoperative Pain recommend educating patients and developing perioperative pain management plans and expectations with patients before surgery.[26]

SUMMARY

Perioperative pain management in surgery of the hand and upper extremity relies on a multimodal approach to be effective. Individualized pain management plans can increase the effectiveness for patients and should take into account the anticipated surgical procedure, medical history, and available evidence to support a pain control modality. The management of pain of patients undergoing upper extremity surgery begins before any surgical intervention and continues postoperatively. Patient education, setting expectations, psychological interventions, and addressing risk factors associated with postoperative pain are critical to successful pain management. Intraoperative anesthesia is accomplished via a variety of means including peripheral nerve blocks, IVRA, continuous infusions, and local infiltration and wide-awake surgery. Cryotherapy, TENS, acupuncture, massage, and localized heat are all physical modalities that are used in concert with pharmacologic therapies postoperatively to continue pain management.

DISCLOSURE

The authors have nothing to disclose.

REFERENCES

1. Pregler JL, Kapur PA. The development of ambulatory anesthesia and future challenges. Anesthesiol Clin North Am 2003;21(2):207–28.
2. Hall MJ, Schwartzman A, Zhang J, et al. Ambulatory surgery data from hospitals and ambulatory surgery centers: United States, 2010. Natl Health Stat Report 2017;(102):1–15.
3. Leblanc MR, Lalonde J, Lalonde DH. A detailed cost and efficiency analysis of performing carpal tunnel surgery in the main operating room versus the ambulatory setting in Canada. Hand (N Y) 2007; 2(4):173–8.
4. Ketonis C, Ilyas AM, Liss F. Pain management strategies in hand surgery. Orthop Clin North Am 2015;46(3):399–408.
5. Lanitis S, Mimigianni C, Raptis D, et al. The impact of educational status on the postoperative perception of pain. Korean J Pain 2015;28(4):265–74.
6. Warrender WJ, Syed UAM, Hammoud S, et al. Pain management after outpatient shoulder arthroscopy: a systematic review of randomized controlled trials. Am J Sports Med 2017;45(7):1676–86.
7. Pozek JJ, De Ruyter M, Khan TW. Comprehensive acute pain management in the perioperative surgical home. Anesthesiol Clin 2018;36(2):295–307.
8. Malik OS, Kaye AD, Urman RD. Perioperative hyperalgesia and associated clinical factors. Curr Pain Headache Rep 2017;21(1):4.
9. Wu CL, Berenholtz SM, Pronovost PJ, et al. Systematic review and analysis of postdischarge symptoms after outpatient surgery. Anesthesiology 2002;96(4):994–1003.
10. Jin F, Chung F. Multimodal analgesia for postoperative pain control. J Clin Anesth 2001;13(7):524–39.
11. Centers for Disease Control and Prevention. Understanding the epidemic. 2018. Available at: https://www.cdc.gov/drugoverdose/epidemic/. Accessed June 6, 2019.
12. Florence CS, Zhou C, Luo F, et al. The economic burden of prescription opioid overdose, abuse, and dependence in the United States, 2013. Med Care 2016;54(10):901–6.

13. Morris BJ, Mir HR. The opioid epidemic: impact on orthopaedic surgery. J Am Acad Orthop Surg 2015;23(5):267–71.

14. Tawfic QA, Faris AS. Acute pain service: past, present and future. Pain Manag 2015;5(1):47–58.

15. Tawfic Q, Kumar K, Pirani Z, et al. Prevention of chronic post-surgical pain: the importance of early identification of risk factors. J Anesth 2017;31(3):424–31.

16. Argoff CE. Recent management advances in acute postoperative pain. Pain Pract 2014;14(5):477–87.

17. Budiansky AS, Margarson MP, Eipe N. Acute pain management in morbid obesity: an evidence based clinical update. Surg Obes Relat Dis 2017;13(3):523–32.

18. Mitra S, Carlyle D, Kodumudi G, et al. New advances in acute postoperative pain management. Curr Pain Headache Rep 2018;22(5):35.

19. Cashman JN. The mechanisms of action of NSAIDs in analgesia. Drugs 1996;52(Suppl 5):13–23.

20. Huang YM, Wang CM, Wang CT, et al. Perioperative celecoxib administration for pain management after total knee arthroplasty: a randomized, controlled study. BMC Musculoskelet Disord 2008;9:77.

21. Giuliani E, Bianchi A, Marcuzzi A, et al. Ibuprofen timing for hand surgery in ambulatory care. Acta Ortop Bras 2015;23(4):188–91.

22. Bowers MR, Pulos N, Pulos BP, et al. Opioid-sparing pain management in upper extremity surgery. Part 2: surgeon as prescriber. J Hand Surg Am 2019;44(10):878–82.

23. Thomas DA, Boominathan P, Goswami J, et al. Perioperative management of patients with addiction to opioid and non-opioid medications. Curr Pain Headache Rep 2018;22(7):52.

24. Gonano C, Latzke D, Sabeti-Aschraf M, et al. The anxiolytic effect of pregabalin in outpatients undergoing minor orthopaedic surgery. J Psychopharmacol 2011;25(2):249–53.

25. Taylor CP. Mechanisms of action of gabapentin. Rev Neurol (Paris) 1997;153(Suppl 1):S39–45.

26. Chou R, Gordon DB, de Leon-Casasola OA, et al. Management of postoperative pain: a clinical practice guideline from the American Pain Society, the American Society of Regional Anesthesia and Pain Medicine, and the American Society of Anesthesiologists' Committee on Regional Anesthesia, Executive Committee, and Administrative Council. J Pain 2016;17(2):131–57.

27. Pulos BP, Bowers MR, Shin AY, et al. Opioid-sparing pain management in upper extremity surgery. Part 1: role of the surgeon and anesthesiologist. J Hand Surg Am 2019;44(9):787–91.

28. McNicol ED, Schumann R, Haroutounian S. A systematic review and meta-analysis of ketamine for the prevention of persistent post-surgical pain. Acta Anaesthesiol Scand 2014;58(10):1199–213.

29. Rana MV, Desai R, Tran L, et al. Perioperative pain control in the ambulatory setting. Curr Pain Headache Rep 2016;20(3):18.

30. Eipe NG S, Penning J. Intravenous lidocaine for acute pain: an evidence-based clinical update. BJA Educ 2016;16(9):292–8.

31. Bovill JG. Mechanisms of actions of opioids and non-steroidal anti-inflammatory drugs. Eur J Anaesthesiol Suppl 1997;15:9–15.

32. Ruetzler K, Blome CJ, Nabecker S, et al. A randomised trial of oral versus intravenous opioids for treatment of pain after cardiac surgery. J Anesth 2014;28(4):580–6.

33. Hah JM, Bateman BT, Ratliff J, et al. Chronic opioid use after surgery: implications for perioperative management in the face of the opioid epidemic. Anesth Analg 2017;125(5):1733–40.

34. Harrison RK, DiMeo T, Klinefelter RD, et al. Multimodal pain control in ambulatory hand surgery. Am J Orthop (Belle Mead NJ) 2018;47(6).

35. Lee SK, Lee JW, Choy WS. Is multimodal analgesia as effective as postoperative patient-controlled analgesia following upper extremity surgery? Orthop Traumatol Surg Res 2013;99(8):895–901.

36. Gauger EM, Gauger EJ, Desai MJ, et al. Opioid use after upper extremity surgery. J Hand Surg Am 2018;43(5):470–9.

37. Dwyer CL, Soong M, Hunter A, et al. Prospective evaluation of an opioid reduction protocol in hand surgery. J Hand Surg Am 2018;43(6):516–522 e511.

38. Labrum JTT, Ilyas AM. Preemptive analgesia in thumb basal joint arthroplasty: immediate postoperative pain with preincision versus postincision local anesthesia. J Hand Microsurg 2017;9(2):80–3.

39. Welton KL, Kraeutler MJ, McCarty EC, et al. Current pain prescribing habits for common shoulder operations: a survey of the American Shoulder and Elbow Surgeons membership. J Shoulder Elbow Surg 2018;27(6S):S76–81.

40. Sabatino MJ, Kunkel ST, Ramkumar DB, et al. Excess opioid medication and variation in prescribing patterns following common orthopaedic procedures. J Bone Joint Surg Am 2018;100(3):180–8.

41. Brandal D, Keller MS, Lee C, et al. Impact of enhanced recovery after surgery and opioid-free anesthesia on opioid prescriptions at discharge from the hospital: a historical-prospective study. Anesth Analg 2017;125(5):1784–92.

42. Kim N, Matzon JL, Abboudi J, et al. A prospective evaluation of opioid utilization after upper-extremity surgical procedures: identifying consumption patterns and determining prescribing guidelines. J Bone Joint Surg Am 2016;98(20):e89.

43. Bruce BG, Green A, Blaine TA, et al. Brachial plexus blocks for upper extremity orthopaedic surgery. J Am Acad Orthop Surg 2012;20(1):38–47.

44. Mian A, Chaudhry I, Huang R, et al. Brachial plexus anesthesia: a review of the relevant anatomy, complications, and anatomical variations. Clin Anat 2014;27(2):210–21.

45. Gulur P, Nishimori M, Ballantyne JC. Regional anaesthesia versus general anaesthesia, morbidity and mortality. Best Pract Res Clin Anaesthesiol 2006;20(2):249–63.

46. Nadeau MJ, Levesque S, Dion N. Ultrasound-guided regional anesthesia for upper limb surgery. Can J Anaesth 2013;60(3):304–20.

47. Abrahams MS, Aziz MF, Fu RF, et al. Ultrasound guidance compared with electrical neurostimulation for peripheral nerve block: a systematic review and meta-analysis of randomized controlled trials. Br J Anaesth 2009;102(3):408–17.

48. Leone S, Di Cianni S, Casati A, et al. Pharmacology, toxicology, and clinical use of new long acting local anesthetics, ropivacaine and levobupivacaine. Acta Biomed 2008;79(2):92–105.

49. Desroches J. The infraclavicular brachial plexus block by the coracoid approach is clinically effective: an observational study of 150 patients. Can J Anaesth 2003;50(3):253–7.

50. Lenters TR, Davies J, Matsen FA 3rd. The types and severity of complications associated with interscalene brachial plexus block anesthesia: local and national evidence. J Shoulder Elbow Surg 2007;16(4):379–87.

51. Neal JM, Gerancher JC, Hebl JR, et al. Upper extremity regional anesthesia: essentials of our current understanding, 2008. Reg Anesth Pain Med 2009;34(2):134–70.

52. Brown AR, Weiss R, Greenberg C, et al. Interscalene block for shoulder arthroscopy: comparison with general anesthesia. Arthroscopy 1993;9(3):295–300.

53. McCartney CJ, Brull R, Chan VW, et al. Early but no long-term benefit of regional compared with general anesthesia for ambulatory hand surgery. Anesthesiology 2004;101(2):461–7.

54. Wu CL, Rouse LM, Chen JM, et al. Comparison of postoperative pain in patients receiving interscalene block or general anesthesia for shoulder surgery. Orthopedics 2002;25(1):45–8.

55. Huang Y, Chiu F, Webb CA, et al. Review of the evidence: best analgesic regimen for shoulder surgery. Pain Manag 2017;7(5):405–18.

56. Blackburn EW, Shafritz AB. Why do Bier blocks work for hand surgery ... Most of the time? J Hand Surg Am 2010;35(6):1022–4.

57. Arslanian B, Mehrzad R, Kramer T, et al. Forearm Bier block: a new regional anesthetic technique for upper extremity surgery. Ann Plast Surg 2014;73(2):156–7.

58. Rodola F, Vagnoni S, Ingletti S. An update on intravenous regional anaesthesia of the arm. Eur Rev Med Pharmacol Sci 2003;7(5):131–8.

59. Brown EM, McGriff JT, Malinowski RW. Intravenous regional anaesthesia (Bier block): review of 20 years' experience. Can J Anaesth 1989;36(3 Pt 1):307–10.

60. Viscomi CM, Friend A, Parker C, et al. Ketamine as an adjuvant in lidocaine intravenous regional anesthesia: a randomized, double-blind, systemic control trial. Reg Anesth Pain Med 2009;34(2):130–3.

61. Sen H, Kulahci Y, Bicerer E, et al. The analgesic effect of paracetamol when added to lidocaine for intravenous regional anesthesia. Anesth Analg 2009;109(4):1327–30.

62. Abdallah FW, Halpern SH, Aoyama K, et al. Will the real benefits of single-shot interscalene block please stand up? A systematic review and meta-analysis. Anesth Analg 2015;120(5):1114–29.

63. Ilfeld BM, Morey TE, Wright TW, et al. Continuous interscalene brachial plexus block for postoperative pain control at home: a randomized, double-blinded, placebo-controlled study. Anesth Analg 2003;96(4):1089–95. table of contents.

64. Axley M, Horn JL. Indications and management of continuous infusion of local anesthetics at home. Curr Opin Anaesthesiol 2010;23(5):650–5.

65. Fredrickson MJ, Krishnan S, Chen CY. Postoperative analgesia for shoulder surgery: a critical appraisal and review of current techniques. Anaesthesia 2010;65(6):608–24.

66. Kulkarni M, Elliot D. Local anaesthetic infusion for postoperative pain. J Hand Surg Br 2003;28(4):300–6.

67. Joshi GP, Hawkins RJ, Frankle MA, et al. Best practices for periarticular infiltration with liposomal bupivacaine for the management of pain after shoulder surgery: consensus recommendation. J Surg Orthop Adv 2016;25(4):204–8.

68. Matsen FA 3rd, Papadonikolakis A. Published evidence demonstrating the causation of glenohumeral chondrolysis by postoperative infusion of local anesthetic via a pain pump. J Bone Joint Surg Am 2013;95(12):1126–34.

69. Lalonde DH, Wong A. Dosage of local anesthesia in wide awake hand surgery. J Hand Surg Am 2013;38(10):2025–8.

70. Lalonde D, Martin A. Epinephrine in local anesthesia in finger and hand surgery: the case for wide-awake anesthesia. J Am Acad Orthop Surg 2013;21(8):443–7.

71. Lalonde DH, Martin AL. Wide-awake flexor tendon repair and early tendon mobilization in zones 1 and 2. Hand Clin 2013;29(2):207–13.

72. Lalonde DH. Wide-awake extensor indicis proprius to extensor pollicis longus tendon transfer. J Hand Surg Am 2014;39(11):2297–9.

73. Huang YC, Chen CY, Lin KC, et al. Comparison of wide-awake local anesthesia no tourniquet with general anesthesia with tourniquet for volar plating of

distal radius fracture. Orthopedics 2019;42(1): e93–8.

74. Sluka KA, Walsh DM. Transcutaneous electrical nerve stimulation and interential therapy. In: Sluka KA, Walsh DM, editors. Mechanisms and management of pain for the physical therapist. 1st edition. Seattle (WA): International Association for the Study of Pain; 2009. p. 167–90.

75. Bjordal JM, Johnson MI, Ljunggreen AE. Transcutaneous electrical nerve stimulation (TENS) can reduce postoperative analgesic consumption. A meta-analysis with assessment of optimal treatment parameters for postoperative pain. Eur J Pain 2003; 7(2):181–8.

76. Amin-Hanjani S, Corcoran J, Chatwani A. Cold therapy in the management of postoperative cesarean section pain. Am J Obstet Gynecol 1992;167(1): 108–9.

77. Barber FA, McGuire DA, Click S. Continuous-flow cold therapy for outpatient anterior cruciate ligament reconstruction. Arthroscopy 1998;14(2):130–5.

78. Bert JM, Stark JG, Maschka K, et al. The effect of cold therapy on morbidity subsequent to arthroscopic lateral retinacular release. Orthop Rev 1991;20(9):755–8.

79. Gupta S, Francis JD, Tillu AB, et al. The effect of preemptive acupuncture treatment on analgesic requirements after day-case knee arthroscopy. Anaesthesia 1999;54(12):1204–7.

80. Kotani N, Hashimoto H, Sato Y, et al. Preoperative intradermal acupuncture reduces postoperative pain, nausea and vomiting, analgesic requirement, and sympathoadrenal responses. Anesthesiology 2001; 95(2):349–56.

81. Tsang RC, Tsang PL, Ko CY, et al. Effects of acupuncture and sham acupuncture in addition to physiotherapy in patients undergoing bilateral total knee arthroplasty: a randomized controlled trial. Clin Rehabil 2007;21(8):719–28.

82. Forchuk C, Baruth P, Prendergast M, et al. Postoperative arm massage: a support for women with lymph node dissection. Cancer Nurs 2004;27(1):25–33.

83. Hattan J, King L, Griffiths P. The impact of foot massage and guided relaxation following cardiac surgery: a randomized controlled trial. J Adv Nurs 2002;37(2):199–207.

84. Deng G, Rusch V, Vickers A, et al. Randomized controlled trial of a special acupuncture technique for pain after thoracotomy. J Thorac Cardiovasc Surg 2008;136(6):1464–9.

85. Grabow L. Controlled study of the analgetic effectivity of acupuncture. Arzneimittelforschung 1994; 44(4):554–8.

86. Martelete M, Fiori AM. Comparative study of the analgesic effect of transcutaneous nerve stimulation (TNS); electroacupuncture (EA) and meperidine in the treatment of postoperative pain. Acupunct Electrother Res 1985;10(3):183–93.

87. Lin JG, Lo MW, Wen YR, et al. The effect of high and low frequency electroacupuncture in pain after lower abdominal surgery. Pain 2002;99(3):509–14.

88. Felhendler D, Lisander B. Pressure on acupoints decreases postoperative pain. Clin J Pain 1996;12(4): 326–9.

89. Bot AG, Bekkers S, Arnstein PM, et al. Opioid use after fracture surgery correlates with pain intensity and satisfaction with pain relief. Clin Orthop Relat Res 2014;472(8):2542–9.

90. Baert IA, Lluch E, Mulder T, et al. Does pre-surgical central modulation of pain influence outcome after total knee replacement? A systematic review. Osteoarthritis Cartilage 2016;24(2):213–23.

91. Powell R, Scott NW, Manyande A, et al. Psychological preparation and postoperative outcomes for adults undergoing surgery under general anaesthesia. Cochrane Database Syst Rev 2016;(5): CD008646.

92. Louw A, Diener I, Butler DS, et al. Preoperative education addressing postoperative pain in total joint arthroplasty: review of content and educational delivery methods. Physiother Theory Pract 2013; 29(3):175–94.

93. Lemay CA, Lewis CG, Singh JA, et al. Receipt of pain management information preoperatively is associated with improved functional gain after elective total joint arthroplasty. J Arthroplasty 2017;32(6): 1763–8.

Printed and bound by CPI Group (UK) Ltd, Croydon, CR0 4YY

08/05/2025

01864691-0016